Small Animal Therapeutics

Small Animal Therapeutics

R. J. Martin, BVSc, PhD, MRCVS
Lecturer in Veterinary Pharmacology,
Royal (Dick) School of Veterinary Studies,
University of Edinburgh

WRIGHT
London Boston Durban Singapore Sydney Toronto Wellington

PART OF REED INTERNATIONAL P.L.C.

Wright
is an imprint of Butterworth Scientific

First published 1989

British Library Cataloguing in Publication Data

Martin, R. J.
Small animal therapeutics.
1. Livestock: Small animals. Veterinary care,
— Manuals
I. Title
636.089

ISBN 0-7236-0930-6

Library of Congress Cataloging in Publication Data

Martin, R. J., BVSc.
Small animal therapeutics/R. J. Martin.
p. cm.
Contents: Bibliography: p.
Includes index.
ISBN 0-7236-0930-6:
1. Veterinary pharmacology. I. Title.
SF915.M29 1989
636.089'58 — dc 19

Photoset by Butterworths Litho Preparation Department
Printed and bound in Great Britain by Anchor Press Ltd, Tiptree, Essex

Preface

The aim of this text is to provide a modern account of small animal therapeutics. The basic scientific principles have been kept to a minimum and only included when they give rise to a better understanding of the clinical use of the drugs mentioned.

Suggested drug dosages are also included as a guide for therapy but recent data sheets should always be checked. Doses are quoted for body weights measured in pounds as well as kilograms.

I wish to express my appreciation to Dr Geoffrey Smaldon of Butterworths who suggested the writing of the text and who has continued throughout to offer advice. Neal King, the series editor, has also been involved, suggesting suitable topics of particular interest to the practitioner. Mary Elizabeth Raw, a fellow Liverpool graduate, has also helped by reading the manuscript critically. I also wish to express my thanks to Dr Alan Kifton and Professor Frank Alexander who have, over the years, encouraged me into the area of veterinary therapeutics.

Contents

Chapter 1

General Principles of Drug Distribution and Dosage

This chapter describes the principles of pharmacokinetics, i.e. factors which control and influence the distribution and excretion of drugs within the body. The various parameters used to estimate the duration of action of individual drugs, together with their dose frequency and amplitude, are described. Although most clinicians will use the data sheets to determine dose amplitude and frequency, the description of the way in which these are determined should be of interest.

Drug translocation

Figure 1.1 summarizes drug translocation, i.e. the distribution routes of a drug within the body following administration. The drug could be administered orally, intramuscularly or sub-

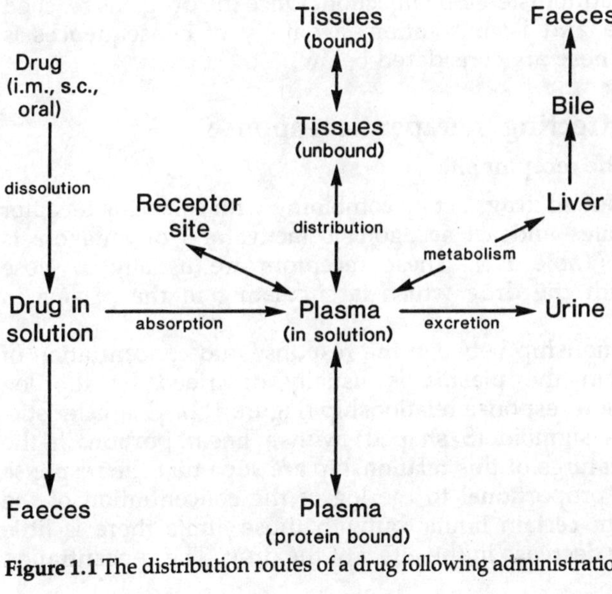

Figure 1.1 The distribution routes of a drug following administration

cutaneously. Following administration it undergoes a process of dissolution so that it passes into solution: the drug may then be absorbed or, if it is administered orally, remain unabsorbed and pass out into the faeces. The fraction absorbed is known as the bioavailability of the drug. If the bioavailability of the drug is 100% then it is completely absorbed. A variety of factors influence the bioavailability, including the nature of the preparation: a finely divided or micronized preparation is more likely to be completely absorbed following oral administration than an undivided pellet.

A variety of other factors influence absorption: these include the local pH, the degree of ionization of the preparation and its lipid solubility. Lipid-soluble drugs which are not highly ionized tend to be more readily absorbed. Drugs which have been administered intramuscularly or subcutaneously will pass, after absorption, directly into the circulating bloodstream. Drugs which have been administered orally are absorbed in the gut and passed via the hepatic portal system to the liver. Once they reach the liver they may be metabolized or passed directly into the circulating bloodstream by the hepatic veins: the passage of the drug through the liver after oral administration and the possibility of metabolism is known as 'the first-pass effect'. This means that some drugs may reach the bloodstream and achieve much lower concentrations when administered orally and may have to be administered by injection. Once the drug has reached the plasma and is in solution, a variety of consequences is possible. These are considered below.

Factors affecting therapeutic response

Action at the receptor site

Most but not all drugs act by combining with a specific receptor in the tissues and act as agonists (activators) or antagonists (blockers) (Table 1.1). These receptors are usually in close contact with the drug which is circulating in the plasma in solution.

The relationship between the response and concentration of the drug in the plasma is usually described by the log concentration response relationship (Figure 1.2). Characteristically this is sigmoid (S shaped) with a linear portion in the middle. Features of this relationship are such that the response is directly proportional to the log of the concentration of the drug within certain limits: outwith those limits there is little increase or decrease in the effect of the drug. The concentration

Table 1.1 Some receptor types, distribution, agonists and antagonists

Receptor type	*Subtype*	*Natural agonist*	*Synthetic agonists*	*Antagonists*	*Tissue location*
Cholinergic	Muscarinic	Acetylcholine	Carbachol arecoline	Atropine	Parasympathetic
	Nicotinic	Acetylcholine	Carbachol nicotine	Curare	Neuromuscular junction
				Hexamethonium	Ganglia
Adrenergic	α_1	Noradrenaline	Methoxamine	Prazosin	Sympathatic + CNS
		Adrenaline			
	α_2	Noradrenaline	Xylazine	Yohimbine	Sympathetic + CNS
		Adrenaline	Detomidine	Idazoxan	
	β_1	Noradrenaline	Isoprenaline	Propranolol	Heart blood vessels
		Adrenaline	Dobutamine	Practolol	
	β_2	Adrenaline	Clenbuterol	Propranolol	Bronchi
			Salbutamol	Butoxamine	Uterus
			Isoprenaline		
Opioid	μ	β-endorphin	Pethidine	Naloxone	CNS
		Metenkephalin	Morphine		Spinal cord
			Etorphine		Gut
	δ	Leuenkephalin	Etorphine	Naloxone	CNS
		Metenkephalin			Spinal cord
	κ	Dynorphin	Buprenorphine	Naloxone	CNS
			Etorphine		Spinal cord
			β-Allyl normetazocine		CNS
Histamine	H_1	Histamine	2-Methyl histamine	Mepyramine	Blood vessels
				Tripelennamine	Bronchi
				Promethazine	
	H_2	Histamine	4(5)-Methyl histamine	Cimetidine	Stomach
				Ranitidine	
GABA	$GABA_A$	GABA	Muscimol	Bicuculline	CNS
			Diazepam	Picrotoxin	
	$GABA_B$	GABA	Baclofen		CNS
Glutamate	NMDA		*N*-methyl D-aspartate	Ketamine	CNS

of the drug producing 50% of the maximum response is usually referred to as the ED_{50} (ED, effective dose). Also shown in Figure 1.2 is the log concentration response relationship of a deleterious (toxic) effect: the response may be the percentage of animals killed or some other untoward effect. The aim of any therapy, then, is to exceed a minimum plasma concentration (Cp_{min}, see below) to obtain a beneficial effect but keeping below a maximum plasma concentration (Cp_{max}, see below) which may produce a deleterious effect.

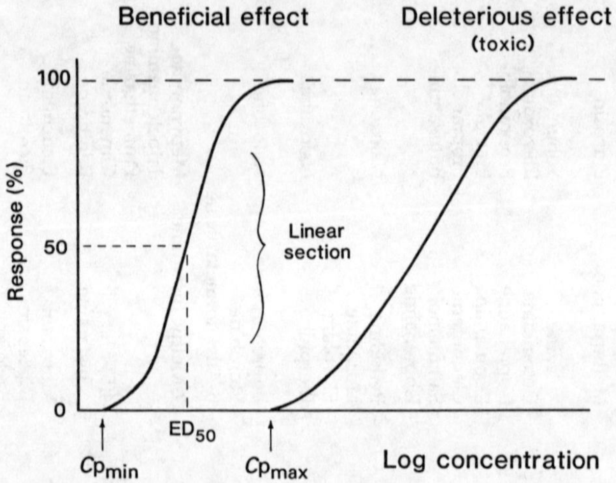

Figure 1.2 Log dose/response relationship showing how Cp_{min} and Cp_{max} are determined

This description is clearly simplified but does illustrate the requirement to maintain the concentration of therapeutic agent above a minimum level but not to exceed a maximum level. It also serves to illustrate the fact that the response to a therapeutic agent is usually related to the log of the plasma concentration within certain limits.

The action of most drugs at the receptor is selective and specific (only acting on one receptor) and gives rise to the description 'the magic bullet'. Drug receptors are typed and subtyped pharmacologically (Table 1.1).

Plasma protein binding

Most drugs are carried in the blood either bound to plasma albumin or in their free state (see Figure 1.1). It is only in the free state that they are available to enter the tissues and act with appropriate receptors. Drugs which are highly bound (greater than 80%) are not available for excretion and metabolism, nor are they available to act as a therapeutic agent. Sulphamethoxypyridazine is an example of a sulphonamide which is highly bound to plasma proteins: it has a very long half-life and stays in the body for a considerable period of time. The high degree of protein binding limits the free concentration of the drug as well as its distribution in the body and also reduces the therapeutic value of the substance. Oxytetracycline is only about 20% bound to the plasma proteins whereas the longer acting derivatives doxycycline and metacycline are bound to a great extent (90%) at similar concentrations. Cloxacillin is also highly bound (75%) whereas benzyl penicillin and phenoxymethyl penicillin are only bound to a limited extent (30–60%); ampicillin is bound to a lesser extent (18%). As a general rule it is only where agents are more than 80% bound that the distribution of the drug is limited.

The level of protein binding may vary according to the condition of the animal. Acidic drugs like phenylbutazone are highly bound to plasma proteins and may be displaced by other acidic drugs like aspirin or in conditions of uraemia where there is a metabolic acidosis. The half-life (the duration of effect) of these agents is decreased in these conditions but their toxic effects are increased, since their free plasma concentration is elevated.

Tissue distribution

Once a drug has entered the plasma and is not bound to protein it is then available for carriage around the body and distribution to the tissues. In general, those tissues which are highly vascular, like the kidney, liver, brain and heart, receive the drug first and it is in these tissues that there is an initial rise in the concentration of the drug. Tissues like the fat and skin, which are poorly vascularized, receive the drug at a slower rate. This means that tissue concentrations in the kidney, liver, heart and brain will rise more rapidly after the intravenous administration of the drug than in the skin, fat and connective tissues.

Some drugs remain fairly tightly localized in the circulating blood system. Other drugs move out of the plasma and are well distributed throughout the tissues. A measure of the degree with which the drug is distributed is the volume of distribution (V_d). The volume of distribution is an important concept characterizing the pharmacokinetics of drugs. It is defined as the volume of fluid which would be required to contain the amount of the drug in the body if it were uniformly distributed at a concentration equal to that found in the plasma. It is assumed that the body behaves as a homogeneous compartment with respect to the drug and that the drug is equally distributed. Although it is a theoretical concept, it can be measured experimentally and serves to illustrate the degree with which the drug is distributed in the body. A large volume of distribution implies a wide distribution of the drug in the body. Organic bases like morphine, quinidine, lignocaine and diazepam are widely distributed in the body fluids and tissues and have large volumes of distribution (1 litre/kg). Organic bases which have a low lipid solubility, like the aminoglycosides (streptomycin and neomycin), have low volumes of distribution (less than 0.3 litre/kg). Highly ionized organic acids like the penicillins and phenylbutazone have small volumes of distribution (less than 0.25 litre/kg) and are not well distributed in the body. Weakly ionized organic acids like the sulphonamides and barbiturates exist in both ionized and non-ionized forms and so can penetrate the biological membranes of the cells with relative ease: as a consequence they have volumes of distribution that are between 0.3 and 0.8 litres/kg; they are fairly well distributed. In summary, the volume of distribution is a useful pharmacokinetic term: it does not correspond to a physiological volume; it is useful for calculating the dose of substances that are used therapeutically.

pH

Most drugs which are used therapeutically are either weak acids or weak bases: as a consequence they exist in the ionized and unionized forms. The barriers which separate the compartments of the body are composed of cell walls made up of phospholipids. This means that it is only the unionized form of the drug which crosses the barrier between the body compartments: the ionized form of the drug remains trapped and cannot cross the barrier (Figure 1.3). If there is a pH difference across the barrier then this will give rise to differences in the total concentration of the drug on either side of the membrane: basic drugs accumulate where the pH is low (under acidic conditions); acidic drugs accumulate in conditions where the pH is high (in alkaline conditions). The formalization of the effect of pH on the distribution of drugs is also known as 'the pH partition hypothesis'.

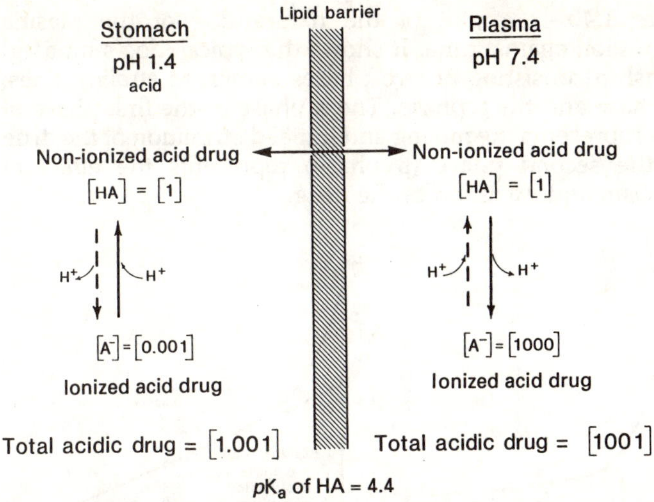

Figure 1.3 Diagram illustrating the absorption of an acidic drug (e.g. aspirin) from the stomach and ion trapping.

The pH of the stomach of the cat and dog is low, about pH 3.0. Under these conditions, acidic drugs like salicylic acid are poorly ionized and so are well absorbed from the stomach. In the kidney acidic drugs will accumulate in an alkaline urine while basic drugs will accumulate in acidic urine. To facilitate the secretion of phenobarbitone (a long-acting sedative and a weak acid) the urine may be made alkaline with the administration of sodium bicarbonate to the cat or the dog. If a diuretic like frusemide is also given to stimulate diuresis, the clearance of the weak acid will be markedly increased. This is an appropriate step for the treatment of phenobarbitone poisoning. Milk is slightly acid (pH 6.4) relative to plasma (pH 7.4) so that weak bases like lincomycin and tylosin will accumulate; strong acids like benzyl penicillin will accumulate in the milk at lower concentrations than found in the plasma.

Plasma concentration/time relationship

Figure 1.4a illustrates a typical plasma concentration/time relationship following the intravenous injection of a therapeutic agent. After an initial very rapid rise in plasma concentration, the level of the drug in the blood progressively falls in a geometric manner suggestive of a decaying process.

Figure 1.4b is a plot of the natural log of the plasma concentration against time. It shows the typical 'dog's hindleg' relationship consisting of two phases shown as straight lines: the α phase and the β phase. The α phase or the first phase of the line represents the mixing and initial distribution of the drug while the second phase (β phase) represents the effect of metabolism and excretion of the drug.

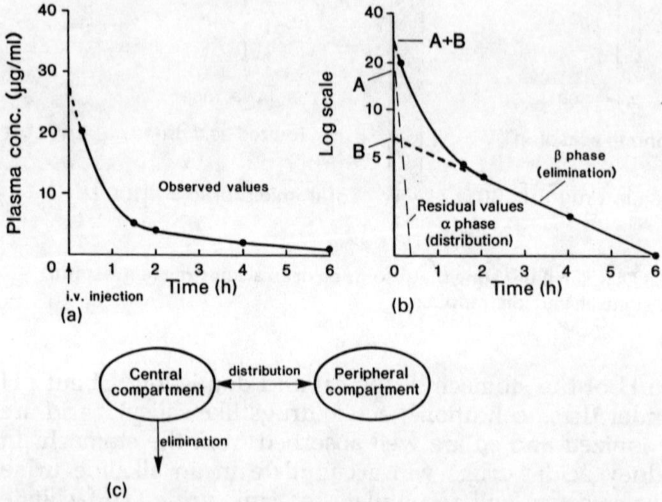

Figure 1.4 (a) The plasma concentration/time relationship and (b) the log concentration/time relationship. (c) The 'two compartment open' model. A and B are concentrations measured by extrapolation to time zero; plasma concentration = $Ae^{-\alpha t} + Be^{-\beta t}$

A popular model of the fate of drugs in the body is the 'two compartment open' model (Figure 1.4c). This model assumes that the drug enters the body and distributes instantaneously in the central compartment. The central compartment consists of the blood plasma and the extracellular fluid of tissues that are highly vascular, such as the lungs, heart, liver and kidneys. The distribution into the remaining space of the body (known as the peripheral compartment) takes place more slowly. Usually the peripheral compartment (the tissues) consists of the less vascular organs such as the muscle, skin and fat. The apparent volume of the central and peripheral compartments will vary from drug to drug in the same animal, depending on the drug's ability to gain access to the tissues from the circulating blood system and on the extent of binding to tissues.

Another way of representing the plasma concentration/time relationship is to describe it by mathematical equations.

$$Cp = A_e^{-\alpha t} + B_e^{-\beta t}$$

If t = 0,

$$Cp = A + B$$

If α is very high (rapid distribution),

$$Cp \sim B_e^{-\beta t}$$

In the first equation, A and B are the units of concentration and are determined from the intersect on the *y* axis: α and β are the distribution and elimination rate constants respectively and have the units of reciprocal time (usually min^{-1}); the lower this number the slower the rates of distribution and elimination. The first part of the plasma concentration/time relationship (the α phase) is dominated by the distribution of the drug from the central compartment to the peripheral (tissue) compartment. After this, where there has been the establishment of an equilibrium, the rate of decline of the drug concentration in the plasma is dominated by the elimination of the drug from the central compartment and is termed the β or the elimination phase. The β phase is usually the most important phase since it lasts much longer and is used to determine the half-life of the drug.

The half-life of a drug is determined as the time required for the drug to fall to half of its value during the β phase; numerically it is calculated from the slope of the graph in the β phase. The half-life of a drug is a particularly important descriptive quantity since it describes the rate of elimination of a drug from the body. A short half-life means a rapid elimination; a long half-life means the elimination of the drug is slow. Suppose the half-life of a drug equals two hours and if, at one hour after administration of a drug, the plasma concentration equals 4 μg/ml (after distribution is complete); then at three hours the plasma concentration will be 2 μg/ml; at five hours the plasma concentration will be 1 μg/ml; at seven hours the plasma concentration will be 0.5 μg/ml. Table 1.2 shows the half-life ($T_{1/2}$) of a number of commonly used antibacterial agents in the cat and dog.

Metabolism

It has already been pointed out that a variety of factors influence the plasma concentration of the drug just after administration.

Table 1.2 Pharmacokinetic parameters of antibacterial drugs used in the dog and cat

Drug	$T_{1/2}$ (h)	V_d (ml/kg)	Cp_{min} (μg/ml)
Sodium penicillin	0.5	156	0.1
Procaine penicillin	0.5	156	0.1
Sodium ampicillin	1.0	350	1.0
Amoxicillin	1.0–1.5	200	1.0
Cloxacillin	0.5	200	0.1
Cephalexin	1.3–2.6	270	8.0
Gentamicin	1.0–1.25	300	4.0
Kanamycin	0.75–1.0	250	–
Streptomycin	2.5	200	–
Trimethoprim	2.5	150	2.0
Sulphadiazine	10.0	100	–
Chloramphenicol	4.5	180	8.0
Oxytetracycline	6.0	210	1.0
Erythromycin	1.0–1.5	2000	0.5
Tylosin	1.0	1700	–
Lincomycin	5.0	500	–

One of the important factors is metabolism (see Figure 1.1). Drugs undergo metabolism (also known as biotransformation) to products that are usually more polar and less lipid soluble than their original products. Usually the products that are produced following metabolism are less active pharmacologically, although this is not invariably the case. Sometimes prodrugs are given therapeutically which are initially inactive but are converted to active drugs as a result of metabolism: hetacillin is an example of an antibiotic compound which is converted to the active prodrug ampicillin. Most drugs are metabolized in the liver in two phases, phase I and phase II.

Phase I reactions usually involve oxidation of the drug during metabolic transformation. They usually increase the degree of ionization of the drug and permit the subsequent synthetic reactions (generally coupling with endogenous compounds like glucuronic acid, acetate, glycine or sulphate). Phase I reactions are carried out in the smooth endoplasmic reticulum of the liver by a wide range of oxidation reactions due to enzymes known as mixed function oxidases. These reactions require the P_{450} system, oxygen, energy, and the drug as the substrate. The products of the phase I reactions are then available for phase II reactions.

$$\text{Drug} \xrightarrow[\text{reactions}]{\text{Phase I}} \text{Oxidation products} \xrightarrow[\text{reactions}]{\text{Phase II}} \text{Conjugated products}$$

The *phase II* reactions (synthetic reactions) take the products of phase I and conjugate them with glucuronic acid, glycine, cysteine, methionine or a variety of other metabolites. The most common reaction in the dog is conjugation with glucuronic acid under the influence of the specific enzyme glucuronyl transferase. This enzyme is deficient in the cat so that glucuronic acid conjugation is not available in this animal. It also means that drug metabolism in the cat is lower as a result. The products of conjugation are much more water soluble and highly ionized so that their distribution is restricted and they are excreted more readily in the urine (or occasionally in the bile).

Most glucuronides or other conjugated substances pass back into the bloodstream from the liver and are filtered in the kidney by glomerular filtration and pass into the urine. Some drugs are excreted by the liver into the bile where they pass into the small intestine. Once they reach the small intestine, the glucuronide form of the drug may be hydrolized by the digesting enzymes and the drug reabsorbed. This reabsorption of the drug is known as enterohepatic cycling. If it occurs, it prolongs the action of the therapeutic agent. It is seen with morphine and the strong opiate analgesic etorphine (Immobilon).

It has been pointed out that in cats glucuronide synthesis is slow or absent and this means that lipid-soluble compounds may be excreted very slowly and have an extended duration of action. In general, may drugs have longer half-lives in the cat for this reason. The particular example where the half-life of the drug is dramatically different is aspirin: in cats the half-life is about 36 hours compared with 12 hours in the dog.

Conjugation by acetylation also occurs for drugs like the sulphonamides. In the dog the acetylation process is deficient. This has a clinical consequence in that crystalline urea is more likely to occur in the dog because the sulphonamides are converted to a limited number of metabolites. The concentration of individual sulphonamide metabolites is, therefore, higher in the dog. In the cat, because acetylation is available, the sulphonamides may be excreted in the urine in a variety of metabolites and so decrease the risk of crystalline urea. The risk of producing a crystalline urea may be reduced in the dog (and in the cat) by making the urine alkaline: the metabolites of the sulphonamides are more soluble in alkaline urea. Sodium bicarbonate may be given by mouth to make the urine more alkaline.

Drug induced changes in metabolism: enzyme induction and antagonism

The use of formal mathematical descriptions of the duration of drug action in the body (e.g. the use of the half-life) leads falsely to the conclusion that this quantity is fixed and does not vary. The duration of many drugs is determined by their metabolism and the enzymatic processes in the liver microsomes which may be modified by other drugs. For example, phenobarbitone, if given for a long period of time (say 2 weeks), will increase the activity of the liver microsomes. This will lead to a reduction in the half-life of a variety of other drugs including phenylbutazone, other barbiturates and cortisone. The generalized increase in drug metabolism is known as enzyme induction. It can lead to the development of tolerance and the loss of the therapeutic benefit of any drug.

The opposite process, which is less common, is known as enzyme antagonism; it occurs with chloramphenicol. Chloramphenicol will antagonize the action of liver microsomes after a single injection, so leading to the increase in half-life of drugs which are metabolized by the liver. Thus, a dog anaesthetized with pentobarbitone will remain anaesthetized for much longer if it has received an injection of chloramphenicol within an hour of the administration of the anaesthetic.

Factors affecting dose frequency

Delayed absorption depot therapy

A variety of therapeutic agents are prepared by the pharmaceutical industry in such a way that they are released slowly from a depot which is deposited intramuscularly or, occasionally, subcutaneously. These preparations consist of insoluble esters, which are hydrolysed slowly, or therapeutic agents given in oily bases (e.g. oestradiol). As a consequence, the therapeutic agent is released slowly from the depot so that the absorption phase is prolonged. This means that the concentration of the drug in the plasma is not dominated and determined by the excretion rate. It provides a convenient way of maintaining effective plasma concentrations.

Therapeutic plasma concentrations (Cp_{min} and Cp_{max})

For most drugs to be effective a minimum plasma concentration (Cp_{min}) must be maintained throughout therapy: should concentrations drop below this level, no therapeutic benefit from the drug would be seen. A maximum plasma concentration (Cp_{max}) should not be exceeded because toxic effects could be produced. Table 1.3 illustrates some examples where the therapeutic ranges (Cp_{min} and Cp_{max}) have been defined in human patients based on clinical experience. The general aim of drug administration is, then, to maintain concentrations above a minimum plasma concentration and not to exceed a maximum plasma concentration.

Table 1.3 Concentration ranges for some therapeutic agents

Agent	Cp_{min} (μg/ml)	Cp_{max} (μg/ml)
Sulphonamides	50	150
Trimethoprim	2	6
Penicillin	0.1	25
Gentamicin	4	16
Erythromycin	2	8
Oxytetracycline	1.5	4
Chloramphenicol	5	15
Propranolol	0.02	0.08
Digoxin	0.001	0.003
Phenytoin	10	20

Duration of action after a single dose

Many drugs in veterinary medicine are administered as a single dose, e.g. acetylpromazine, ketamine, atropine, morphine and naloxone. They are often given by intramuscular injection so that the absorption and distribution phase is rapid compared with the elimination. The plasma concentration/time relationship is then described by a single exponential governed by the rate constant β. The duration of action of this drug (Figure 1.5a) is then described by the equation

$$T_{ther} = \frac{\log_e (D_0/D_{min})}{\beta}$$

T_{ther} is the duration of a therapeutic level of the drug (i.e. above Cp_{min}). The just effective dose (D_{min}) is defined as that dose (mg/kg) which gives the minimum plasma concentration. The just-effective dose is equal to the product of Cp_{min} and the volume of distribution. β is the rate constant of elimination.

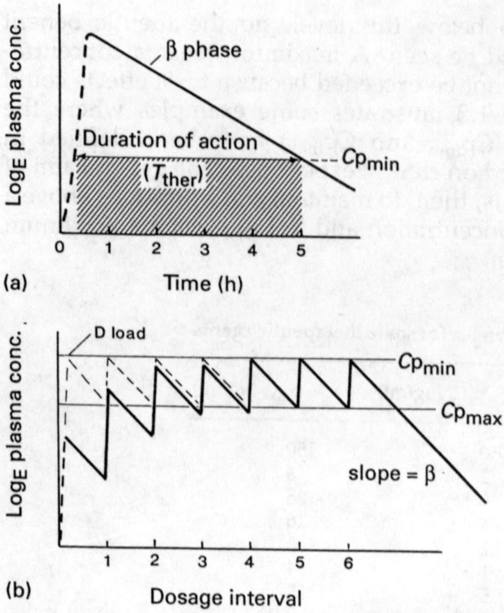

Figure 1.5 (a) Duration of action after a single injection;

$$T_{ther} = \frac{\log_e(\text{dose given} \div \text{just effective dose})}{0.693 \div T_{1/2}}$$

(b) Plasma concentration/time relationships during a multiple dosage schedule. Dotted line shows the effect of a loading dose and maintenance doses. Solid line shows the effect of maintenance-only doses. D load, the loading dose

Incidentally, β is directly related to the half-life of the drug ($T_{1/2}$) by the equation

$$\beta = \frac{0.693}{T_{1/2}}$$

Thus the duration of action of a drug increases with the log of the dose of the drug administered (D_0). Administration of twice the just-effective dose produces a duration of action which is equal to the half-life of the drug. In order to produce a duration of action three times the length of the drug's half-life, it is necessary to administer eight times the amount of the just-effective dose.

In conclusion, we can say that it is the margin of safety which determines the maximum dose which may be given and it is the half-life of the drug which then determines the duration of action following administration of a single dose by intravenous or intramuscular injection when the drug is rapidly absorbed and distributed. If drugs are more slowly absorbed compared to their elimination, the rate of absorption will determine the duration of action as long as sufficient amounts are absorbed to give effective plasma levels.

Dose schedule

Rather than administering a single dose, most therapeutic agents are given as multiple doses at regular periods. A dose schedule contains two variables: the magnitude of each dose and the frequency with which the dose is repeated. The objective of a dose schedule is to maintain the plasma concentrations above the minimum effective level and below the maximum safe concentration (i.e. between Cp_{min} and Cp_{max}). In designing dose schedules it is usually assumed that the bioavailability, volume of distribution and half-life of the drug (as determined from single dose studies) are not altered during the course of administration in a diseased animal. Clearly this is not invariably the case since animals may have impaired hepatic and renal function and in those cases it would be reasonable to expect the half-life of drugs to be increased. The following account is applicable to drugs which are rapidly absorbed and distributed when compared to their rate of elimination. It is not applicable to drugs which are slowly absorbed.

Figure 1.5b illustrates the drug concentration in the plasma, plotted on a log scale against time, following repeated administration of a therapeutic agent. Two approaches can be used for dosing. The first approach is to use one loading dose which quickly establishes an effective concentration in the plasma and this is maintained by the repeated administration of a maintenance dose at fixed intervals thereafter. The second approach involves the repeated administration of only the maintenance dose at fixed intervals. This provides an effective plasma concentration after a period of equilibration; initially there are periods where an effective plasma concentration is not achieved.

Normally, dosage intervals are chosen to be 4, 6, 8, 12 or 24 hours. Table 1.4 illustrates the relationship between the half-life of the drug, the dose interval and the percentage change in plasma concentration. This table also illustrates the fact that the longer the half-life of the drug, the smaller is the fluctuation between successive doses. Similarly, the shorter the dose interval, the smaller is the fluctuation in the plasma concentration between successive doses.

It is the half-life of the drug and the safety margin (the difference between Cp_{min} and Cp_{max}) which can determine the dose interval of the drug. For example, if a maintenance dose is given at regular intervals equal to the half-life of the drug, then there will be a 50% change in the concentration of the drug in the plasma. The level of fluctuation in concentration of the drug in the plasma can be reduced by reducing the maintenance dose and by reducing the interval between doses; if the maintenance dose is halved, then the dosage interval should also be halved.

Table 1.4 Half-life ($T_{1/2}$):dose interval % fluctuation relationship for drugs that are rapidly absorbed and distributed

	Dose interval (h)				
$T_{1/2}$ (h)	*24*	*12*	*8*	*6*	*4*
24	50	30	20	16	11
12	75	50	37	30	20
8	87.5	64.5	50	40	20
6	93.75	75	60	50	37
4	98.44	87.5	75	64.5	50
2	99.23	98.44	93.75	87.5	75

Calculation of dose

If an initial priming dose is to be given then that dose (D_{prime}) may be calculated from the equation:

$D_{prime} = Cp_{max} \times$ volume of distribution

Once again Cp_{max} is the maximum concentration of the drug desirable in the plasma and if exceeded is likely to precipitate untoward effects. Again the volume of distribution is a constant that relates the plasma concentration of the drug to the amount present in the body and is obtained from single dose studies.

After this priming dose has been administered, repeated doses are then administered at constant intervals known as the dose interval (previously described). The aim of the maintenance dose is to replace the drug which has been eliminated by excretion during the preceding dosage interval. The maintenance dose is calculated from the equation

$$D_{\mathrm{maintenance}} = D_{\mathrm{prime}} \times \text{fraction eliminated}$$

This equation appears simple enough except that the fraction eliminated has to be determined from a more complicated equation, namely

$$\text{Fraction eliminated} = 1 - \exp\left(\frac{-0.693 \times \text{time}}{T_{1/2}}\right)$$

In this equation $T_{1/2}$ is the half-life of the drug and time is the dose interval. This equation may appear formidable at first sight but is easily calculated using a microcomputer: it starts with a value of zero at time = 0 and increases exponentially as time increases up to the value of 1; 50% of the drug would be eliminated after an interval equal to the half-life; 75% of the drug would be eliminated after an interval of twice the half-life; 87.5% of the drug would be eliminated after three times the half-life.

Therapeutic considerations

A loading dose is usually necessary for drugs which have long half-lives, like digitoxin and digoxin, and for compounds which have a low safety margin ($Cp_{max} - Cp_{min}$ is small) like lignocaine and procainamide. It is also an advantage to use a loading dose followed by a maintenance dose for bacteriostatic compounds like the tetracyclines and sulphonamides. A simple and effective approach is to use a loading dose followed by a maintenance dose calculated as one half of the loading dose and given at intervals equal to the half-life of the drug. Under this dose schedule there is no period of inadequate therapy and there is a minimum toxic risk. The loading dose can be calculated as before.

It is unnecessary to use a loading dose with drugs that have short half-lives like penicillin, cephalosporins and gentamicin. These compounds are bactericidal and the peak serum levels or tissue levels may be more important for these drugs than maintaining plasma levels that have a bactericidal activity throughout the course of treatment. It is known that the penicillins are more potent and bactericidal on bacteria which are in their active growth phase.

Variation occurs from animal to animal

A variety of factors can influence the main pharmacokinetic parameters ($T_{1/2}$ and volume of distribution). The half-life of the drug may be influenced by liver and kidney disease since these organs are involved in the elimination of the drug. Induction of hepatic microsomal enzymes also occurs, so that in some cases the half-life of the drug progressively shortens with chronic therapy. Other disease states, including uraemia and hyperproteinaemia, are also going to adjust the pharmacokinetic parameters. The pharmacokinetic parameters are also established on a limited number of animals and provide for no variability between the animals that the veterinary surgeon has to treat. It is therefore imperative that the clinician uses his judgement to make appropriate corrections in dose amplitude and interval to take account of varying circumstances.

Example: dose determination

Determine a suitable dose schedule for a 20 kg dog for gentamicin. Given: $V_d = 300$ ml/kg; $T_{1/2} = 1$ h; $Cp_{max} = 16$ µg/ml; $Cp_{min} = 4$ µg/ml; assume rapid absorption and distribution.

$$\text{Total volume of distribution} = \text{Weight} \times V_d = 20 \times 300\ \text{ml} = 6000\ \text{ml}$$

$$D_{prime} = Cp_{max} \times V_d \times \text{fraction absorbed} = \frac{16 \times 6000 \times 1}{1000}\ \text{mg} = 96\ \text{mg}$$

Duration of action of D_{prime}

$$T_{ther} = \frac{\log_e (D_{prime} \div D_{min})}{0.693 \div T_{1/2}}\ \text{h} = \frac{\log_e (Cp_{max} \div Cp_{min})}{0.693 \div T_{1/2}}\ \text{h} = \frac{\log_e (16 \div 4)}{0.693 \div 1}\ \text{h} = 2\ \text{h}$$

$$
\begin{aligned}
\text{Let dose interval} &= 1\,\text{h} \\
D_{\text{maintenance}} &= \text{fraction eliminated} \times D_{\text{prime}} \\
&= 1 - \exp\left(\frac{-0.693 \times 1}{1}\right) \times D_{\text{prime}} \\
&= 1 - \exp(-0.693) \times D_{\text{prime}} \\
&= (1 - 0.5) \times D_{\text{prime}} \\
&= 0.5 \times D_{\text{prime}} \\
&= 48\,\text{mg hourly}
\end{aligned}
$$

$$
\begin{aligned}
\text{Let dose interval} &= 1.5\,\text{h} \\
\text{Then } D_{\text{maintenance}} &= 1 - \exp\left(\frac{-0.693 \times 1.5}{1}\right) \times D_{\text{prime}} \\
&= (1 - 0.354) \times D_{\text{prime}} \\
&= 0.646 \times 96\,\text{mg} \\
&= 62\,\text{mg every } 1.5\,\text{h}
\end{aligned}
$$

Note that because $T_{1/2}$ is short and Cp_{max}/Cp_{min} is small, maintenance doses have to be given frequently.

Further reading

Gibaldi, M. and Perrier, O. (1975) *Pharmacokinetics*, Dekker, New York

Baggot, J. D. (1977) *The Principles of Drug Distribution in Domestic Animals: The Basis of Veterinary Clinical Pharmacology*, Saunders, Philadelphia, London and Toronto

Marriner, S. E. (1986) How drugs act in the body. *Veterinary Record*, **119**, 132–135

Chapter 2

Antibiotics

Most but not all antibacterial agents are antibiotics derived from fungal moulds. Penicillin was the first to be isolated by Florey and Chain from *Penicillium notatum*. Many others have been isolated and are now available for therapeutic purposes. This chapter considers the antibacterial agents and their properties, the factors which influence their selection for therapeutic purposes and the treatment of some general conditions seen in small animal practice.

The properties of antibacterial drugs

Penicillins

Benzyl penicillin (penicillin G)

This acidic antibiotic (Figure 2.1), or a derivative, is frequently used in veterinary practice. With calcium, sodium or potassium it forms very soluble salts in water; it also forms a procaine salt which is relatively insoluble. The sodium and calcium salts are stable when dry but gradually lose their strength in aqueous

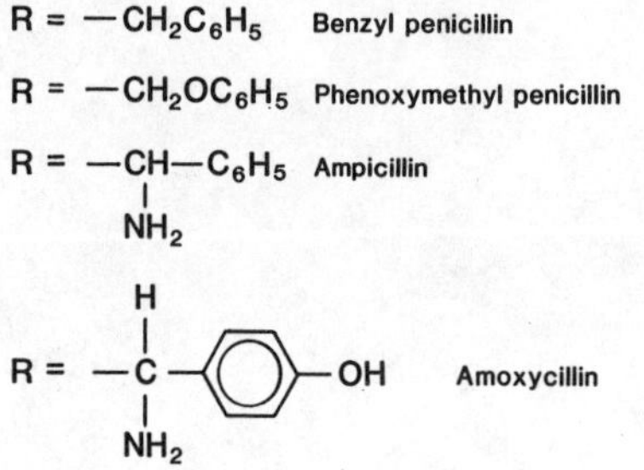

Figure 2.1 The structure of penicillins

solution: oily solutions are stable. It is important not to contaminate the oily solutions with water since this results in hydrolysis. Aqueous solutions of penicillin are quickly absorbed if they are given by intramuscular or subcutaneous injection. They cannot be given orally since they are not stable at the acid pH of the stomach and are broken down. The half-life of benzyl penicillin is short (about 30 minutes); it is quickly excreted in the urine.

In general, benzyl penicillin is distributed in the extracellular fluids; this includes joints, wound fluids, and the fetus in the pregnant animal. However, penicillin does not enter the cerebrospinal fluid when given parenterally, nor does it penetrate the eye. In order to maintain serum concentrations of benzyl penicillin, manufacturers prolong the absorption of the antibiotic by preparing a suspension of the insoluble procaine penicillin salt in oil or water for administration by intramuscular or subcutaneous injection. Absorption is further delayed by using a water repellent, such as aluminum stearate, in the preparation. Unfortunately, preparations such as these may provide only a low blood level of the drug and may not be useful when high concentrations are required therapeutically.

Penicillin is effective against most Gram-positive bacteria such as staphylococci and streptococci (see Table 2.1) but it is ineffective against Gram-negative bacteria like *E. coli* and salmonellae. Penicillin interferes with the synthesis of the bacterial cell wall and as a result is bactericidal. It interferes with the synthesis of polypeptide required for the cell wall and is most effective against rapidly growing bacteria. It has no effect on formed cell walls and has little effect on mature non-dividing bacteria. Penicillin has little effect against L forms of bacteria which are deficient in the cell wall polypeptide. Certain strains of staphylococcal bacteria produce a penicillinase (β-lactamase) which converts penicillin to the inactive penicilloic acid.

Penicillins, unlike the sulphonamides, are not inactivated by blood, pus, tissue autolysates or large numbers of bacteria. Hypersensitivity reactions, which include urticaria, pruritus and, *in extremis*, acute anaphylaxis may be seen. Guinea pigs and hamsters are particularly sensitive to penicillins and may develop fatal diarrhoea at therapeutic doses.

Phenoxymethyl penicillin (penicillin V)

This compound has the same action as benzyl penicillin but is more stable following oral absorption because it is resistant to

Table 2.1 Sensitivity of bacteria to antibacterials

Antibacterial	Mode of action	*Staphylococcus aureus*	*Staphylococcus* (β-lactamase producers)	*Streptococcus*	*E. coli*	*Proteus*	*Pseudomonas*	*Pasturella*	*Spirochaetes*	*Klebsiella pneumoniae*	*Corynebacterium*	*Micrococcus*	*Bacteroides*	*Alcaligenes*	*Salmonella*	*Mycobacterium*	*Haemophilus*	*Fusobacterium*	*Enterobacter*	*Diplococcus*	*Chlamydia*	*Aerobacter*	*Serratia*	*Rickettsia*	*Mycoplasma*	*Leptospira*	*Clostridium*	*Bordetella*	*Actinomyces*	*Vibrio*
Penicillins (benzyl penicillin)	C	S		R/S				R/S	R/S		S	S	S				R/S			S						R/S	S		S	
Ampicillin	C	S		S	S	R/S		S		R/S	S	S	S	S	S		S	S	R/S	S						S	S	S		R/S
Amoxycillin	C	S		S	S	R/S		S			S	S	S	S	S		S	S	S	S						S	S	S		R/S
Clavulanate + amoxycillin	C	S	S	S	S	R/S		S	S	S	S	S	S	S	S		S	S	S	S						S	S	S		S
Streptomycin	C	R/S	R/S	R/S	R/S	R/S		R/S		R/S	S			S	R/S	S	S		S	R/S						S			R/S	
Neomycin	C	S	S	R/S	S	S	R/S	S	S		S	S		S	S	R/S	S			S	R/S	S			S				R/S	
Framycetin	C	S	S	R/S	S	S	R/S	S		S	S	S		S	S	R/S	S		S	R/S								R/S		
Gentamicin	C	S	S	S	S	S	R/S	S		S	S	S		S	S	R/S	S		S	R/S								R/S	R/S	
Spectinomycin	C	R/S	R/S	R/S	S			S		S					S		R/S	S	S				R/S		S					
Novobiocin	C	S	S	S				R/S			S						S			S								S		
Tetracyclines	St	R/S	R/S	R/S	R/S	R/S		S	S	S	S		R/S	S	R/S		R/S		S	S	R/S	S		S	S	S	S	R/S	S	S
Chloramphenicol	St	R/S	R/S	S	S	S			S	S	S		S	S	S	S	S	S	S	S	S	S	S	S	S		S	S	S	S
Lincomycin	St/CS		R/S	S					R/S		S	R/S	S			R/S				R/S							S	S		R/S
Erythromycin	St/CS		S	S				S	S	R/S	S	S	R/S			R/S	S	S		S							S	S		S
Tylosin	St/CS		R/S	S				R/S	S		R/S		R/S			R/S	R/S	S		S	S				S	S	S			S
Polymyxin	C				S		S			S					S		S											S		
Bacitracin	St/CS		S	S							S	S								S							S			
Sulphonamides	St	R/S			R/S	S		R/S		R/S	S		S	S	S		R/S	S	S			S	S		R/S		S	S		
Trimethoprim + sulphonamides	St/CS		R/S	S	S	S		S		S	S		S	S	S		S	S	S			S	S		S		S	S		S
Metronidazole	C			R/S									S					S									S		S	S
Sodium fusidate	C	S	S	R/S							S			R/S													S	S		
Nalidixic acid	C				S	S				S					S															
Nitrofurantoin	C	S	S	S	S	S				S	R/S																R/S	R/S	S	
Nitrofurazone	C	S	S	S	S	S				S	R/S																R/S	R/S	S	
Nitroxoline	C	S	S	S	S	S	S	S			S																			
Cephalexin	C	S	S	S	S	R/S		S		R/S	S	S	S	S	S		S	S	S	S			S	S	S		S	S		R/S

St = bacteriostatic; C = bactericidal; S = likely to be sensitive to antibiotic; R/S = sometimes resistant to antibiotic.

destruction by the gastric acid. It is usually given orally after another penicillin has been given parenterally to initiate treatment.

Benethamine and benzathine salts of penicillin

Both of these compounds are long-acting preparations which, when given intramuscularly, will release benzyl penicillin slowly. Benzathine penicillin also has the advantage of being acid stable and may therefore be given to dogs and cats by mouth.

Ampicillin

This is a semi-synthetic penicillin which has an extended spectrum of activity against Gram-negative organisms including *E. coli* and proteus. Like benzyl penicillin, the half-life of ampicillin is short (approximately 1 hour); it is available as the sodium or the trihydrate salt. Although prolonged concentrations may result from the administration of the trihydrate, plasma levels are often insufficient to control many bacteria.

Amoxycillin

This also is a semi-synthetic penicillin and has an antimicrobial spectrum similar to ampicillin: it is more readily absorbed and persists for longer times, having a half-life of about 1.5 hours.

β-Lactamase inhibitors

β-Lactamase inhibitors have been synthesized. Such a compound is clavulanic acid which is administered with amoxycillin and as such is effective against staphylococcal organisms producing the lactamase enzymes.

Cloxacillin

Cloxacillin is a semi-synthetic penicillin but is resistant to penicillinase produced by strains of staphylococcus. It is stable in acid conditions. It has a half-life of about 30 minutes.

Cephalosporins

This group of compounds is closely related to the penicillins and has a 7-amino-cephalosporanic acid nucleus. They have a very similar mode of action, physiological disposition and toxicity. In general they have a greater resistance to inactivation by the β-lactamase enzymes produced by staphylococcus. They may sometimes be given to patients sensitive to the penicillins because the opening of the β-lactam ring of cephalosporin gives rise to an unstable product which cannot combine with protein to become antigenic.

Cephalexin

This is a first generation cephalosporin which has an action against Gram-positive cocci as well as some Gram-negative organisms like *E. coli*, salmonella, proteus and pseudomonas.

Aminoglycosides

These compounds are so called because they are composed of amino sugars connected by glycosidic linkages. They are organic bases and are highly water soluble. They should not be mixed with the penicillins since they are inactivated in solution (except for streptomycin and dihydrostreptomycin). Their mode of action includes an inhibition of bacterial protein synthesis due to binding to the 30S ribosomal subunit of the bacteria. The aminoglycosides are taken up actively by the bacteria by a process which requires aerobic conditions: this means that the aminoglycosides are inactive against anaerobic organisms. The spectrum of activity of the aminoglycosides includes aerobic Gram-negative bacteria. Bacterial resistance to these antibiotics develops quickly and occurs as a result of enzymic alteration of the drug at several sites. An organism resistant to one aminoglycoside may still be sensitive to another. The aminoglycosides are most active at alkaline pH but are inactivated by high concentrations of pus. These antibiotics are not well absorbed following oral administration. They remain in the gastrointestinal tract. Absorption from intramuscular or subcutaneous sites is rapid. These compounds are distributed in the extracellular fluid with little accumulation taking place in the cerebrospinal fluid (CSF).

Since the aminoglycosides are excreted unchanged in the urine, the half-life depends on the glomerular filtration rate. The half-life may be as little as 1.5 hours but can increase dramatically in cases of renal dysfunction (up to 2 days). It is obvious that the dose schedule must be altered to take account of renal dysfunction. Toxicity of the aminoglycosides includes damage to the auditory and vestibular branches of the eighth cranial nerve, producing changes in balance and hearing. This ototoxicity is particularly likely to occur if there is a failure to detect pre-existing renal dysfunction or if the aminoglycoside is given concurrently with furosemide. Nephrotoxicity is also a potential hazard of these compounds.

Streptomycin and dihydrostreptomycin

These compounds are the oldest aminoglycosides. The dihydrostreptomycin derivative should be used with particular care since it has a more toxic effect on the vestibular nerve. Resistance to these compounds is known to develop rapidly. Penicillin is often used with streptomycin since, in combination, these compounds show synergism. Streptomycin is active against most penicillin-sensitive organisms and some Gram-negative bacteria, including *E. coli*, proteus and pseudomonas.

Neomycin

Neomycin is poorly absorbed from the gut and is useful for the treatment of enteric infections. Neomycin is the most toxic of the aminoglycosides and should not be used systemically, its use being limited to topical, ophthalmic and irrigating preparations. The prolonged use of neomycin for the treatment of enteric infections may lead to malabsorption or suprainfections.

Framycetin

This compound is very similar to neomycin but is too toxic to be used systemically. Its use is in topical enteric applications.

Kanamycin

This is more effective against a wider spectrum of bacteria than streptomycin but is less effective than gentamicin.

Gentamicin

This compound is a useful aminoglycoside in veterinary practice. It is a broad spectrum aminoglycoside, having an effect against Gram-negative and some Gram-positive organisms. Because bacterial resistance to this compound develops relatively quickly, it would be sensible to limit its use to minimize the spread of resistance.

Spectinomycin

The main action of this compound is against Gram-negative organisms and mycoplasma. Although this compound acts by inhibition of protein synthesis as the other aminoglycosides, it is bacteriostatic rather than bactericidal in its action.

Novobiocin

This antibiotic is similar in its spectrum of action to benzyl penicillin. It also appears to act by interfering with the synthesis of the bacterial cell wall. It is bactericidal and has an action against Gram-positive cocci but little effect against Gram-negative organisms. Resistance to this antibiotic develops fairly quickly.

Tetracyclines

This broad spectrum group of antibiotics includes oxytetracycline, chlortetracycline and tetracycline. They have the broadest spectrum of all antibiotics and affect Gram-positive cocci, Gram-negative bacilli and rickettsia and psittacosis (Table 2.1).

Tetracyclines act by interfering with protein synthesis at the 30S ribosomal unit and, to a lesser extent, interfere with oxidative phosphorylation, glucose oxidation and cell membrane permeability.

The tetracyclines can be given orally and, in the dog and cat, peak concentrations in the blood occur after three hours. Levels persist for up to six hours. The tetracyclines are widely distributed; they cross the placenta and enter the CSF. Excretion is in the bile and also in the urine. There is some degradation in the body. A dose administered orally takes up to four days for complete excretion. An oral dose is incompletely absorbed leaving a high concentration of the antibiotic in the faeces. They have a chelating action, binding metallic ions, particularly calcium, magnesium and manganese, and so inhibit a number of essential enzymes. However, this chelating action can also lead to tetracyclines being deposited in the bones and teeth as a bright yellow fluorescent calcium complex. As a result it has been suggested that in young animals tetracyclines may prevent or inhibit the growth of teeth and bones. Tetracyclines are irritant and it is necessary to inject them by deep intramuscular injection to minimize the effects of sterile abscesses. Procaine hydrochloride is usually incorporated to minimize the sensation of pain at the injection site. In general, tetracyclines have a low toxicity. Adverse effects are seen following oral administration and result from suprainfection. This may give rise to symptoms of vomiting and diarrhoea in dogs. Cats tolerate the tetracyclines less well.

Oxytetracycline

This is the most commonly used tetracycline and is available in tablet form and a preparation suitable for intravenous injection. Like the other tetracyclines, this compound is bacteriostatic rather than bactericidal and is effective against a broad spectrum of bacteria.

Doxycycline and minocycline

These are the newer tetracyclines which have not been used extensively in veterinary practice. They show a greater spectrum of action *in vitro* compared with the other tetracyclines.

Chloramphenicol

This antibiotic has a relatively simple structure and is readily synthesized. It is stable in acid and can withstand boiling. It is a broad spectrum bacteriostatic compound and has an action against Gram-positive and Gram-negative bacilli. It is active against *Salmonella typhi* and *S. paratyphi*. It has an action against protein synthesis by blocking synthesis at the ribosome. It combines competitively with the 50S subunit of the ribosome and can then block amino acid uptake on the growing peptide chain. It is well absorbed from the gut, peak plasma levels taking about 2 hours to reach a maximum. It is well distributed throughout the body and is found in adequate concentrations in the CSF and in the eye. Conjugation of chloramphenicol takes place in the liver and excretion is then mainly via the urine. The half-life of chloramphenicol is 4 hours in the dog and 5 hours in the cat. Chloramphenicol is prepared as a salt of the palmitate or sodium succinate. Topical preparations are frequently used and applied to the conjunctivae for treatment of bacterial infections.

The use of chloramphenicol is now limited in the UK because of reports of toxic reactions, particularly in causing blood dyscrasias. It is also known that chloramphenicol inhibits microsomal drug metabolism in the liver and thus prolongs the effects of other drugs normally removed from the body by oxidation. The effect of barbiturates on dogs undergoing treatment with chloramphenicol is extensively prolonged. In addition to these toxic effects, the use of chloramphenicol is restricted because of its involvement in transmissible resistance. It is possible that chloramphenicol may produce a resistant strain of *E. coli* which may transmit its resistance to other enterobacter (including salmonella).

In man chloramphenicol is an important specific treatment for typhoid and the increase in chloramphenicol-resistant strains of the organism causing this disease has given rise to concern. Because of this risk and the possible toxic effects of chloramphenicol, it is suggested that this drug is restricted to conditions for which no other antimicrobial agent is available. Thus the use of chloramphenicol in small animal practice appears to be justified for the treatment of feline panleucopenia and infections of the eye.

Lincomycin

Lincomycin is a naturally occurring antibiotic. A synthetic variant has been marketed: this is called clindamycin. The latter compound is not used frequently in small animal practice.

These compounds have an effect against Gram-positive cocci and bacteroides. Penicillinase-producing staphylococci are often sensitive, although some reports of resistance to lincomycin have occurred. Acquired resistance can develop after prolonged use for the treatment of staphylococci. The lincomycin interferes with protein synthesis at the level of the ribosome. It acts in the same way as erythromycin and some cross-resistance may occur for this reason. Lincomycin is not completely absorbed from the gut and plasma levels are reduced if food is taken with the drug. This latter effect is less marked with clindamycin. The half-life of lincomycin in the dog is 5 hours; the half-life of clindamycin is 14.5 hours. Lincomycin is used as a bacteriostatic against streptococci and penicillinase-producing staphylococci but not against Gram-negative organisms. It is found in particularly high concentrations in the bone and so is useful for treating osteomyelitis of the acute or chronic form. Lincomycin produces minimal side-effects. Occasional diarrhoea and, very rarely, jaundice are seen.

Macrolides

This is a large group of antimicrobial compounds and is so called because they possess a large lactone ring. They are active against most Gram-positive organisms and in addition pleuro-pneumonia-like organisms including rickettsia and psittacosis. Most of the macrolides are bacteriostatic but in high concentrations and against certain bacteria may be bactericidal. Their mode of action is to interfere with protein synthesis by disrupting bacterial ribosomes.

Erythromycin

Erythromycin is well absorbed from the gut but the stearate requires an enteric coat to resist digestion by gastric acid. Plasma levels reach a peak in about 2 hours and the drug is cleared with a half-life of 1–1.5 hours. The drug reaches most tissues, except the brain, and only 20% is excreted in the kidneys. Most is metabolized and appears in the bile, where it is highly concentrated. Erythromycin is indicated for penicillin-resistant Gram-positive infections or in patients where penicillin sensitivity has been seen. Toxicity with this compound is low: only delayed hypersensitivity of Type IV is seen occasionally. Allergic skin rashes are more common with the ester form of the drug than with alternate forms.

Tylosin

This is another macrolide antibiotic and is absorbed from the gut and excreted in the urine and bile. It is active against a large number of Gram-positive organisms, a few Gram-negative organisms and mycoplasma. It is also useful for treatment of chlamydia infestations of the gut. It is therefore useful for certain enteric infections.

Polypeptides

Polymyxins

These are polypeptide antibiotics. There are several polymyxins. Polymyxin B is the least toxic and the only member of the group used clinically. It is water soluble and stable in acids but is destroyed by alkalis. It has a selective action against Gram-negative bacteria including *E. coli*, salmonella, haemophilus, pasteurella and chlamydia (Table 2.1). Polymyxin is usually restricted to local or topical application because it is regarded as too toxic to administer parenterally. It is not absorbed from the gut and so is used very occasionally for the treatment of gastrointestinal infections. It may have a use in the treatment of infection in the urinary tract where an organism is resistant to other antibiotics. It is effective for this treatment since it is excreted in the urine.

Polymyxin is bactericidal and acts on growing as well as non-growing cells. It appears that polymyxin makes the bacterial cell well permeable so that cytoplasmic constituents are lost. It also has an inhibitory action on oxidative metabolism. Since resistance to polymyxin is rare, this drug is often used in combination with other antibiotics. In small animal practice it can be used for local applications to the skin, external ear, mucous membranes and similar surfaces.

Bacitracin

Bacitracin is another polypeptide antibiotic. It is active against Gram-positive organisms including some clostridia and actinomyces organisms. It is poorly absorbed from the gut and is in fact destroyed in the alimentary tract. The mode of action of this compound is to block the incorporation of nucleotides into the cell wall. It may be useful for topical application.

Sulphonamides

The sulphonamides have been used as antibacterial agents since the 1930s. They are weak acids and moderately soluble. Sodium salts of these compounds are most frequently used. Since these solutions are alkaline they may produce sloughing if injected perivascularly. These compounds are usually metabolized in the body after acetylation and become less soluble than the parent compound. These acetylated forms of sulphonamide may be precipitated in the urine and form crystalline urea. Precipitation is particularly likely in acid urine. To minimize this effect triple sulphonamide mixtures may be used, since the presence of one sulphonamide does not appreciably affect solubility of another similar sulphonamide. The sulphonamides act by interfering with the synthesis of folic acid from para-aminobenzoic acid (PABA). Because the sulphonamides work in this way it means that organisms which can utilize preformed folic acid are insensitive. It also means that the onset of the action of the sulphonamide is slow (up to 5 hours) while the preformed folic acid present in the bacteria is used up.

Since the synthesis of folic acid is necessary in a wide range of bacteria, the sulphonamides have a broad spectrum of action.

Their spectrum includes Gram-negative and Gram-positive organisms. Previous frequent use of the sulphonamides has led to many resistant organisms. However, this can be circumvented by incorporating trimethoprim which acts synergistically with the sulphonamide to block folic acid synthesis. As a result, the combination of trimethoprim and the sulphonamide (often sulphadiazine) is effective against a wide range of organisms (Table 2.1).

In general the absorption of the sulphonamides is very good: they become well distributed throughout the body. The exception to this general rule are the so-called enteric sulphonamide preparations (phthalylsulphathiazole) which are confined to the intestine following oral administration. The half-lives of the sulphonamides vary from about 4 hours to 12 hours. The main route for excretion is via the kidney, the long acting sulphonamides undergoing extensive tubular reabsorption.

Sulphacetamide

This compound forms a neutral sodium salt so that it is not irritant and may be used as an antiseptic in the eye. Sulphacetamide is like sulphathiazole and is short acting, lasting less than 12 hours.

Sulphadiazine

This sulphonamide compound has an intermediate duration of action lasting 12–24 hours. It is probably the most active sulphonamide and is well absorbed from the gut. The high concentration produced in the urine is useful for the treatment of urinary infections. The substantial proportion which is reabsorbed in the renal tubules is responsible for its longer action.

Sulphamethoxypyridazine and sulphamethylphenazol

In recent years chemists have synthesized various sulphonamides in an attempt to find those compounds which are well absorbed from the gut and are excreted slowly. As a result they produced these compounds which have a high concentration in the plasma and which persist for more than one day. These compounds suffer the disadvantage that they are slowly absorbed so the onset of their action is slow. Also their excretion is slow and there is a longer time where concentrations may fall below the bacteriostatic levels and this may result in the appearance of resistant strains.

Sulphonamide synergists

When it was found that the sulphonamides interfered with the conversion of para-aminobenzoic acid to folic acid, a search was made for further compounds which would interfere with the synthesis. It was found that an intermediate stage between para-aminobenzoic acid and folic acid was a reaction which involved reduction of dihydrofolate to tetrahydrofolate. This conversion was carried out under the influence of the enzyme dihydrofolate reductase, which could be blocked to potentiate the action of sulphonamides.

Trimethoprim

Trimethoprim antagonizes dihydrofolate reductase in a selective manner. It is effective against bacterial dihydrofolate reductase in a concentration tens of thousands times less than that required to antagonize the enzyme in mammalian tissues. In the dog the half-life of trimethoprim is about three hours. It is interesting to compare this with the half-life of sulphadiazine which is ten hours. It can be seen that if these two compounds are used together in an attempt to obtain a synergistic effect, steps must be taken so that the compounds are present simultaneously. There is another complication in using trimethoprim as a synergist and that is that it is not found evenly distributed in the tissues. It is found in high concentrations in the kidney and liver but in lower concentrations in the other tissues. Organisms which have shown a resistance to sulphonamides are frequently susceptible to the mixture of sulphonamide and trimethoprim. The sequential block which trimethoprim and the sulphonamide have on the synthesis of folic acid in the bacteria make the development of resistance unlikely. The main disadvantage of their use is that trimethoprim and the sulphonamide may not be simultaneously present in the same concentrations at the site of action because of their different distributions and half-lives.

Metronidazole

Metronidazole is a nitroimidazole and is a synthetic compound. The action of this compound is mainly against anaerobic organisms. The nitro group of metronidazole is reduced by susceptible organisms and as a result it inhibits deoxyribonucleic acid (DNA) synthesis. Metronidazole has a broad spectrum of action against pathogenic protozoa. As a bactericidal compound it is effective against anaerobic bacteria including bacteroides, enterobacter, fusobacterium and vibrio. It is well distributed following oral administration and is found in the CSF. It is excreted primarily by the kidney after extensive metabolism. Adverse effects are not considered to be important.

Sodium fusidate

Sodium fusidate has a simple steroid structure. It is bacteriostatic and has an action against Gram-positive and Gram-negative cocci. It is useful against penicillinase-producing staphylococci and is frequently used in ointments for skin infections. When it is administered topically it can penetrate the skin, particularly if it is given dissolved in dimethyl sulphoxide. If it is given orally, it is absorbed from the gut and is widely distributed but does not enter the CSF or cross serous membranes. It can be used to treat infections of the bone since it will diffuse into bone fragments.

Nitrofurans

These compounds are synthetic compounds derived from 5-nitrofuran. They are readily absorbed following oral administration and are widely distributed in the body but concentrations are very low. Concentrations sufficient for systemic antimicrobial action would be too toxic. The drugs are usually metabolized and excreted by the kidney with 50% appearing in the active form. Acidification of the urine promotes tubular reabsorption, thereby increasing the duration of the action of the drug and decreasing urine concentrations. Despite this, however, urine concentrations are sufficiently high, permitting these compounds to be used for the treatment of cystitis. The urine should be made acid to enable the drug to diffuse across the bacterial cell membrane. These compounds appear to act by blocking oxidative decarboxylation of pyruvate to acetyl CoA. The spectrum of action of the nitrofurans includes an action against Gram-positive and Gram-negative organisms as well as some protozoa.

Nitrofurazone

This compound is usually used topically and has an action against Gram-positive organisms as well as some Gram-negative organisms. It has little effect against proteus and pseudomonas.

Nitrofurantoin

This compound is usually used in small animal practice as a treatment for urinary tract infection. It is quite effective for this condition but is contraindicated if there is pre-existing renal dysfunction. Toxic effects have been reported which include peripheral neuritis, pulmonary complications and hepatitis. Gastrointestinal side-effects are fairly frequently seen.

Nalidixic acid

This drug is useful for the treatment of urinary tract infections caused by Gram-negative organisms, especially those caused by pseudomonas. Toxic signs in cats and dogs are characterized by neurological reactions and epileptiform seizures. Doses of 3 mg/kg, however, have been reported to be safe in dogs and cats if administered every six hours. Nalidixic acid works by inhibiting nucleic acid synthesis.

Amphotericin B

Amphotericin B is a polyene antibiotic. It is poorly absorbed following oral administration and as a result is only given orally for the treatment of fungal infections in the gastrointestinal tract. Although preparations are available for intravenous administration, adverse reactions, including nephrotoxicity and other life-threatening reactions like cardiac arrhythmia and acute hepatic failure, are likely to occur. Other problems include nausea and haemolytic anaemia. Amphotericin B is frequently used as a topical application. The mechanism of action involves a combination of the antibiotic with the sterols of cell membranes of susceptible fungi. As a result, ion channels are formed in the membrane: these leak potassium and sodium. This prevents the cell from controlling its intracellular environment and thus produces its death. Amphotericin B has a broad spectrum action against pathogenic fungi, including those causing histoplasmosis, blastomycosis, cryptococcosis, candidiasis, aspergillosis and sporotrichosis. The basis of its selective action is that it is has no effect on membranes that do not contain sterols. The cholesterol in mammalian cell membranes form less susceptible binding sites than the sterols of the pathogenic fungi.

Nystatin and natamycin

Nystatin is also a polyene antibiotic and has a similar mode of action to amphotericin B. It is not used parenterally because of its systemic toxicity. Preparations for oral and topical administration are available. It is frequently used for the treatment of candidiasis. Natamycin is also a polyene antibiotic and is used for topical application as a fungicidal compound. It is not absorbed through the skin and so there is no likelihood of systemic toxicity.

Griseofulvin

This compound is used for the treatment of ringworm infection. It is very insoluble in water and it is important that the absorption is increased using micronized preparations. The drug is given orally and only a small amount is absorbed. It is known that a diet high in fat will facilitate absorption. Once the drug has entered the bloodstream it is laid down selectively in the keratin of the skin, hair and nails. Initially it is laid down in the stratum germinativum, the growing layer of the skin. It then grows out gradually with the new layers of skin and hair. It may take several weeks to reach the outer keratin layers of the skin or the distal portions of the nails. Griseofulvin is metabolized by methylation and only a small proportion (1%) is excreted unchanged in the urine. The mechanism of the antifungal action is that it enters the susceptible fungi and inhibits division by attacking the mitotic spindles. It arrests the cells in the metaphase of division. Toxic effects include gastrointestinal upsets, photosensitization and occasionally depressed spermatogenesis. It has been shown to be teratogenic to cats. Phenobarbitone is known to depress the absorption of griseofulvin.

Miconazole

This compound is a β-substituted benzimidazole which is active against ringworm (trichophyton and microsporum) or candida infections. It may be applied topically or given by mouth. It appears, at least in the case of yeast, to inhibit the uptake of nucleic acid. Other related compounds (clotrimazole and etisazole) are also used for the local treatment of ringworm in small animals.

Factors which influence the selection of an antibacterial agent

Bacterial sensitivity

It is obvious that any antibacterial agent used must be effective against the infecting organism. If it is not, then such use will be without result. There are two major ways in which bacterial sensitivities may be estimated.

The first approach is to use sensitivity tests whereby the bacteria are cultured on to suitable agar media on which filter papers soaked in various antibiotics have been placed. If an antibiotic is effective against the organism it will inhibit growth around the edge of the filter paper and leave a clear zone. The clear zones therefore show sensitivity to the antibiotic. The lack of a clear zone right up to the filter paper suggests that the organism is not sensitive to that particular antibiotic. Antibiotic sensitivity tests like these usually take up to two days to produce results and this can limit their effectiveness.

In small animal practice the most commonly used approach to estimating sensitivity is to establish the likely organisms involved on a basis of the clinical history which indicates the affected organ or tracts. Table 2.2 shows the likely pathogenic organisms which are recovered from the various tissues or organs. For example, streptococcal and staphylococcal infections occur in most tissues, whereas organisms like vibrio are only commonly recovered from the gastrointestinal tract. Once the likely organism has been identified on this basis, it is then possible to use Table 2.1 which shows the sensitivity of bacteria to antibacterial agents and suggests suitable antibacterial agents for therapy. Table 2.1 shows, for example, that the penicillins are often effective against staphylococcal organisms which do not produce β-lactamase enzymes but that there are many organisms which are not sensitive to its action. In contrast, it can be seen that trimethoprim in conjunction with sulphadiazene is active against a wide range of bacteria. Tables 2.1 and 2.2 therefore provide useful guides for the selection of antibacterial agents. It is clear that many infections may be treated

Table 2.2 Likely tissue locations of pathogenic bacteria

Location	Wounds	Skin	Ears	Eyes	Mouth	GI tract	Respiratory tract	Urinary tract	Genital tract	Mammary gland	Bones and joints	CNS	Bacteraemia
Vibrio	–	–	–	–	–	✓	–	–	–	–	–	–	–
Actinomyces	✓	–	–	–	–	–	–	–	–	–	–	–	–
Bordetella	–	–	–	–	–	–	✓	–	–	–	–	–	–
Clostridium	✓	–	–	–	–	–	–	–	–	–	–	–	–
Leptospira	–	–	–	–	–	–	–	✓	–	–	–	–	–
Mycoplasma	–	–	–	–	–	–	✓	–	–	–	–	–	–
Rickettsia	–	–	–	–	–	✓	✓	✓	–	–	–	–	✓
Serratia	–	–	–	–	–	–	–	✓	–	–	–	–	–
Aerobacter	–	–	–	–	–	–	✓	✓	–	–	–	–	–
Chlamydia	–	–	–	✓	–	–	✓	–	–	–	–	–	–
Diplococcus	–	–	–	–	–	–	✓	–	–	–	–	–	✓
Enterobacter	–	–	–	–	–	✓	–	✓	–	–	–	–	–
Fusobacterium	✓	–	–	–	✓	–	–	–	–	–	–	–	–
Haemophilus	–	–	–	–	–	–	✓	–	–	–	–	✓	–
Mycobacterium	–	–	–	–	–	✓	✓	–	–	–	–	–	–
Salmonella	–	–	–	–	–	–	✓	–	–	–	–	–	✓
Alcaligenes	✓	–	–	–	–	–	–	✓	–	–	–	–	✓
Bacteroides	✓	–	–	–	✓	–	–	–	–	–	–	–	✓
Micrococcus	–	–	–	✓	–	–	✓	✓	–	–	–	–	–
Corynebacterium	✓	–	–	–	–	✓	–	–	–	✓	–	–	–
Klebsiella pneumoniae	–	–	–	–	–	✓	✓	✓	–	–	–	–	✓
Spirochaetes	✓	–	–	–	✓	✓	–	–	✓	–	–	–	–
Pasturella	✓	–	–	–	✓	–	✓	✓	–	–	–	–	✓
Pseudomonas	✓	✓	✓	–	–	✓	✓	✓	–	–	–	–	–
Proteus	✓	✓	✓	–	–	✓	✓	✓	–	–	–	–	✓
E. coli	✓	✓	✓	–	–	✓	✓	✓	✓	✓	–	–	✓
Streptococcus	✓	✓	✓	✓	✓	✓	✓	✓	✓	✓	✓	✓	✓
Staphylococcus aureus	✓	✓	✓	✓	✓	✓	✓	✓	✓	✓	✓	✓	✓

successfully with more than one antibacterial agent and it is therefore imperative that further criteria are used to select the appropriate agent.

Antibacterial distribution

The distribution of the antibacterial agent to the site of infection in an adequate concentration is necessary for the successful treatment of the disease. Antibacterial agents like the penicillins, which are highly ionized, are relatively poorly distributed throughout the body. In contrast, substances like the sulphonamides and chloramphenicol, which are not highly ionized, are well distributed throughout the body and are found in high concentrations in the CNS as well as the eye when they are administered parenterally. It must also be appreciated that the access of an antibacterial agent to the invading organism may be reduced in the presence of oedema, fibrinous tissue or purulent material which can be associated with the infectious process.

Bactericidal or bacteriostatic?

In general it is better to use bactericidal rather than bacteriostatic agents since the host animal's immune response may be impaired in the presence of an overwhelming infection. The common bactericidal antibiotics are the penicillins, streptomycin and polymixin. The common bacteriostatic agents are the sulphonamides, tetracyclines, chloramphenicol, erythromycin and novobiocin.

Narrow or broad spectrum?

The prime function of an antibacterial agent is to kill the invading pathogenic organism. It is not intended that the antibacterial agent should kill non-pathogenic organisms often found in the intestine and on the skin. The exposure of the non-pathogenic organisms to the antibacterial agent may result in diarrhoea, or development of resistance which may be passed on to other bacteria.

Duration of action

If antibacterial agents are used in combination then it is appropriate that their duration of action should be similar. For example, penicillin and streptomycin are often used in combination since the two antibiotics show a synergistic effect. Penicillin (benzyl penicillin), however, is rapidly cleared from the body, having a half-life of only 30 minutes. Streptomycin, on the other hand, has a half-life of 2.5 hours. Trimethoprim and sulphadiazene (Tribrissen) are often used in combination. Trimethoprim however, has a half-life of 3 hours but sulphadiazene has a half-life of 10 hours in the dog. There is, therefore, a considerable period of time when these two drugs are not present together in adequate concentrations.

Local conditions

The presence of large amounts of pus will not permit the rapid bacterial growth which is necessary for the bactericidal action of penicillin and the cephalosporins. Pus will also lead to an accumulation of para-aminobenzoic acid which will antagonize the action of the sulphonamides.

pH

Weak acids like the penicillins, the sulphonamides, nitrofurantoin, novobiocin and tetracycline accumulate in alkaline conditions. Weak bases like the aminoglycosides and the macrolides accumulate in conditions where the pH decreases. Acidic urine will therefore favour the secretion of weak bases. An alkaline urine will favour the excretion of weak acids.

Development of resistance

It has been shown in the laboratory that repeated exposure of an organism to antibiotics may induce resistance. The speed of onset of the resistance depends to a certain extent on the antibiotic used. Penicillin, for example, does not easily produce resistance. Streptomycin, erythromycin and novobiocin fairly easily induce resistance. It is therefore considered better if those compounds which easily induce resistance are used in conjunction with at least one other drug which is effective against that particular organism being treated.

Synergism

Some antibiotics may act together and show synergism. This means that in combination they are much more effective than used separately. For example, antibiotics which are bactericides

Table 2.3 Oral antibiotics

Generic and trade names	Presentation	Dose		
		Dog (10 lb)	*Dog (40 lb)*	*Cat*
Amoxycillin				
Clamoxyl Palatable Tablets	Tabs 40 mg	½–1 b.i.d.	–	½–1 b.i.d.
Clamoxyl Palatable Tablets	Tabs 200 mg	–	½–1 b.i.d.	–
Clamoxyl Palatable Drops	Drops 50 mg/ml	½–1 ml b.i.d.	–	½–1 ml b.i.d.
Ampicillin				
Amfipen	Tabls 50 mg	½–2 b.i.d.	–	½–2 b.i.d.
Amfipen	Tabs 125 mg	½ b.i.d.	3 b.i.d.	½ b.i.d.
Amfipen	Caps 250 mg	–	1 b.i.d.	–
Amfipen	Tabs 500 mg	–	½ b.i.d.	–
Penbritin	Caps 50 mg	1 b.i.d.	4 b.i.d.	1 b.i.d.
Penbritin Capsules	Caps 250 mg	–	1 b.i.d.	–
Penbritin Oral Doser	Paste 50 mg/ml (1 dose)	1 dose b.i.d.	4 doses b.i.d.	1 dose b.i.d.
Cephalexin				
Ceporex Tablets	Tabs 50 mg	1 b.i.d.	–	1 b.i.d.
Ceporex Tablets	Tabs 250 mg	–	1 b.i.d.	–
Ceporex Oral Drops	Drops 100 mg/ml	½–1 ml b.i.d.	3 ml b.i.d.	½–1 ml b.i.d.
Chloramphenicol				
Chloramphenicol	Tabs 50 mg	4–6	–	4–6
Chloramphenicol	Tabs 100 mg	1 b.i.d.	4	1 b.i.d.
Chloromycetin	Caps 250 mg	1	4	1
Chloromycetin Palmitate	Suspn 125 mg/5 ml	5 q.i.d.	20 q.i.d.	5 q.i.d.

Clavulanate potentiated amoxycillin				
Synulox Palatable Tablets and Drops	Tabs 50 mg	1 b.i.d.	–	1 b.i.d.
	Tabs 250 mg	–	1 b.i.d.	–
	Drops 50 mg/ml	1 ml b.i.d.	5 ml b.i.d.	1 ml b.i.d.
Erythromycin				
Erycen	Tabs	½–1	2–3	½–1
Lincomycin				
Lincocin	Tabs 100 mg	1 b.i.d.	4 b.i.d.	1 b.i.d.
Lincocin	Tabs 500 mg	–	1 b.i.d.	–
Lincocin Aquadrops	Drops 50 mg/ml	2–3 ml b.i.d.	–	2–3 ml b.i.d.
Metronidazole				
Flagyl	Tabs 200 mg	½	2	½
Torgyl	Solution	4 ml/kg	4 ml/kg	4 ml/kg
Neomycin				
Neobiotic	Tabs 100 mg	¼ b.i.d.	1 b.i.d.	¼ b.i.d.
Neobiotic Liquid	Soln 50 mg/ml	1	4	1
Neobiotic-P Aquadrops	Drops 50 mg/ml	1 ml b.i.d.	4 ml b.i.d.	1 ml b.i.d.
Neo-sulphentrin	Tabs	1	4	1
Neo-sulphentrin	Suspn	5 ml	20–25 ml	5 ml
Nitrofurantoin				
Furadantin	Tabs 50 mg	½ t.i.d.	2 t.i.d.	½ t.i.d.
Furadantin	Tabs 100 mg	–	1 t.i.d.	–
Nitroxoline				
Nibiol-V	Tabs 50 mg	1	4–6	1–2
Nibiol-V Forte	Tabs 100 mg	NR	2–3	NR
Streptomycin				
Neo-sulphentrin	Tabs 21 mg	1	4	1
Neo-sulphentrin	Suspn 200 mg/30 ml	5 ml	20–25 ml	5 ml

Generic and trade names	Presentation	Dose: Dog (10 lb)	Dose: Dog (40 lb)	Dose: Cat
Sulphonamides				
Kaobiotic (+Neomycin)	Tabs	½ b.i.d.	2 b.i.d.	½ b.i.d.
Kaobiotic (+Neomycin)	Suspn	3 b.i.d.	10 ml b.i.d.	3 b.i.d.
Keosul (+Neomycin)	Tabs	1 b.i.d. then ½ b.i.d.	3 b.i.d. then 1 b.i.d.	½ b.i.d.
Keosul (+Neomycin)	Suspn	5 ml b.i.d. then 2½ b.i.d.	10–20 ml b.i.d. then 10 b.i.d.	5 ml b.i.d. then 2½ b.i.d.
Neo-sulphentrin (+Neomycin +Streptomycin)	Tabs	1	4	1
Neo-sulphentrin (+Neomycin +Streptomycin)	Suspn	5 ml	20–25 ml	5 ml
Tetracycline				
Berkmycen	Tabs 250 mg	–	2 t.i.d.	–
Berkmycen	Caps 250 mg	–	2 t.i.d.	–
Berkmycen	Syrup 125 mg/5 ml	2½ ml t.i.d.	5 ml q.i.d.	2½ ml t.i.d.
Dio Oxytet Powder	Powder 13.77 g/250 g	5 g	20 g	3–5 g
Oxytetracycline	Tabs 250 mg	–	2 b.i.d.	–
Oxytetracycline	Tabs 100 mg	1 b.i.d.	–	1 b.i.d.
Oxytetracycline Tablets B.P.	Tabs 50 mg	1–5	–	1–5
	Tabs 100 mg	1–2	2–10	1–2
	Tabs 250 mg	1	1–4	1
Panmycin Aquadrops	Drops 100 mg/ml	2½ ml q.i.d.	–	2½ ml q.i.d.
Rondomycin	Caps 150 mg (methacycline)	–	2 b.i.d.	–
Trimethoprim + Sulpha				
Tribrissen 20	Tabs T.20 mg S.100 mg	½ b.i.d. or 1 once daily	2 b.i.d. or 4 once daily	½ b.i.d. or 1 once daily
Tribrissen 80	Tabs T.80 mg S.400 mg	–	½–1 b.i.d. or 1–2 once daily	–
Tylosin				
Tylan Tablets	Tabs 200 mg	¼–½ b.i.d.	1–2 b.i.d.	¼–½ b.i.d. or once daily

such as penicillin, neomycin and streptomycin can potentiate each other. However, they should not be used with bacteriostatic compounds like tetracyclines and chlorampenicol because they may produce antagonism.

Duration of therapy

The treatment of simple acute infections can be discontinued if the animal has been free of clinical signs for three days. In practice, this means that a course of antibacterial agents lasts three to five days. Chronic bacterial infections may require several weeks of therapy.

Treatment of some specific bacterial infections

Tables 2.1 and 2.2 illustrate the likely pathogenic bacteria infecting particular tissues and the appropriate antibacterial agent suitable for treatment. Tables 2.3 and 2.4 show the preparations and doses of most antibacterials which are available for administration orally or by injection. Further comment is now made on the treatment of infections of particular tissues.

Infections of the ear

Bacterial otitis externa is particularly common in the dog; it is also seen in the cat but at a lower frequency. Table 2.5 illustrates the likely pathogens that are found in this condition. *Staphylococcus aureus* with *Pityrosporum canis* are common isolates recovered from dogs with affected ears. In cats, similar pathogens are found. *Staph. aureus* is less common (*Otodectes cynotis* is the commonest cause of otitis in cats). β-Haemolytic streptococcal organisms are also recovered commonly from otitis externa. Pseudomonas and proteus are recovered commonly from dogs with chronic infections. The condition is evident following examination of the external ear canal.

Before the administration of an appropriate antibiotic it is important that the ear canal is thoroughly cleansed by flushing rather than wiping with cotton tipped swabs. It is also important to examine the tympanic membrane since chronic infections can be associated with rupture of the membrane and secondary otitis media. Topical applications of benzyl penicillin, neomycin, polymyxin and gentamicin are particularly useful in the

Table 2.4 Injectable antibiotics†

Generic and trade names	*Presentation*	*Route of administration*	*Dose* (ml) *Dog (10 lb)*	*Dog (40 lb)*	*Cat*
Amoxycillin					
Clamoxyl Ready to Use	150 mg/ml	i.m., s.c.	0.25	1	0.25
Clamoxyl LA	150 mg/ml	i.m., s.c.	0.5	2	0.25–0.5
Ampicillin					
Penbritin Injectable Suspension	150 mg/ml	i.m., s.c.	0.25	1	0.25
Penbritin Veterinary Injectable	500 mg	i.v., i.m.	0.25	1	0.25
Chloramphenicol					
Chloramphenicol	150 mg/ml	i.m.	0.25–0.5	1–2	0.25–0.5
Chloramphenicol Suspension	10%	s.c.	0.25	1–1.5	0.25
Chloramphenicol Suspension	150 mg/ml	i.m.	0.25	1	0.25
Chloromycetin Succinate	10%	i.v., i.m.	1	4	1
Intramycetin Aqueous Suspension	15%	i.m.	0.25–0.75	2–3	0.5–0.75
Erythromycin					
Erythrocin Injectable	200 mg/ml	i.m.	0.25	1–1.5	0.25
Erythrocin i.v.	Powder for reconstitution	i.v.		See data sheet	
Framycetin					
Framomycin Injection	5%	i.m.	1	3–4	1
Framomycin Injection	15%	i.m., i.v.	–	1–1.5	–
Gentamicin					
Gentovet	50 mg/ml	i.m., s.c.	0.5	2	0.25–0.5
Lincomycin					
Lincocin Sterile Solution	100 mg/ml	i.v., i.m., s.c.	1	4	1

Metronidazole					
Torgyl	5 mg/ml	i.v., i.m., s.c.		4 mg/kg	
Neomycin					
Neobiotic Sterile Solution	50 mg/ml	i.v., i.m.	1	4	1
Neobiotic Sterile Solution	200 mg/ml	i.v., i.m.	–	1	–
Penicillin					
Crystapen	5 mega sod. pen.	i.m.	0.25–0.5	1–2	0.25–0.5
Mylipen	*300 000 IU/ml	i.m.	0.5–1	2	0.5–1
Penillin	*300 000 IU/ml	i.m.	0.25	1	0.25
Penillin L.A.	proc. 150 000 benz. 150 000 IU/ml	i.m.	0.5	1	0.5
Propen (LA)	proc. 150 000 benz. 150 000 IU/ml	i.m.	0.5	2	0.5
Penicillin/Streptomycin					
B-Pen-S (LA)	100 ml strep. 250 mg proc. 100 000 benz. 100 000	i.m.	0.5	1–2	0.5
Penicillin/Streptomycin	proc. 200 000 IU/ml strep. 250 mg	i.m.	0.25	1	0.25
Pen & Strep	proc. 200 000 IU/ml strep. 250 mg				
Spectinomycin					
Spectam Injectable	100 mg/ml	i.m.	0.5–1	2–3	0.5–1
Streptomycin (with dihydrostreptomycin)					
Dimycin	1 g/3 ml	i.m.	0.25–0.5	1	–
Ilcocllin S	1 g/4 ml	i.m.	0.5	2–3	0.25

Generic and trade names	Presentation	Route of administration	Dose (ml) Dog (10 lb)	Dog (40 lb)	Cat
Sulphonamides					
Intradine	33⅓%	s.c., i.v., i.m., i.p.	1	4	1
Sulphamezathine Sodium Solution 33⅓	33⅓%	s.c.	–	Init. 10 then 5	–
Vesulong	20%	s.c., i.m.	0.75–1	3–5	0.5–1
Oxytetracycline					
DioTet	50 mg/ml	i.v. (cats only), i.m., s.c.	1	4	0.5–2
Duphacycline 50	50 mg/ml	i.m., i.v., s.c.	0.5–1	2	0.5
Engemycin	50 mg/ml	i.m., i.v., s.c.	0.5–1	2–4	0.5–1
Occrycetin Injection	100 mg/ml	i.m., i.v., s.c.	0.5–1	2–2.5	0.5
Oxytetracycline HCl	50 mg/ml	i.m., s.c., i.p.	1	4	0.5–2
Oxytetrin	50 mg/ml	i.m., i.v., s.c.	0.5–1	2–3	0.5–1
Oxyvet	50 mg/ml	i.m., s.c., i.p.	0.5–1	2–3	0.5–1
Oxytracyl	50 mg/ml	i.m., i.v., s.c.	0.5–1	2–3	0.5–1
Trimethoprim + Sulpha					
Borgal	trim. 12.5 mg sulph. 62.5 mg	s.c., i.m.	1	4	1
Tribrissen 24% Injection	trim. 40 mg sulph. 200 mg	s.c.	0.5–0.75	2–3	0.5–0.75
Trivetrin	trim. 4% sulph. 20%	i.v.	0.25	1	Ci
Tylosin					
Tylan 50 Injectable	50 mg/ml	i.m.	0.5–1	1–3	0.5–1

*Procaine penicillin only.
Ci – contraindicated.
†Table modified from the *Henston Veterinary Vade Mecum – Small Animals*.

Table 2.5 Microorganisms recovered from normal and diseased ears (dogs)

	Recovered (%)	
Microorganism	*Normal ears*	*Diseased ears*
Pityrosporon canis	27	83
Staphylococcus aureus	3	38
Other staphylococci	5	21
Streptococci	–	8
Pseudomonas	–	15*
Proteus	–	4*
Other Gram-negative bacteria	–	2*

*More common in chronic and severe cases.

treatment of bacterial infections associated with otitis externa. The success of the treatment depends on the ability of the antibiotic to make contact with the infected areas in the ear canal. Thus it is important that all the wax associated with the inflammation, the blood or other debris is removed prior to the application of the antibiotic. Corticosteroids are often combined with antibiotics in commercial ear preparations. The aim of this is to reduce the tissue inflammation and scratching associated with the infection. As yet there appears to be no evidence suggesting that the use of topical corticosteroids impairs the antimicrobial effect of the antibiotic.

It is usual to apply the antibiotic twice or sometimes three times daily in order to control the bacterial infection. It is important to point out, however, that ototoxicity in animals has been associated with the administration of streptomycin and neomycin and other aminoglycosides where there is a ruptured tympanic membrane. Infection of the middle ear may follow and develop as a secondary problem to chronic otitis externa if the tympanic membrane becomes ruptured. Damage to the fifth and seventh nerves may become evident clinically. In extreme cases the inner ear may also become infected in dogs and cats which have a ruptured tympanic membrane. Bacterial meningitis can then develop subsequently but this appears to be more common in cats than dogs.

Infections of the gastrointestinal tract

There are many causes of acute diarrhoea in dogs and cats. Bacterial infections are uncommon and probably limited to only a few species of bacteria which are not normally found in the gut. The diagnosis of a specific pathogen causing enteritis in dogs or cats can only follow bacterial sampling of the faeces. Salmonella species (often *Salmonella typhimurium*) and *Campylobacter jejuni* are the organisms most likely to cause bacterial enteritis. It is difficult to establish clear-cut guidelines for treatment in the case of salmonella enteritis since the treatment of the animal with an antibiotic may lead to chronic shedding and the development of resistant strains. It may be better, therefore, to use non-antibacterial treatment for the treatment of salmonella enteritis. *Campylobacter* spp. are sensitive to erythromycin and tylosin so that it is appropriate to use these compounds for the treatment of enteritis due to this organism. In general, it is wise not to rely on antibacterial treatment alone (without fluid treatment) for enteritis.

Infections of the respiratory tract

Primary bacterial infection of the respiratory tract is not common in small animal practice. Bacterial infections usually follow as a secondary infection to viral infections of the respiratory tract. Usually diagnosis is made on the history of sneezing and serosanguineous discharge or mucopurulent nasal discharges associated with marked respiratory sounds. The treatment of these conditions will to some extent depend on the severity of the condition. Fluid therapy or the treatment of any dehydration and the administration of topical decongestants may be appropriate. Antibiotic therapy is only appropriate if a bacterial infection is likely to be present. In dogs and cats a mixed population of staphylococcal species and streptococcal species are most likely to be involved. There are, however, a large number of possible bacterial organisms which may cause the problem (see Table 2.1). As a result it may be appropriate to use a broad spectrum antibacterial treatment like ampicillin, trimethoprim/sulphadiazine or oxytetracycline. The specific organisms for *Bordetella bronchiseptica* and mycoplasma have been recovered from dogs with chronic respiratory tract infections. Tetracycline is the preferred antibiotic against these organisms. In kittens, bacterial pneumonia is a particularly nasty complication of virus infections of the upper respiratory tract.

Bone infection

Bacterial osteomyelitis is not easy to manage. It is most commonly caused by staphylococcal and streptococcal organisms (see Table 2.2). Signs of osteomyelitis include heat and swelling over the infected bone, draining tracts (sinus) and lameness. X-ray, together with a positive culture from swabs, can confirm the diagnosis of osteomyelitis. Treatment must involve surgery with drainage of the affected side. Antibiotic therapy is therefore considered as only part of the treatment of osteomyelitis. Lincomycin and clindamycin are both noted for their ability to penetrate bone. Since they are effective against the common Gram-positive organisms associated with osteomyelitis, these compounds are specifically indicated for the treatment of this problem. They must be given early while the blood supply is maintained. Fusidic acid (a small steroid) will diffuse into bone sequestra; it is the only antibacterial agent to do so and should also be considered for therapy.

Bacteraemia

Table 2.2 shows that a variety of organisms, including Gram-positive and Gram-negative organisms, may produce a bacteraemia. The colonization of one or more of the body tissues may produce a septicaemia. The clinical signs associated with this are variable, depending on the organisms and the tissues involved. Obvious features include a continuously raised temperature, anorexia, lethargy, a leucocytosis with a shift to the left. Other signs will depend on the tissues affected. Treatment must include fluid therapy aimed at treating the shock (see Chapter 10) together with appropriate antibiotic therapy. It is imperative that animals suffering septicaemia are treated with bactericidal rather than bacteriostatic antibiotics. Gram-positive septicaemia associated with staphylococcal or streptococcal infections can be treated with benzyl penicillin, ampicillin, erythromycin or cephalexin. Gram-negative infections may be suitably treated with gentamicin, ampicillin or amoxycillin.

Infections of the central nervous system

Antibacterial treatment of the central nervous system is only effective if the agent crosses the blood–brain barrier. The normal meninges are not permeable to erythromycin or the penicillins but in meningitis they do become permeable. It is best to select a therapeutic agent which will permeate the meninges so that the antibacterial agent continues to be effective as the condition subsides. Chloramphenicol and the potentiated sulphonamides (trimethoprim and sulphadiazine) are the drugs of choice.

Further reading

Adams, H. R. (1975) Acute adverse effects of antibiotics. *Journal of the American Veterinary Medical Association*, **166**, 983

English, P. B. (1965) The therapeutic use of penicillin: the relationship between dose rate and plasma concentration after parenteral administration of benzyl penicillin (Penicillin G). *Veterinary Record*, **77**, 810

Garrod, L. L. and O'Grady, F. (1971) *Antibiotic and Chemotherapy*, 3rd edn, Livingstone, Edinburgh

Milner, N. A. (1975) Penicillin toxicity in guinea pigs. *Veterinary Record*, **96**, 554

Owen, L. N. (1963) The effects of administering tetracyclines to young dogs with particular reference to localization of the drugs in the teeth. *Archives of Oral Biology*, **8**, 715

Rowley, R. A. and Rubin, L. F. (1969) Penetration of penicillin into aqueous humour of the dog. *American Journal of Veterinary Research*, **30**, 1945

Verwey, W. F., Williams, H. R. and Kalsow, P. (1966) Penetration of chemotherapeutic agents into tissues. *Antimicrobial Agents and Chemotherapy*, **1965**, 1016

Watson, A. D. J. (1972) Chloramphenicol plasma levels in the dog: a comparison of oral, subcutaneous and intramuscular administration. *Journal of Small Animal Practice*, **13**, 147

Chapter 3

Glucocorticoids

Glucocorticoids are very potent drugs commonly used in small animal practice. Proper use requires a knowledge of their physiology and pharmacology. The aim of this chapter is to describe a logical basis for their use: it also illustrates the use of glucocorticoids in a number of clinical conditions.

Glucocorticoid secretion (Figure 3.1)

Glucocorticoids are secreted in the dog at a rate equivalent to 1 mg/kg/day of cortisol. Similar rates of secretion are presumed to occur in the cat. The cortisol is released from the zona reticularis of the adrenal cortex under the influence of adrenocorticotrophic hormone (ACTH). ACTH interacts with receptors on the surface of the adrenal cortical cells to stimulate and increase the level of cortisol secretion. The central nervous

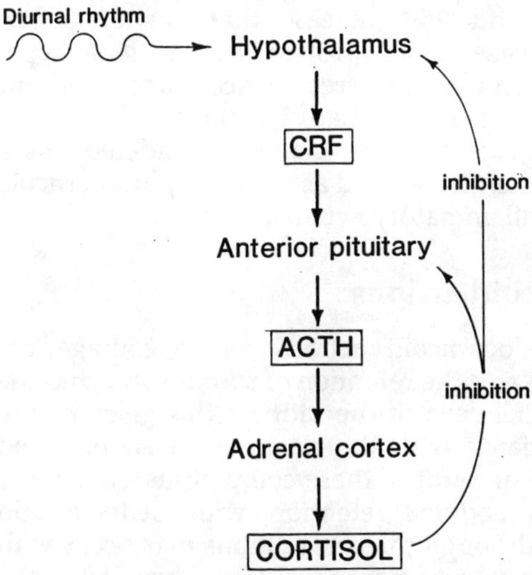

Figure 3.1 The control of glucocorticoid secretion. CRF, corticotrophin releasing factor; ACTH, adrenocorticotrophic hormone

system is able to control and monitor the level of cortisol production and to vary the amount according to conditions (temperature, stress, trauma, etc.). There is a natural diurnal rhythm in cortisol secretion: in dogs the peak level of secretion occurs in the morning; in cats the peak level of secretion is seen in the evening. The hypothalamus releases corticotrophin releasing factor (CRF) which acts on the anterior pituitary to stimulate the production of ACTH. ACTH in its turn will stimulate the adrenal cortex to increase the production of cortisol. There is an important inhibitory feedback effect of cortisol which, on release from the adrenal cortex, will inhibit further production of ACTH in the anterior pituitary and further production of CRF in the hypothalamus. This inhibitory feedback mechanism may also be activated by synthetic glucocorticoids during therapy. It will suppress the natural production of cortisol and could lead, if glucocorticoid therapy were prolonged, to a secondary adrenocortical insufficiency.

Glucocorticoid steroids are secreted directly into the blood: some are bound to plasma proteins and some remain unbound, free in the plasma. There is a specific protein (transcortin) in the plasma which is responsible for carrying the glucocorticoid; it is only the free, unbound glucocorticoid which is able to exert a therapeutic effect. Disease states which decrease the amount of the glucocorticoid bound will increase the potency of the glucocorticoid: a decrease in the protein binding in a hypoproteinaemia will increase the free concentration of the glucocorticoid and so increase its relative potency.

The actions of the glucocorticoids may be considered under three headings: the mineralocorticoid actions, the glucocorticoid actions and the anti-inflammatory actions.

The mineralocorticoid actions

Steroids with mineralocorticoid actions will encourage the excretion of potassium and the retention of sodium and chloride by the tubular epithelial cells of the kidney: this gives rise to water retention associated with the retention of sodium and chloride. An excessive amount of these compounds can lead to abnormal water and sodium retention with oedema and circulatory changes. Although these conditions may occur with Cushing's disease, they are more likely to occur after the administration of glucocorticoids which have pronounced mineralocorticoid activity; such glucocorticoids include hydrocortisone, cortisone and 11-deoxycorticosterone (Table 3.1). The

Table 3.1 Some properties of glucocorticoids

Glucocorticoid	*Relative glucocorticoid activity*	*Relative mineralocorticoid activity*	*Equivalent dose for 20 kg dog*	*Half-life* (h)
Short acting				
Hydrocortisone (cortisol)	1	1	20	12
Cortisone	0.8	1	25	12
11-Deoxycorticosterone	0	40	na	na
Medium acting				
Prednisolone	4	0.6	5	12–36
Methylprednisolone	5	0	4	12–36
Triamcinolone	5	0	4	12–36
Flumethazone	5	0	4	12–36
Long acting				
Betamethazone	35	0	0.6	48
Dexamethazone	30	0	0.75	48

na – doses not available.

other glucocorticoids, which have little mineralocorticoid action, may have the opposite effect and give rise to a diuresis, probably because they increase glomerular filtration. This means that polydipsia and polyuria are often seen during the early stages of corticosteroid therapy but these effects often decrease with time. Long courses of treatment with hydrocortisone and cortisone can lead to a hypernatraemia, a hypokalaemia and oedema. Such effects are not likely to occur with the synthetic glucocorticoids like methylprednisolone.

A deficiency in mineralocorticoid hormone levels will give rise to an undue loss of sodium and an elevation of potassium in the plasma and extracellular fluid. If this is sufficiently severe it will give rise to dehydration and circulatory collapse. The severity of the clinical signs will depend on the dietary intake of sodium and potassium: if there is a high sodium intake it is likely that less mineralocorticoid hormone is required.

Mineralocorticoids are only required for therapy in patients suffering from adrenocortical insufficiency. This is discussed later in this chapter.

The glucocorticoid actions

Glucocorticoids increase the plasma concentration of glucose, producing a hyperglycaemia, by stimulating lipolysis and protein catabolism. There is also an anti-insulin effect which adds to the hyperglycaemic effect. The anti-insulin effect occurs as a result of decreasing glucose metabolism in the peripheral tissues and is associated with an increase in the glycogen synthesis in the liver: long-term administration of glucocorticoids tends to produce hepatomegaly. It is known that glucocorticoid administration itself does not cause diabetes mellitus but can precipitate or unmask the disease. The anti-insulin effect should be remembered during insulin therapy for diabetes mellitus and adjustments in dosage made if glucocorticoids are administered simultaneously.

Protein synthesis, which is decreased as a result of glucocorticoid action, is exhibited clinically as thinning of the skin, often associated with a bilateral symmetrical alopecia, delayed healing, muscle atrophy and decreased protein synthesis. The breakdown of connective tissue may lead to softening of the bones (osteoporosis) and an increase in the serum calcium level. If calcium is deposited in the thin skin it gives rise to the condition known as calcinosis cutis. Fat metabolism is affected with long chain fatty acid synthesis being inhibited, together with immobilization and redistribution of the fat stores: dogs on long-term glucocorticoid therapy develop 'pot bellies'.

The anti-inflammatory actions

Glucocorticoids possess an anti-inflammatory and immunosuppressant action. This action is connected directly with their glucocorticoid action and cannot be separated using steroids of different chemical structures. This contrasts with the mineralocorticoid actions which can be separated using different steroid structures.

Anti-inflammatory actions and their effects include:

1. The inhibition of capillary dilatation and reduction of capillary permeability.
2. The reduction of plasma extravasation.
3. The reduction of the movement of neutrophils and monocytes into the area of inflammation.
4. The reduction of macrophage activation by inhibition of lymphokine production by lymphocytes.
5. The reduction of collagen and mucopolysaccharide formation. This impairs healing.
6. Cell membranes of lysosomes and mast cells are stabilized and so reduce the release of the mediators of inflammation.
7. The glucocorticoids induce the release of a specific protein, lipocortin (also known as lipomodulin), from leucocytes. Lipocortin then inhibits the action of the enzyme phospholipase A_2 (Figure 3.2) which is responsible for the production of arachidonic acid from cell membranes. Arachidonic acid is further metabolized and converted to produce the prostaglandins and the leukotrienes. The prostaglandins and the leukotrienes are major mediators of the inflammatory process. By inhibiting the production of these substances, glucocorticoids control and inhibit inflammation.

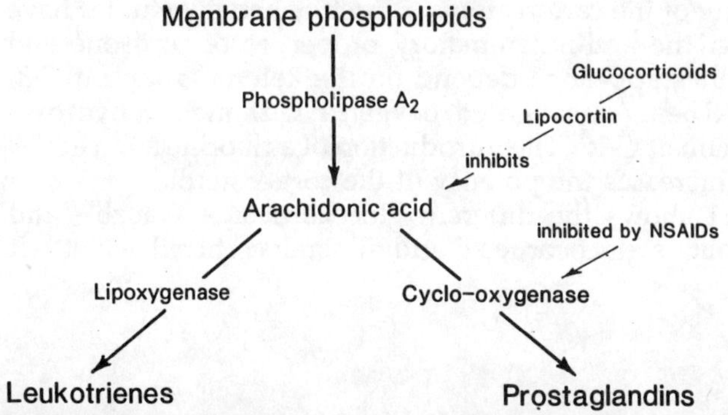

Figure 3.2 Glucocorticoids release lipocortin and inhibit leukotriene and prostaglandin production

The glucocorticoids depress the immune response, as they depress the inflammatory response, acting as follows:

1. They increase the release of neutrophils from bone marrow but reduce the entry of the neutrophils into the sites of inflammation.
2. The eosinophils are directed away from the peripheral circulation and away from the sites of inflammation, so giving rise to an eosinopenia.
3. Monocytes are no longer released from the bone marrow and this leads to a monocytopenia.
4. Lymphocytes no longer enter the inflamed tissues.
5. Interleukin 2 (a growth factor for T cells) production is inhibited and this gives rise to a reduction in T cell proliferation.
6. Antibody production by the B cells appears to be unaffected in the dog since the glucocorticoids do not reduce the response to distemper vaccination or to subsequent challenge.

Glucocorticoids and vaccination

Data sheet information states that animals which have received immunosuppressive drugs (e.g. glucocorticoids) should not be vaccinated until an interval of four weeks has elapsed. Experimental studies support this approach to a degree: in steroid-treated dogs there is a degree of immunosuppression; the immunosuppression is not absolute and depends on the dose and type of the glucocorticoid used with many but not all animals still responding to vaccination.

Synthetic glucocorticoids

Figure 3.3 shows the structure of a number of glucocorticoids and mineralocorticoids. It also shows the pregnane nucleus and the labelling of the carton atoms. Structure activity studies have shown that the anti-inflammatory properties of cortisone and the cortisones appear to depend on the ketone group on C-3, C-4 and C-5 being unsaturated, oxygen at C-11 and a dehydroxyacetone chain at C-17. The introduction of a fluorine atom at C-9 markedly increases the potency of the corticosteroid.

Table 3.1 shows the different glucocorticoids available and lists the relative glucocorticoid and mineralocorticoid activity. It

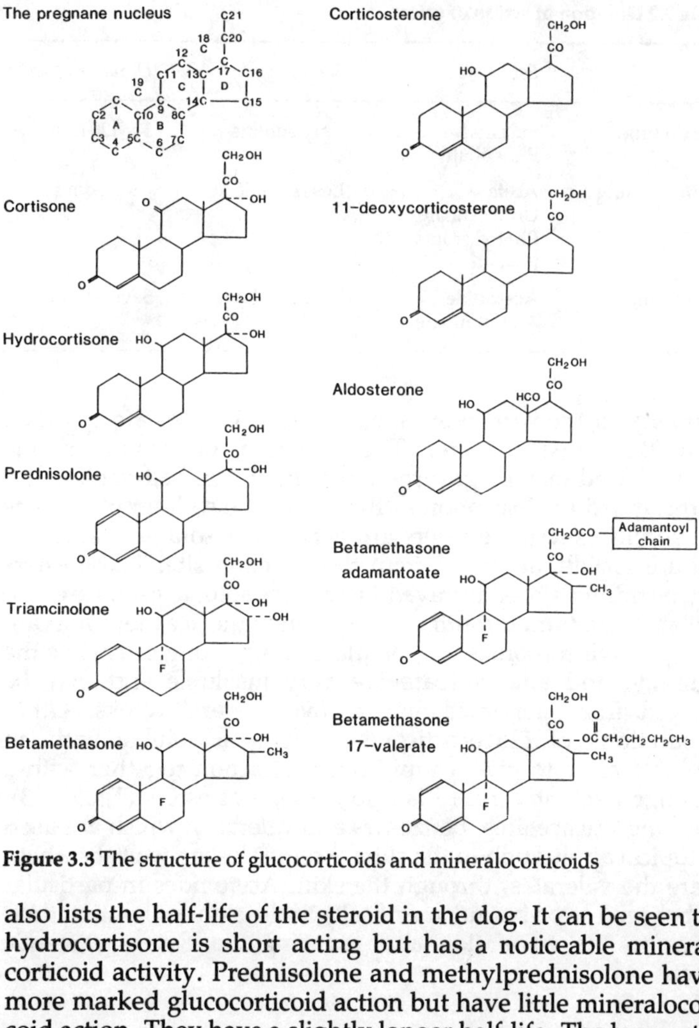

Figure 3.3 The structure of glucocorticoids and mineralocorticoids

also lists the half-life of the steroid in the dog. It can be seen that hydrocortisone is short acting but has a noticeable mineralocorticoid activity. Prednisolone and methylprednisolone have a more marked glucocorticoid action but have little mineralocorticoid action. They have a slightly longer half-life. The long acting and very potent glucocorticoids like betamethasone and dexamethasone have a marked glucocorticoid activity with no detectable mineralocorticoid action. Their half-life is greater than two days.

Ester preparations

The glucocorticoids are free alcohols so that they may be modified and presented as esters. Esters vary in their water

Table 3.2 Duration of action of esters

Type	*Ester*	*Solubility*	*Duration of action*
Short acting	Succinate Phosphate	Very soluble	30–120 min
Medium acting	Acetate Undecanoate Phenylpropionate Pivalate	Less soluble	2–14 days
Long acting	Acetonide Adamantoate	Very insoluble	Several weeks

solubility and so vary in the speed with which they are absorbed from the injection site. The duration of action of the corticosteroid may be governed not only by its half-life but also by the speed of absorption of the ester. The sodium phosphate and sodium succinate esters are very water soluble (Table 3.2) and are rapidly absorbed from the injection site. These esters may be administered intravenously. Less soluble esters are also available: medium duration esters include the acetate, undecanoate, phenylpropionate and pivulate. Long acting esters like the acetonide and adamantoate are very insoluble and may be released from the injection site over several weeks. Other preparations of glucocorticoids combine a soluble with an insoluble ester to give a rapid onset of action together with a prolonged activity. There is also a range of esters (Table 3.3), including the acetates, benzoates and valerates, which are used for topical application to the skin. Acetonides are well absorbed, as are the valerates, through the skin. Acetonides in particular are believed to be bound specifically to the skin, so limiting their access to the circulation and reducing the risk of systemic effects.

Uses of glucocorticoids

Primary adrenocortical insufficiency (Addison's disease)

This is associated with a reduction in cortisol and aldosterone secretion from the adrenal cortex. It is not seen frequently in practice but may be produced by poisoning with DDD, a DDT derivative. For treatment it is necessary to replace the natural glucocorticoid and mineralocorticoid production of the adrenal

Table 3.3 Ester preparations available in the UK

Base	*Oral*	*i.v., rapid i.m.*	*i.m., intra-articular depot, etc.*	*Topical*
Hydrocortisone	–	–	Acetate	Base, acetate
Prednisolone	Free base[a]	–	Free base,[b] pivalate[c]	Free base, metasulphobenzoate, acetate
Methyl prednisolone	–	Sodium succinate[d]	Acetate[e]	–
Triamcinolone	–	–	–	Acetonide
Fluocinolone	–	–	–	Acetonide[f]
Flumethazone	Free base[g]	–	Free base[h]	+ DMSO[i]
Betamethazone	Free base[j]	Sodium phosphate[k]	Adamantoate,[ℓ] dipropionate	Sodium phosphate, 17-valerate[m]
Dexamethazone	Free base[n]	Sodium phosphate[o]	-21-undecanoate,[p] phenylpropionate, acetate,[q] free base, pivalate, -21-isonicotinate[r]	

[a]Prednivet Tablets, Prednisolone Tablets BP.
[b]Prednivet Injection, Nisolone.
[c]Vecortenol.
[d]Solu-medrone V.
[e]Depo-medrone V.
[f]Vetalog Long-acting.
[g]Fluvet Tablets.
[h]Fluvet-Depot.
[i]Fluvet DMSO.
[j]Betsolan Tablets.
[k]Betsolan Soluble.
[ℓ]Betsovet Injection.
[m]Vetsovate Cream.
[n]Opicorten Tablets.
[o]Dexadreson.
[p]Dectan.
[q]Dexamethazone Aqueous Suspension.
[r]Voren 14.

cortex. This may be achieved by subcutaneous implantation of desoxycorticosterone acetate pellets or the intramuscular injection of a depot preparation of desoxycorticosterone pivalate every 25 days. In some cases additional glucocorticoid medication, or oral prednisolone or hydrocortisone may be required. If the animal is collapsed, an initial intravenous injection of soluble glucocorticoid is indicated to improve the circulation.

Secondary adrenocortical insufficiency

This occurs as a result of inadequate ACTH secretion which may be suppressed iatrogenically or due to disease of the pituitary gland. Since ACTH secretion only controls the secretion of glucocorticoids but not mineralocorticoids, it is only necessary to use glucocorticoids for the treatment of secondary adrenocortical insufficiency. The glucocorticoids should mimic the natural secretion of glucocorticoids as closely as possible. This may be achieved using the following approach:

1. Using short-acting hydrocortisone or prednisolone to minimize the suppression of the hypothalamus–pituitary–renal (HPA) axis.
2. Using low doses which correspond to endogenous cortisol secretion, i.e. prednisolone 0.2 mg/kg per day.
3. Administering the glucocorticoid at the right time of the day to mimic the natural diurnal rhythm (morning in the dog, evening in the cat).
4. Increasing the dose during stress situations, e.g. during surgery.

Musculoskeletal conditions

Glucocorticoids are often used for the treatment of a variety of inflammatory musculoskeletal conditions including bursitis, arthritis, myositis and tendonitis. If compounds are used early in the disease, they can produce a marked remission of the signs of inflammation. However, there is a danger that if the animal continues to use the damaged limb or organ it will put unnecessary strain on it and so lead to an aggravation of the clinical condition.

Intra-articular administration

Long-acting glucocorticoid preparations are administered intrasynovially into an inflamed joint to control and minimize arthritis in dogs. Although this method of administering the glucocorticoids appears to be useful and beneficial to the animal in a number of cases, it has been noticed that there can be a postinjection flare in the joint and other pathological changes can follow, giving rise to a steroid arthropathy. The long-term administration of the glucocorticoids will inhibit the synthesis of new articular cartilage and give rise, after erosion, to a dry joint. The risk of degenerative changes occurring intra-articularly may be reduced by the concurrent injection of hyaluronate. Intra-articular injection of the glucocorticoids is contraindicated if there is a pre-existing erosion of the articular cartilage, an intra-articular fracture, a septic arthritis, or if there is an extensive degenerative bony lesion.

Skin conditions

Glucocorticoids are often administered systemically or topically for the control of inflammatory conditions of the skin. A particularly frequent condition is flea bite allergy. Glucocorticoids are useful in reducing the self-inflicted damage by reducing the irritation. If glucocorticoids are used for a long time in the dog they may give to thinning of, and calcium deposits in the skin, leaving a condition known as calcinosis cutis. A bilateral and symmetrical hair loss may also be seen.

Keratitis (eye)

One indication for glucocorticoids is in the treatment of cases of non-ulcerative keratitis to reduce the inflammation and minimize the risk of corneal opacity. Glucocorticoids are contraindicated if there is a superficial corneal ulceration because they will retard the re-epithelialization and vascularization of the lesion. If bacteria are present, corticosteroids must be administered with antibiotics, preferably bactericidal antibiotics. Viral infections of the eye such as feline viral rhinotracheitis (FVR) in cats may be aggravated by the topical application of corticosteroids. Long-term administration of glucocorticoids can lead to blocking of the canal of Schlemm and give rise to glaucoma as a result.

Shock

High doses of soluble glucocorticoids are used for short periods of about two days for the treatment of acute shock. Glucocorticoids are thought to be particularly useful in inhibiting pulmonary oedemas resulting from smoke damage or harm due to inhalation of noxious gases. They may also be useful in suppressing the harmful effects of the endotoxins produced by enterobacter. The protective effect of the glucocorticoids has been illustrated for haemorrhagic and endotoxaemic shock when given to the animal prior to the exposure to the shock stimulus. This particular type of study is not identical to that of the clinical situation where an animal is presented after the administration of the shock stimulus. In fact the available evidence concerning the beneficial use of the glucocorticoids in shock under clinical conditions has not been conclusively demonstrated. Short-term use of high doses of glucocorticoids are, however, unlikely to produce harmful effects.

Asthma-like conditions

Asthma-like conditions in the cat can be treated with glucocorticoids but may be more specifically treated with bronchodilators (clenbuterol) and mycolytics (bromhexine). Non-steroidal anti-inflammatory drugs are definitely contraindicated in these conditions because they increase the production of leukotrienes which are bronchoconstrictors.

Autoimmune diseases

A variety of autoimmune diseases may be treated with glucocorticoids. It is suggested that high doses of prednisolone (2–4 mg/kg daily in divided doses) are required to treat conditions such as systemic lupus, autoimmune haemolytic anaemia and bullous pemphigoid. The dosage should be reduced after symptoms have been turned back and eventually reduced to alternate day administration. If the prednisolone by itself is not successful it is suggested that the treatment is supplemented with a cytotoxic drug such as cyclophosphamide. Eventually it is hoped that the dose of both these compounds can be reduced to a level which will control the disease when they are given on alternate days. Glucocorticoids are not the drugs of choice for the treatment of rheumatoid arthritis because of their lytic effect on bone cartilage. In dogs, chronic colitis which is associated with an autoimmune condition may respond to prednisolone therapy.

Neoplasia

Glucocorticoids have been used together with cytotoxic drugs such as cyclophosphamide and vinblastine in the treatment of leukaemia in dogs and cats.

Complications of chronic glucocorticoid administration

HPA axis suppression

The potent synthetic glucocorticoids will suppress the production of CRF and ACTH. They give rise to a secondary suppression of the adrenal cortex. Long-acting preparations (because they exert continued depressant action on the HPA axis) are more prone to produce secondary adrenocortical insufficiency. There is evidence to suggest, for example, that prednisolone acetate will depress the response of the adrenal cortex to ACTH for a period of up to four weeks. It is difficult to assess the significance of this action when using long-acting glucocorticoid preparations since it is difficult to estimate the time for which the animal remains 'uncovered' by the persistent glucocorticoid given in the injection. However, there is evidence to show that the withdrawal of glucocorticoids following a continuous dose for a 4-month course may precipitate acute collapse and require the intravenous administration of glucocorticoid therapy. The onset of secondary adrenocortical insufficiency may be minimized by gradually reducing the daily dose or using alternate day therapy with prednisolone.

Alternate day therapy

Many attempts have been made to reduce the adrenal suppression that results from chronic glucocorticoid administration. Apparently a critical factor in the long-term use of glucocorticoids is the maintenance of the normal diurnal cortisol secretory pattern. In the dog, the plasma cortisol levels are highest in the morning and lowest at night. The blood levels of ACTH vary inversely with the plasma concentration of cortisol. In the cat, the cortisol levels are highest at night and lowest in the morning. An alternate day steroid scheme has been developed to preserve this natural diurnal cortisol rhythm. This can only be achieved with glucocorticoids which have a short half-life (like prednisolone and methylprednisolone). These glucocorticoids are given to the dog in the morning or the cat at night when the plasma cortisol levels are normally at their highest and when the ACTH release is already inhibited by the natural negative feedback. On a subsequent day when the glucocorticoid is not administered, it will allow the hypothalamus and anterior pituitary axis to function normally and to release ACTH. Thus for long-term therapy in the dog it may be useful to administer prednisolone or methylprednisolone every second day in the morning, while in the cat to administer these compounds every second day between 10 p.m. and midnight.

A useful alternate day steroid routine is as follows: for the first 5–7 days during induction, a daily dose of prednisolone 0.5–1 mg/kg is given orally. Induction is necessary because alternate day steroid therapy is better at maintenance rather than inducing remissions. Subsequently, after the induction, an oral dose of prednisolone 1–2 mg/kg is given orally every other morning at 8 a.m. After this the dose may be reduced by 50% at weekly intervals until the lowest maintenance dose is reached which is compatible with remission of symptoms. Although this dose varies considerably from dog to dog, it often averages out at 0.5 mg/kg every other morning. In the cat the steroid is given at night.

The alternate day steroid therapy has been designed for maintenance therapy and is intended to minimize the suppression of the secretion of ACTH from the anterior pituitary. However, it has been established that although this approach does not eliminate adrenocortical atrophy and hypofunction, suppression is less and much slower in onset when alternate day therapy is used and compared with a standard daily maintenance dose.

Other complications

Table 3.4 summarizes some of the effects of chronic glucocorticoid administration. These include:

1. *Catabolic effects* The glucocorticoids lead to muscle weakness, thinning of the skin in which calcium may be deposited (calcinosis cutis), an alopecia, growth reduction and possible liver damage. A particular effect is noted at the injection site of long-acting glucocorticoids in the dog where alopecia and extensive skin thinning over the injection site may appear.
2. *Diabetes mellitus* The anti-insulin effect of glucocorticoids may lead to a glycosuria and the unmasking of latent diabetes

Table 3.4 Side-effects of glucocorticoid therapy

	Side-effect(s)
Skin	Calcinosis cutis
Muscle/bone	Weakness, osteoporosis
Metabolic effects	Hyperglycaemia, growth reduction
Digestive effects	Ulceration, pancreatitis, liver damage
Eye	Cataracts
CNS	Mood change
Endocrine organs	Secondary hypoadrenocorticism, diabetes mellitus

mellitus. The elevation of the blood glucose may also lead to eye cataracts.

3. *Water and salt movement* Polydipsia and polyuria are often seen after glucocorticoid therapy but adaptation usually takes place after about three days. It also depends on which glucocorticoid is used. Continued high doses of glucocorticoids may produce a hypokalaemia and alkalosis.
4. *Digestive effects* Glucocorticoids reduce the rate of growth of the superficial epithelial cells in the gastrointestinal tract and so may lead to ulcers. There may also be an associated pancreatitis. The liver is affected due to the stimulated gluconeogenesis and becomes enlarged. If this is sufficiently serious, liver damage ensues.
5. *Osteoporosis* The decreased protein synthesis leads to a reduction in the osteoblasts in bone and the resorption of bone. Long-term glucocorticoid therapy may lead to softening of the bone and the production of osteoporosis.
6. *Teratogenic effects* Glucocorticoids administered during pregnancy may cause cleft palate in man and laboratory animals. It is possible that similar effects may occur in the dog and the cat.

Immunosuppressants other than glucocorticoids

In addition to glucocorticoids, cytotoxic drugs have been used to treat a variety of autoimmune diseases. These drugs include cyclophosphamide (Endoxana), chlorambucil (Leukeran) and azathioprine (Imuran). Cyclophosphamide and chlorambucil are alkylating agents and act by a different molecular action to the purine analogue azathioprine. They are all immunosuppressive, cytotoxic drugs which decrease antibody formation and the production of leucocytes. They are often used with glucocorticoids.

Cyclophosphamide

This may be given by mouth on 4 consecutive days followed by 3 days rest (no drug) for up to 3 weeks at a dose rate of 1.5 mg/kg for dogs greater than 25 kg, or 2.2 mg/kg for 5–25 kg in dogs or 25 mg/kg for dogs and cats less than 5 kg. As an alternative a once weekly i.v. dose of 7 mg/kg may be given. Leukopenia should be checked for; haemorrhagic cystitis is another possible side-effect. Therapy should be ceased if the white blood cell count goes below 5000 cells/mm^3.

Azathioprine

This drug is less immunosuppressive but is less toxic. A daily dose of 2.2 mg/kg orally may be used. The white blood cell levels should be monitored and if counts fall below 6000 cells/mm^3 the dose should be reduced to 0.5 mg/kg. If the white blood cell levels fall lower than 5000 cell/mm^3, treatment should be stopped.

Chlorambucil

This drug is often restricted to use with dyscrasias of plasma cells.

Further reading

Burke, T. J. (1982) Hormone and corticosteroid therapy. *Veterinary Clinics of North America*, **12**, 1

Keen, P. M. (1986) The uses and abuses of corticosteroids. *Veterinary Annals*, **45**

Scott, D. W. (1982) Dermatologic use of glucocorticoids. *Veterinary Clinics of North America*, **12**, 19

Chapter 4

Vaccination

Dogs can be vaccinated against distemper, infectious canine hepatitis, two types of leptospirosis, canine parvovirus infection, *Bordetella bronchiseptica*, parainfluenza, tetanus and rabies. Cats can be vaccinated against feline panleucopenia, feline calicivirus and feline viral rhinotracheitis. The primary vaccination course usually consists of two or three injections when the animal is six to sixteen weeks of age and may be followed by an annual booster. This chapter considers vaccination of the dog and cat.

The immune response

The immune response to an invading agent may be local or general. Local responses consist of a limited and localized (secretory) antibody response and a local cell-mediated response, with circulating serum antibody having little effect. This localized immune response is seen against pathogens which invade only the surface mucosa. These include the respiratory pathogens like canine parainfluenza, feline calicivirus and *Bordetella bronchiseptica*. This means that local administration of a vaccine by intranasal instillation or aerosol will provide a better antigenic stimulus than may be provided by the administration of the vaccine parenterally.

Generalized immune responses occur in response to invading pathogens which travel though the bloodstream and lymphatics to reach their target sites. These pathogens include canine distemper, infectious canine hepatitis, canine parvovirus infection, feline panleucopenia and canine leptospirosis. The generalized immune response consists of production of serum antibodies, which are readily produced when the antigen is injected subcutaneously. The immune response may also consist of a cell-mediated response of sensitized T lymphocytes which eliminate the virus by attacking the cells occupied by it. This means that an animal may be immune and withstand an infection without requiring the presence of high serum antibody titres. This cell-mediated immunity can provide a long-term protection which lasts long after the serum antibody titre has fallen below detectable levels.

Inactivated vaccines

Formalin-inactivated vaccines were the first vaccines used from experimentally infected animals. They were made from a formalin-treated suspension of tissues from these animals and contained considerable unwanted host protein. Subsequently tissue cultures became available for the growth of viruses: these provided a simple and much more controllable method of producing vaccines. The vaccines could then be standardized and assayed with respect to their virus concentration prior to inactivation.

Two injections of inactivated vaccines are required to simulate the immune response: the second dose given after a suitable interval (typically two to three weeks) produces a 'secondary response' which is typified by a rapid rise in the serum antibody titres. The second vaccination also invokes the immunological memory and cell-mediated immunity; the latter is usually rather poor. In general the dose of the inactivated vaccine is important: the greater the antigenic mass of the vaccine on the repeated injection, the greater the subsequent serum antibody titre.

Inactivated vaccines are not able to produce 'interference' since they are not able to multiply following administration and occupy receptor sites which may be attacked by the invading pathogen. Inactivated vaccines contain no multiplying viruses and are considered safer than live vaccines. In order to increase the potency of inactivated vaccines they are usually adjuvanted, a process which increases the potency of the vaccine by sensitizing the immune system and stimulating the production of serum antibody titres.

Live vaccines

Live virus vaccines are made from attenuated or modified strains of virus. The virus is attenuated by prolonged, repeated passage through tissue culture in the laboratory. Live vaccines once inoculated can multiply in the tissues of the host animal and stimulate the same immunological reactions that would occur following exposure to the natural virulent virus. It also means that a single dose of the vaccine is sufficient to produce an adequate immune response. The immune response to these vaccines is both cell mediated and humoral. If the attenuated virus can reach the mucous membranes it may also stimulate the production of local antibody which is important for the protection of the animal against many respiratory pathogens. This means that an attenuated or modified vaccine may produce an effective immunity without the production of large quantities of circulating humoral antibody.

Modified or attenuated strains of virus used as a vaccine may produce early protection by 'interference'. This is achieved by the multiplication of the vaccine virus and the occupation of receptor sites which would normally be occupied by the invading pathogenic virus. It is known that distemper and measles virus vaccines can produce an early protection because of this effect. A dog vaccinated against distemper with a live attenuated vaccine may show protection within two or three days.

The attenuated vaccine is able to multiply in the inoculated animal so that the immune response (titre of antibody) is independent of the antigenic mass of the vaccine. However, if any mechanism interferes with the ability of the attenuated vaccine to multiply in the body it will give rise to a reduction in the effectiveness of the vaccine. For example, chemical or physical damage of the vaccine (heat or disinfectants) which inactivates the virus will make it ineffective because it will not be able to multiply in the host animal and reach a sufficient antigenic mass to produce immunity. The inactivation of live vaccines constitutes one of the major causes of vaccine breakdown.

Inactivation of live vaccines

Any mechanism which interferes with the ability of the attenuated vaccine to multiply will damage the effectiveness of the vaccine. Types of virus vary in their ability to resist physical and chemical assault. Viruses which are contained in lipid envelopes such as canine distemper virus and canine parainfluenza virus are particularly delicate structures which can be damaged by environmental factors such as ultraviolet light, heat and even sunlight. The half-life of canine distemper virus at 20°C may be as little as four hours. Canine parvovirus and feline panleucopenia virus, on the other hand, are more resistant to heat damage.

Generally viruses, particularly those with a lipid-containing envelope, are more resistant when contained in a lyophilized suspension rather than an aqueous suspension. Manufacturers produce freeze-dried infected tissue cultures contained in sealed glass ampoules. They are contained in an inert gas in the absence of moisture and air to ensure maximum survival of the virus. These vaccines should also be stored refrigerated between 2°C and 8°C; they should not be frozen or exposed to unnecessary heat. In the summer high temperatures may give rise to inactivation of the vaccine. The vaccine should, therefore, be stored in refrigerated compartments and removed immediately prior to use. The vaccine should also be used immediately after the addition of water for injection. Disposable plastic syringes without any traces of disinfectant should also be used. Small quantities of detergent in poorly rinsed syringes will also result in inactivation of the virus.

Sub-unit vaccines

Sub-unit vaccines are produced from viral capsid or envelope proteins instead of the intact virus. Multiple subunit vaccines may contain more than one type of antigen. The feline leukaemia vaccine is an example: it has a viral envelope protein GP70 and feline oncornavirus-associated cell membrane antigen (a tumour specific antigen). The GP70 induces antibody formation to neutralize feline leukaemia virus (FeLV) in the blood while the feline oncornavirus-associated cell membrane antigen induces immunity against FeLV neoplasms.

The advantage of this type of vaccine is safety, with no replication being possible and little hyposensitivity likely. The disadvantages include cost of production and, more importantly, efficacy. FeLV vaccination is still not regarded as being effective. Subunit vaccines are used for protecting cats against feline rhinotracheitis (Feliniffa RC and P).

Maternal antibody

A puppy or kitten receives most of the maternal antibody via the colostrum. These antibodies, which produce passive immunity, decline in concentration with time. The higher the concentration of the antibody in the pup or kitten, the longer will the antibody persist. Persisting maternal antibodies in the young animal may neutralize and render the vaccine ineffective if given too soon.

The duration of the maternal antibodies in the pup or kitten depends on the titres of the antibody in the mother. Viruses which produce high titres in the mother will pass on high titres to the young so that the antibody will persist at longer intervals in offspring of mothers with high serum titres. Particular viruses are more likely to produce higher titres than others. This means that the ideal time for vaccination against one disease may not correspond to the ideal time for vaccination against other diseases.

At 9 weeks, 65% of puppies have less than critical antibody titres to distemper. By 12 weeks virtually 100% of the puppies have less than critical levels of serum antibody. Similar results are obtained in puppies whose mothers are immune to infectious canine hepatitis. With canine parvovirus a similar period of time is required before the antibody titre in the pup declines to adequate levels (typically 12 weeks). In exceptional circumstances, where the infection to canine parvovirus is present in the epizootic form, many bitches will have very high antibody titres. This means that a small proportion of the puppies may be unable to respond to canine parvovirus vaccination at 12 weeks of age and may be unresponsive.

In cats a similar situation exists, with maternal antibodies to feline panleucopenia, feline viral rhinotracheitis and feline calicivirus persisting in the kitten for up to twelve weeks. In exceptional circumstances, where there is an epizootic infection in a breeding cattery, extremely high antibody titres may also be present in the queens so that, as with dogs, kittens may be unresponsive for as long as 15–16 weeks. Many kittens, however, may be responsive as early as nine weeks of age.

Deleterious effects of vaccination

Attenuated and inactivated vaccines contain protein material which is designed to provoke the immune system. In addition, they may very occasionally produce a generalized hypersensitivity reaction. The hypersensitivity reaction may be treated by the administration of adrenaline injected subcutaneously, histamine antagonists like mepyramine, or, in extreme cases, an injection of a soluble glucocorticoid preparation which will antagonize and reduce the development of immunity.

A transient corneal opacity ('blue eye') may be produced by vaccination with canine adenovirus type I (CAV-1). This condition is now avoided by using canine adenovirus type 2 (CAV-2) for vaccination against infectious canine hepatitis.

Table 4.1 Dog vaccines

Vaccine	*Manufacturer*	*Distemper*	*Measles*	*Infectious canine hepatitis*	*Leptospiroses (2)*	*Parvo*	*Bordetella*	*Parainfluenza*	*Rabies*
Boostervac DH	C-vet	L	–	L(2)	–	–	–	–	–
Boostervac DHPi		L	–	L(2)	–	–	–	L	–
Boostervac CPv		–	–	–	–	L(c)	–	–	–
Boostervac CPvL		–	–	–	K	L(c)	–	–	–
Boostervac L		–	–	–	K	–	–	–	–
Boostervac Pv		–	–	–	–	L(f)	–	–	–
Canilep-Parvo	Glaxovet	–	–	–	–	K(c)	–	–	–
Canilep-HL		–	–	K	K	–	–	–	–
Canilep-HLP		–	–	K	K	K(c)	–	–	–
Canilep-DHL		L	–	K	K	–	–	–	–
Canilep-DHLP		L	–	K	K	K(c)	–	–	–
Enduracell Parvo	Smith Kline	–	–	–	–	L(c)	–	–	–
Enduracell Parvo L		–	–	–	K	L(c)	–	–	–
Enduracell dml-pi		L	L	–	K	–	–	L	–
Enduracell 6		L	–	L(2)	K	–	–	L	–
Enduracell 7		L	–	L(2)	K	L(c)	–	L	–
Lepto ci		–	–	–	K	–	–	–	–

Epivax P/Vaxitas K Parvo	Coopers	–	–	–	–	K(c)	–	–	–
Epivax PL		–	–	–	K	K(c)	–	–	–
Epivax D/Vaxitas O		L	–	–	–	–	–	–	–
Epivax KHL		–	–	K	K	K	–	–	–
Epivax KHPL/Vaxitas K Parvo L		–	–	K	K	K(c)	–	–	–
Epivax-plus L/Vaxitas L		–	–	–	K	–	–	–	–
Vaxitas DA_2		L	–	L(2)	–	–	–	–	–
Vaxitas DA_2 Parvo		L	–	L(2)	–	L(c)	–	–	–
Kavak Parvo	Duphar	–	–	–	–	K(c)	–	–	–
Kavak M		–	L	–	–	–	–	–	–
Kavak L		–	–	–	K	–	–	–	–
Kavak D		L	–	–	–	–	–	–	–
Kavak DA_2		L	–	L(2)	–	–	–	–	–
Kavak i-HL		–	–	K	K	–	–	–	–
Kavak i-LP		–	–	–	K	K(c)	–	–	–
Kavak i-HLP		–	–	K	K	K(c)	–	–	–
Maxavac P	Hoechst	–	–	–	–	K(c)	–	–	–
Maxavac L		–	–	–	K	–	–	–	–
Maxavac DHL	L	–	K	K	–	–	–	–	
Nobi-vac Parvo-C	Intervet	–	–	–	–	L(c)	–	–	–
Nobi-vac L		–	–	–	K	–	–	–	–
Nobi-vac D		L	–	–	–	–	–	–	–
Nobi-vac DH_2		L	–	L(2)	–	–	–	–	–
Nobi-vac DH_2P		L	–	L(2)	–	L(c)	–	–	–
Intrac*	Gist-brocades	–	–	–	–	–	L	–	–
Delcavac-r		–	–	–	–	–	–	–	K
Rabiffa	May & Baker	–	–	–	–	–	–	–	K
Rabisin		–	–	–	–	–	–	–	K

* Intranasal.
L, live attenuated; K, killed; c, canine; f, feline; 2, adenovirus-2.
Tetanus toxoid (Hoechst, C-vet, Coopers) can be used against tetanus in the dog and cat.

Live attenuated vaccines may, at least, theoretically, become altered by further passage through the host animal. Thus, an initially avirulent vaccine strain may pass through the host animal and mutate into a more virulent form. The sudden appearance of canine parvovirus in the population of dogs is thought to have occurred as a result of mutation of the feline parvovirus.

Attenuated vaccines are produced by passage of the virus through tissue culture. Originally the virus isolates were obtained from diseased animals. Thus, it is theoretically possible that other adventitious viruses may have been overlooked and passed on through the cell line with the virus intended for the vaccine. This is overcome by the manufacturers using animals in self-contained units and screened for the presence of other unwanted diseases. This is particularly important in cats, where feline leukaemia virus could be transmitted via this mechanism. In practice however, the efficacy and safety of the live vaccine is unaffected by the type of tissue culture used to produce it.

The vaccines

Tables 4.1 and 4.2 show the vaccines produced by various manufacturers in the United Kingdom.

Distemper vaccines

In the UK distemper vaccines are all live attenuated viruses and are of one of three types. The first type is Onderstepoort, which is attenuated in embryonated hens' eggs and grown in embryo tissue culture; the second is the Rockborn strain which is attenuated in dog kidney tissue culture; the third is the Snyder Hill strain, attenuated in monkey kidney cells. These three strains all produce early protection by interference, and a solid immunity, but do not allow excretion of vaccinal virus. Immunity persists until at least middle age in most dogs which receive a single dose of the vaccine. Unfortunately, in a small number of animals antibody titres fall below levels which are regarded as critical after two years. This means that it is advisable to vaccinate against distemper every two years.

Measles vaccine

This vaccine was introduced in an attempt to overcome the problem of maternally-derived antibody in puppies. Although

Table 4.2 Cat vaccines

Vaccine	*Manufacturer*	*Virus enteritis*	*FVR*	*FCV*	*Rabies*
Feli-pan	C-vet	K	–	–	–
Feli-pan MLV		L	–	–	–
C-vet FVR-C		–	L	L	–
Feliflu		K	L	L	–
Felflu Plus		L	L	L	–
Purtect kP	Glaxovet	K	–	–	–
Purtect		L	–	–	–
Purtect RC		–	L	L	–
Purtect RCkP		K	L	L	–
Purtect RC + LP		L	L	L	–
Feliniffa RC + P	Rhône Merieux	K	K*	K	–
Felocine	Smith Kline	K	–	–	–
Felocell		L	–	–	–
Felocell-CVR		L	L	L	–
Vaxicat P	Coopers	L	–	–	–
Vaxicat kP		K	–	–	–
Vaxicat Plus		K	K	K	–
Katavac P	Duphar	L	–	–	–
Katavac IP		K	–	–	–
Katavac CH Nasal		–	L	L	–
Katavac CH Injectable		–	L	L	–
Katavac Plus		K	L	L	–
Felidovac	Hoechst	K	–	–	–
Nobi-vac FPL	Intervet	L	–	–	–
Nobi-vax Tricat		L	L	L	–
Delcavac-r	Gist-brocades	–	–	–	K
Rabisin	May & Baker	K	–	–	K

K, killed; L, live attenuated; * subunit vaccine.

measles virus is not inactivated by antibodies to canine distemper virus, it is able to produce sufficient stimulation of the immune system to produce antibodies against canine distemper virus. Measles virus accelerates the humoral immunity to canine distemper virus.

Infectious canine hepatitis

Inactivated and modified attenuated vaccines are used against infectious canine hepatitis. CAV-1 was originally produced by attenuation using passage in dog kidney tissue culture and subsequently by passage through pig and ferret tissue culture. This vaccine is particularly effective and gives immunity within eight days against infectious canine hepatitis and, in addition, to the respiratory form of the CAV infection. The very occasional occurrence of 'blue eye' led manufacturers to produce the inactivated form of CAV-1. The inactivated vaccine produced adequate immunity against infectious canine hepatitis for twelve months but the duration of immunity is shorter than that produced by the live attenuated vaccine. In addition, the inactivated vaccine fails to produce good immunity to the respiratory adenovirus infection. To help overcome this problem adjuvants were added to the inactivated CAV. Most manufacturers now use CAV-2 vaccine in their live attenuated vaccines: this gives solid immunity without side-effects.

Canine parvovirus

Vaccines against canine parvovirus are of three types: the first is the inactivated adjuvanted canine parvovirus; the second is the live attenuated feline strain of parvovirus; and the third is the attenuated canine parvovirus. The first two are relatively easily inactivated by the presence of maternal antibody. Antibodies to these two types of vaccine disappear after six to twelve months.

The live attenuated canine parvovirus which has been developed produces a more rapid protection with a much higher and longer lasting antibody titre than that available with the other two types of vaccine. This type of vaccine is less susceptible to inactivation, and vaccination may be completed in animals less than twelve weeks of age. Dogs like the Rottweiler are known to be effectively vaccinated by this strain of vaccine.

Leptospirosis

It is usual to vaccinate against *Leptospira canicola* and *Leptospira icterohaemorrhagiae*. An inactivated vaccine is prepared from a whole culture lysate containing approximately equal amounts of both types of bacteria in a medium essentially free of serum. Following the usual two-dose regime of vaccination, titres of agglutinin do not exceed 100 and drop to low levels within three months. However, there is a maintained immunity since the immunological memory is retained for some time after the loss of the circulating humoral antibody.

Kennel cough

Kennel cough is produced by a variety of pathogenic agents; usually there is a mixture. The organisms believed to be responsible are *Bordetella bronchiseptica* (most frequent causal agent), canine parainfluenza virus, canine adenovirus-2 and canine distemper virus.

Bordetella

Bordetella is regarded as the most important pathogen causing kennel cough. The vaccine used is a live avirulent strain (S55) which is intranasally administered. This vaccine multiplies in the respiratory tract and gives rise to the secretion of local IgA antibody in the respiratory tract, conferring the necessary local immunity. Although humoral antibody is also formed there is no correlation between this and the resistance to infection. Initial studies suggest that the immunity lasts for about 10–12 months, with 95% of dogs being resistant to infection 14 days after vaccination.

Canine parainfluenza

A modified strain of canine parainfluenza is not usually produced for kennel cough vaccination on its own. Vaccination involves the use of an attenuated strain of virus grown in kidney cell culture. Two doses of the vaccine are recommended to obtain suitably high antibody titres.

Feline virus enteritis/panleucopenia (parvovirus)

Vaccines used against feline panleucopenia consist of live attenuated feline virus or an inactivated adjuvanted feline virus. Both types are grown on tissue culture of feline origin. The killed vaccine has the advantage that the virus cannot cross the placental barrier in the pregnant queen and replicate in the fetus. There is therefore little risk of cerebellar hypoplasia in the inactivated vaccine. In contrast, the live attenuated vaccine should not be used to vaccinate pregnant female cats. Because of this risk, single doses of the inactivated vaccine and the attenuated vaccine given up to 12 weeks of age are usually satisfactory for producing an immunity which lasts at least one year. Revaccinating annually, with either type of vaccine, is usually recommended by manufacturers.

Feline rhinotracheitis and feline calicivirus

Both inactivated and live attenuated vaccines of these two cat influenza viruses are available. The inactivated vaccine has the advantage that it may be administered to pregnant cats in order to transfer immunity to the kittens following birth. The pregnant queens can be vaccinated two weeks before they are due to kitten. The kittens may then be vaccinated at 6 weeks of age with further doses at 9–10 weeks and 13 weeks of age. Since the vaccine is a dead vaccine it does not multiply in the cat and so may produce a limited local immunity. Exposure to one of the cat flu viruses will, in a small percentage of vaccinated cats, produce mild lingual ulceration. In these cases systemic disease is not likely to occur. The live attenuated feline viral rhinotracheitis and feline calicivirus vaccines are not generally administered to pregnant queens. Because the viruses replicate in the host and reach the respiratory tract they will give rise to an effective local immunity. The live vaccines are better at stimulating local immunity, and mild ulceration of the respiratory tract in the face of severe challenge is unlikely to be seen when the live vaccine has been used.

The vaccination regime

It is clear from the available data that there is no universally applicable vaccination regime. Amongst the pathogens in dogs, canine parvovirus is presently believed to be responsible for the highest mortality although canine distemper is very important. Thus, a puppy which has been purchased from a kennel about which little information is available should be vaccinated at 8 or 9 weeks and subsequently a repeat vaccination given at 12 weeks. This should be adequate to protect most dogs from distemper, parvovirus and canine adenovirus. However, in a limited number of cases high maternal antibodies to canine parvovirus, which can occur as a result of epizootic infection, may prevent effective vaccination. One way round this is to vaccinate again at 16 weeks of age with a parvovirus vaccine. Alternatively, if a vaccine against parvovirus is used based on the parvovirus vaccine of a canine origin (e.g. Nobi-Vac Parvo-C), a third vaccination at 16 weeks will be unnecessary. This vaccine (Nobi-Vac Parvo-C) is believed to be effective in particularly difficult breeds like the Rottweiler.

In cats it is usual to vaccinate first at 12 weeks of age, followed by a second vaccination 3–4 weeks later. Where kittens are exposed to disease before 9 weeks of age, the risk of infection may be reduced by administering a dose of vaccine every 3–4 weeks until they are 12 weeks of age.

Mixing vaccines

Simultaneous administration of the vaccines for the prevention of most of the diseases relevant in the dog and cat is routinely carried out. It is recommended, however, that the manufacturers' instructions are followed, since it is possible that the live attenuated vaccines become inactivated by mixing with an inappropriate vaccine from another manufacturer.

Further reading

Cornwell, H. J. C. and Thompson, H. (1982) Vaccination in the dog. *In Practice,* **September**, 151–158

Dhein, C. R. and Gorham, J. R. (1986) Host response to vaccination. *Veterinary Clinics of North America: Small Animal Practice,* **16**, 1227

Chapter 5

Analgesia

Small animals suffer pain: its relief is the responsibility of the veterinary surgeon but analgesics are not used frequently enough in practice. There are several reasons for this: firstly, opiate analgesics are subject to Controlled Drugs regulations and require the expenditure of time and effort to complete the necessary paperwork; secondly, opiates frequently produce respiratory depression; thirdly, animals in pain are unlike humans and may show no obvious signs. None of these are sufficient reasons for the infrequent use of analgesics in practice. This chapter considers the actions and uses of opiate and non-opiate analgesics.

Pain physiology

The perception of pain (Figure 5.1) involves two processes: the first is the detection of pain, or nociception; the second is the conscious experience associated with the perception of the pain. Special sensory nerves or nociceptive nerve endings are stimulated as a result of painful stimuli. These nerve afferents are unmyelinated or small myelinated A fibres which run to the spinal cord. They then synapse in the dorsal horn of the spinal cord on to a neurone which projects in the contralateral side in the lateral spinothalamic tract. Neural traffic across this synapse in the dorsal horn is controlled by at least two mechanisms.

The first mechanism is a local spinal circuit which can limit the access of the nociceptors to the contralateral spinothalamic tract: this is stimulated or brought into play by low threshold mechanical stimulation or low threshold thermal stimulation. An example of this mechanism in operation is the effect of gentle rubbing of a painful area to ease the pain.

The second mechanism which can inhibit the neural traffic from the nociceptors to the contralateral spinathalamic tracts and from there to the higher centres and consciousness is the descending inhibitory system which originates from the raphé nucleus of the midbrain. This system, which carries 5-

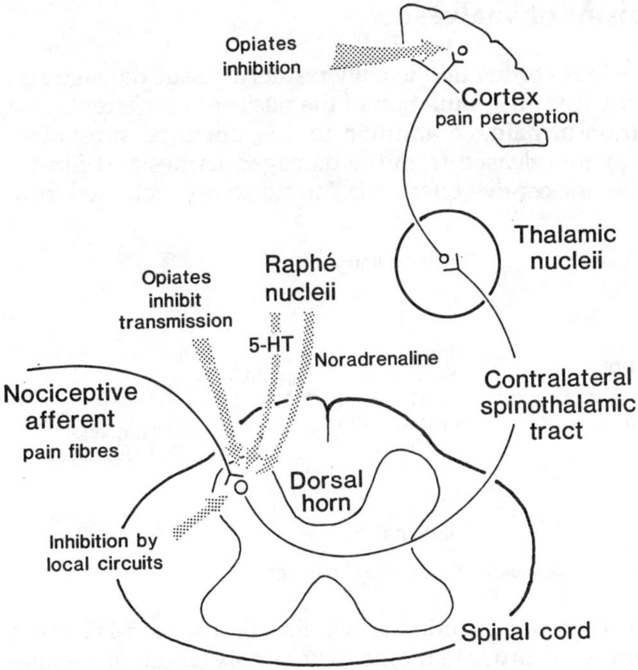

Figure 5.1 Pain pathways in the central nervous system

hydroxytryptamine (5-HT) and noradrenaline containing neurones is capable, when stimulated, of inhibiting nociceptive traffic from the pain afferents to the lateral spinothalamic tract. The increase in the neural traffic in the spinothalamic tract is relayed through the thalamic nuclei to the cortex, where perception of pain occurs.

Cortical activity can also influence the perception of pain; it is often said that pain which occurs as a result of injury during a fight is not experienced until the excitement is over. The mechanism for this is poorly understood.

A recent development in pain physiology has been the discovery of endogenous opioids in the central nervous system. These opioids are referred to as the enkephalins and endorphins. Receptors for these opioids occur throughout the central nervous system and are found in sites where pain processing is believed to occur. It is thought that under appropriate circumstances these endogenous opioids are released and react with receptors on the nerve pathways, modifying the transmission in nociceptive pathways.

Mechanisms of analgesics

Painful noxious stimulation usually results in tissue damage and may directly lead to stimulation of the nociceptive afferents and the sensation of pain. In addition to this, chemical substances (Figure 5.2) are released from the damaged tissues and further activate the nociceptive afferents. The substances released from

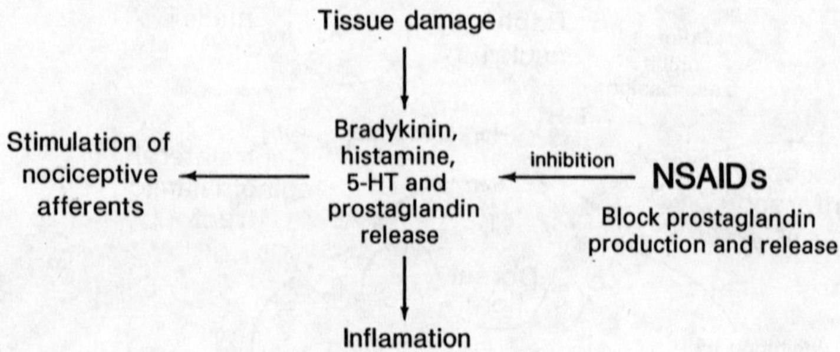

Figure 5.2 Chemicals released during tissue damage

the damaged tissues include bradykinin, histamine, 5-HT and a whole variety of prostaglandins. These substances are sometimes referred to as autocoids. Drugs which inhibit the production of prostaglandins by inhibiting their synthesis have been found to reduce neural traffic in the nociceptive afferents: they therefore act as mild analgesics. Substances which block the effect or release of the other autocoids may be expected to act as analgesics. Despite this, however, compounds like antihistamines are generally not regarded as being very effective. Glucocorticoids, on the other hand, do inhibit the release and production of the autocoids and may have a peripheral analgesic effect.

The transmission of impulses in the nociceptive afferents can be blocked by local anaesthetics. These compounds act by blocking the sodium channels in the nerve fibres and preventing the propagation of an action potential along the afferent fibres. The small myelinated and the unmyelinated nerve fibres are the most sensitive to local anaesthetic action. This means that analgesia can be easily produced by nerve block brought about by local application or nerve trunk block.

It has been pointed out earlier that the perception of pain involves the transmission of neural traffic via the contralateral spinothalamic tract to the thalamus and cortex, where it is believed that pain perception occurs. There are numerous sites where the neural traffic carrying the noxious information may be interrupted. However, in clinical practice only the opiates are used to mimic the action of the intrinsic endorphins and enkephalins. The action of counterirritants (linaments) and acupuncture is probably to stimulate local circuits which release endorphins. It seems quite likely that drugs in addition to the opiates, and having an appropriate central nervous system action, may be used as analgesics in the future.

Analgesic agents

Opiates (Tables 5.1, 5.2)

The opium poppy or *Papaver somniferum* has been used for centuries for the production of opium. Raw opium contains many alkaloids, of which morphine has been used most frequently in the clinical situation. It is now recognized that

Table 5.1 Opiates in the dog

Drug	*Dose*	*Duration*	*Regulations*
Morphine	0.2 mg/kg i.m.	4 h+	Controlled drug
Methadone (Physeptone)	0.1–0.2 mg/kg i.m.	4 h	Controlled drug
Pethidine	2 mg/kg i.m.	2 h	Controlled drug
Pentazocine (Fortral)	2 mg/kg i.m.	4 h	Not controlled
Buprenorphine (Temgesic)	0.01 mg/kg i.m.	4 h	Not controlled
Codeine	2 mg/kg oral	12 h	Not controlled

Table 5.2 Opiates in the cat

Drug	*Dose*	*Duration*	*Regulations*
Morphine	0.1 mg/kg i.m. (excitement in overdose)	4 h	Controlled drug
Pethidine	2.5 mg/kg i.m.	2 h	Controlled drug
Pentazocine (Fortral)	2 mg/kg i.m.	4 h+	Not controlled
Buprenorphine (Temgesic)	0.01 mg/kg i.m. (suggested dose)	4 h	Not controlled
Codeine	1.2 mg/kg oral; care with non-steroidal anti-inflammatory drugs; care overdose!	12 h	Not controlled

morphine and its analogues act at a number of different receptor sites within the central nervous system. These receptor sites include μ, δ, κ and σ sites. At these different receptor sites the opiates may act either as an agonist exciting the receptor or as a competitive antagonist blocking the action of an opiate agonist. An example of an agent which is believed to be a pure agonist at the μ receptors is morphine; an example of a compound which is believed to be a pure antagonist at all the different receptor sites is naloxone. The different opiate alkaloids may act as either agonists or antagonists at the different receptor sites. Compounds which have both agonist and antagonist effects are called partial agonists; some of these can be used to produce analgesia.

Stimulation of the various opiate receptors with different drugs can lead to effects which include analgesia, euphoria, vomiting, respiratory depression and addiction. The pure antagonists like naloxone can be used to reverse the effects of the agonists. The misuse of the opiate alkaloids has led to these compounds being subject to controlled drugs regulations with which veterinary surgeons have to comply.

Morphine

Morphine is a most effective analgesic agent in the dog. In addition to the analgesia, morphine produces sedation for sleep in a dose-dependent manner. Small doses in the cat have a similar effect but larger doses may produce maniacal excitement. This latter effect has led to a reluctance to use morphine in the cat. If appropriate doses are given, however, morphine is acceptable in this species. It is difficult to measure small quantities of the morphine required for the cat without diluting the commercially available preparations.

Morphine depresses the medullary centre and results in respiratory depression. Vomiting may occur in the normal healthy animal as a result of stimulation of the chemoreceptor trigger zone but in the injured or sick animal vomiting is rarely a problem. Stimulation of the gastrointestinal tract with an increase in the tone of the sphincter can lead to constipation. This effect may be useful for the treatment of diarrhoea in the dog.

Methadone

Methadone is a synthetic opiate which is equipotent to morphine. Clinical experience suggests that morphine is a better analgesic because methadone appears to have a shorter duration of action. It has little sedative action; no excitement is usually seen.

Pethidine

Pethidine has about one-tenth the potency of morphine. Clinical experience suggests that pethidine is both shorter acting and inferior to morphine when potent analgesia is required. It has little sedative effect and no sedation has been reported in the cat. Its main action on the gut is spasmolytic and vomiting has not been reported with this compound. Respiratory depression is comparable to that produced by morphine.

Pentazocine (Fortral)

This compound is one of the earliest κ agonist opiate analgesics to be used clinically: it has about a third the potency of morphine but, given in adequate doses, has a comparable analgesic effect. There is little sedative action and no excitement is seen. Since this compound is a κ agonist dysphoria is produced in humans but there is no evidence to suggest that this is a problem in small animals. With little action on the gut, no vomiting is seen. It also produces little respiratory depression compared to that produced by morphine. Pentazocine is not subject, as yet, to controlled drug regulations since it has a low abuse potential.

Buprenorphine (Temgesic)

This is a newer κ agonist and is a synthetic opiate. It has about 30 times the potency of morphine and appears to produce a comparable analgesia. It does have some sedative effect but produces no excitement. Vomiting does not appear to be a problem in animals since the action on the gut is negligible. Like pentazocine, some respiratory depression is produced but this is much less serious than that produced by morphine. Again like pentazocine, buprenorphine has a very low abuse potential and is not subject to controlled drugs regulations.

Fentanyl and etorphine

These compounds are very potent opiates producing marked respiratory depression and hypotension. Because of their marked potency and potentially dangerous side-effects these compounds are usually considered unsuitable as analgesics by themselves.

Codeine

Codeine is a natural alkaloid of opium: it has a much weaker analgesic effect and has negligible side-effects. No vomiting is seen, constipation is mild and respiratory depression absent. It is quite a useful agent for analgesia where there is a low grade pain. Codeine is not subject to controlled drugs regulations.

Non-steroidal anti-inflammatory drugs (NSAIDs)

Non-steroidal anti-inflammatory drugs (Tables 5.3, 5.4) produce their analgesic effect by blocking the action of cyclo-oxygenase which is responsible in part for the production of prostaglandins. In addition to this effect there is also a mild central analgesic effect. Because of their relatively low potency these compounds are useful for mild or chronic low grade pains but are not as effective as the opiates for severe pain.

Table 5.3 Non-steroidal anti-inflammatory drugs in the dog

Drug	*Dose (oral)*	*Duration*
Aspirin	25 mg/kg 4 times daily	6–12 h
Phenylbutazone	20 mg/kg daily, reduced after 3 days	6 h
Ibuprofen (Brufen)	25 mg/kg daily in divided doses; halve dose after 3 days	12 h
Mefenamic acid (Ponstan)	15 mg/kg in divided doses	12 h
Naproxen (Naprosyn)	2 mg/kg once daily	24 h

Table 5.4 Non-steroidal anti-inflammatory drugs in the cat

Drug	*Dose (oral)*	*Duration*
Aspirin	25 mg/kg once daily (care not more frequently; less if possible)	24 h+
Phenylbutazone	10 mg/kg daily in divided doses	12 h
Mefenamic acid (Ponstan)	15 mg/kg daily in divided doses; not yet widely used	12 h

Their action is, in the main, to produce an anti-inflammatory effect. However, in addition to this they have a mild central analgesic effect which is also associated with an antipyretic effect. The various NSAIDs vary in the degree of potency of the central analgesic effect. One of the major problems with their use is the gastric irritation which is produced. This often results in vomiting and diarrhoea and even, occasionally, in gastric haemorrhage. Very occasionally toxic effects on the liver and kidney are seen. The cat is particularly sensitive to the toxic actions of these compounds since the half-life of these drugs is very long in the cat. The reason for this long half-life is the lack of the glucuronyl transferase enzyme which is responsible for conjugating the NSAID to a glucuronide molecule for excretion. Despite their limitations, these compounds have a valuable role as analgesics in the dog and cat.

Acetylsalicylic acid

Acetylsalicylic acid (aspirin) is the most frequently used of the salicylates. Its analgesic action is mediated by peripheral anti-inflammatory and peripheral analgesic actions but there is also believed to be a slight central action. Aspirin causes gastric irritation and may result in vomiting, gastric haemorrhage and abdominal pain. In addition to this effect, it causes platelet aggregation which may prolong clotting time. The side-effects do not prevent the compound from being used in the dog or cat. Because of the very long half-life of aspirin in the cat, dosage should be administered infrequently.

Phenylbutazone

Phenylbutazone is commonly used in veterinary practice. Although in humans a number of toxic effects have been reported, fewer reports of toxic actions have appeared in small animals. Like aspirin, phenylbutazone produces gastric irritation, although it is less severe. Blood dyscrasias are occasionally seen and there is often a tendency for increased sodium and water retention because of depressed tubular reabsorption. Its use is contraindicated in cases of cardiac or renal disease.

Mefenamic acid (Ponstan)

Mefenamic acid has been used as an anti-inflammatory agent for the treatment of arthritis in humans. Although it has been used in the dog and cat to a limited extent, its use is not particularly popular. It produces side-effects similar to phenylbutazone and diarrhoea is a particular problem with this compound.

Naproxen (Naprosyn)

Naproxen is a propionic acid derivative with a long half-life in the dog. Because of this long half-life, fatal doses have been recorded. Like phenylbutazone it produces gastric irritation and blood dyscrasias and should be avoided in cases of cardiac and renal disease.

Ibuprofen (Brufen)

This compound is also a propionic acid derivative and has been used successfully in the dog. It is believed that ibuprofen is one of the safest NSAIDs in this species. Gastric irritation and kidney toxicity are regarded as potential hazards although they are not usually seen at normal therapeutic doses.

Indomethacin

Indomethacin has been used in the dog but gastric irritation is common. It is similar in most respects to the other NSAIDs.

Flunixin

Flunixin is a new NSAID developed primarily for the horse. It has potential as a powerful analgesic agent but has not been used extensively in the dog as yet.

General use of analgesic agents

The opiate analgesics are usually used for the treatment of severe pain while NSAIDs are used for low-grade and chronic pain. In general, NSAIDs should not be used when their anti-inflammatory effect is undesirable, for example after surgery, or when there is cardiac, kidney or liver disease.

Morphine should not be used where there is a raised intracranial pressure, for example after head injury, since it also raises intracranial pressure. The respiratory depressant action of the opiates should also be borne in mind. Since most opiates, including morphine, produce a degree of muscle spasm, they should not be used to treat pain caused by pancreatitis or bile duct obstruction.

Preoperative analgesia

Opiate analgesics should be used as part of any premedication when painful surgery is anticipated. One advantage is that their use reduces the amount of anaesthetic required but their main use must be to alleviate anxiety during consciousness, as well as alleviating pain. The respiratory depression produced by the opiate analgesics is a potential hazard during anaesthesia but is not a significant problem if normal therapeutic doses are used. Morphine is probably the best choice, particularly if there is a severe pain; it also has the advantage of a slight hypnotic effect. Pethidine and methadone can also be used but the animal will need more frequent dosing. The κ opiates pentazocine and buprenorphine are also effective and appear to act for as long as morphine.

Postoperative analgesia

Opiate analgesics are most effective if given prior to the pain experience. They are particularly valuable for the treatment of postoperative pain associated with orthopaedic and thoracic surgery. Again, morphine is probably the best choice as an agent where there is particularly severe pain but the κ agonists pentazocine and buprenorphine are also effective.

Road traffic accidents

Opiate analgesics are particularly useful for the treatment of road traffic accidents: only head injuries with raised intracranial pressure preclude their use. The small effect that the opiates have on the cardiovascular system does not preclude their use, even when haemorrhage has occurred. Opiates are better than acepromazine as sedatives because they do not produce a marked fall in blood pressure in the hypothermic patient. In addition, opiates have a calming effect on the animal and a more potent analgesic action. Morphine again is probably the best choice for treating particularly severe pain but pethidine, methadone and the κ agonists pentazocine and buprenorphine are effective.

Abdominal pain

Abdominal pain associated with marked dilatation or tortion of the intestine can be treated with analgesics and these are indicated on humane grounds. However, they should only be used in conjunction with the necessary diagnostic tests since they will mask any clinical signs. Pethidine as a spasmolytic may be the drug of choice.

Paracetamol poisoning

Paracetamol is used in man as a non-steroidal anti-inflammatory agent. Paracetamol poisoning occurs accidentally and most commonly in the cat. In cats, clinical signs consist of: cyanosis (46%); dyspnoea (14.6%); facial oedema (14.6%); depression (12.3%); hypothermia (8.9%) and vomiting. It is also seen in the dog but is less likely because they can metabolize the paracetamol by forming a non-toxic glucuronide conjugate. In the cat, toxic *N*-acetyl-*p*-benzoquinoneimine is produced in the liver; the removal of this metabolite can be stimulated using *N*-acetylcysteine.

Treatment of paracetamol poisoning

1. If ingestion is within 2 hours, induce vomiting and administer activated charcoal (2 g/kg) and administer a saline cathartic (sodium sulphate; 0.5 g/kg as a 20% slurry).
2. If cyanosis is present, administer oxygen; avoid stress.
3. Intravenous or oral *N*-acetylcysteine at 140 mg/kg. Repeat every 6 h at 70 mg/kg for a total of 36 h (7 treatments).
4. Ascorbic acid 30 mg/kg should be given orally at the same intervals.
5. Fluid therapy with lactated Ringer to correct acidosis.
6. Corticosteroids are contraindicated.

Further reading

Cullison, R. F. (1984) Acetominophen toxicosis in small animals: clinical signs, mode of action and treatment. *Compendium on Continuing Education for the Practicing Veterinarian*, **6**, 315–320.
Hall, L. W. and Clark, K. W. (1983) *Veterinary Anaesthesia*. London, Baillière Tindall
Iggo, A. (1982) The physiological approach to pain and pain relief. *Proceedings of the Association of Veterinary Anaesthetists*, **10** (Supplement), 32
Yoxall, A. T. (1978) Pain in small animals. *Journal of Small Animal Practice*, **19**, 43

Chapter 6

Tranquillizers, Sedatives, and General and Local Anaesthetics

This chapter describes the pharmacology of and suggests therapeutic doses for general tranquillizers, sedatives, and general and local anaesthetics which are commonly used in small animal practice.

Tranquillizers and sedatives

Tranquillizers may be defined as substances which relieve anxiety and tension without causing any signs of drowsiness or sleep. Sedatives have a similar effect but in addition they usually cause some drowsiness. An agent which is described as a hypnotic is a therapeutic substance which induces sleep. It is accepted that these descriptions are simplified and agents which are either tranquillizers, hypnotics or sedatives may have a variety of effects, depending on the animal to which they are given and the dose at which they are given. Higher doses tend to produce a greater degree of CNS depression, seen as sedation or sleep rather than tranquillization.

Phenothiazine ataractics

Acepromazine (Acetylpromazine)

This agent is popular in small animal practice. It produces tranquillization and sedation in a dose-dependent manner and has the additional effect of inhibiting the chemoreceptor trigger zone and, as a result, has an antiemetic action. In addition, acepromazine will produce hypotension due to its strong α-blocking activity and inhibition of the centrally mediated pressor reflexes. Sometimes acepromazine may produce excessive vagal tone and bradycardia. This effect can be controlled by using atropine. Boxer dogs are particularly sensitive to acepromazine and may faint following the administration of a fairly small amount. In animals suffering from hypovolaemia, the administration of acepromazine can produce a severe fall in blood pressure and cardiovascular collapse. When dehydration is suspected it is wise to correct this, using intravenous fluids, prior to the administration of acepromazine. Acepromazine should not be used for the treatment of epilepsy since it may aggravate the condition by its antidopaminergic action.

Dose

Dogs: i.m. injection 0.03–0.2 mg/kg; i.v. dose at a lower rate. Oral route 1–3 mg/kg. Cats: sedation appears to be less reliable and doses of between 0.1 and 0.2 mg/kg by i.m. injection are usually given.

Uses

Acepromazine can be given for tranquillization and sedation to control a nervous or neurotic animal. It appears to be less effective in the cat than the dog. Other uses include: an antiemetic for the prevention of travel sickness; a premedication prior to anaesthesia. Acepromazine will reduce the amount of anaesthetic required to approximately half the original amount. Acepromazine also has a weak antihistaminic action.

Other phenothiazines

1. Chlorpromazine (Largactil).
2. Trimeprazine (Vallergan).
3. Promazine (Sparine).
4. Promethazime (Phenergan).
5. Methotrimeprazine (in small animals, Immobilon).

Butyrophenones

The butyrophenones by themselves are not frequently used in dogs but are usually used in association with opiates for the production of neuroleptanalgesia. The evidence from their use in large animals suggests that intravenous injection in small animals might produce signs of restlessness and excitement: this would seem to suggest that the other agents available are preferable for sedation.

Agents available

1. Droperidol (Droleptan).
2. Azaperone (Stresnil).
3. Fluanisone (in Hypnorm).

Benzodiazepines

In man these agents are commonly used to relieve anxiety and inhibitions without the production of hypnosis. They also have potent anticonvulsant and muscle relaxant action.

Diazepam (Valium)

In wild animals this agent may produce a taming effect when given orally. It has the following uses:

1. *Anticonvulsant and antiepileptic* In dogs given intravenously at a dose rate up to 5 mg/kg it will control a high percentage of convulsions. In cats a dose of 2–10 mg given slowly intravenously can control severe convulsions.
2. *Premedication* If diazepam is used for premedication it may remove anxieties and inhibitions which would make the animal more difficult to control. It has little anaesthetic sparing action but sleeping times are lengthened.
3. *Behavioural problems* Small doses of diazepam given orally have a useful effect in controlling behavioural problems in dogs.

Xylazine (Rompun)

Xylazine is a sedative which has analgesic and central muscle relaxant properties. It has a selective α_2-agonist and local anaesthetic action. The effects of xylazine produce a fall in the peripheral blood pressure and sometimes an atrioventricular block in the heart. It is possible to counteract the bradycardia produced by xylazine by the injection of atropine. In addition to these effects, xylazine usually produces vomiting in the dog and cat and, at higher doses, respiratory depression. Xylazine is contraindicated in the last third of pregnancy because it may induce premature parturition. Because it stimulates vomiting it is contraindicated in cases of intestinal obstruction. It should not be used when there is suspected cardiac or pulmonary disease. Despite these known side-effects, xylazine is a useful agent in small animal practice.

Uses

Xylazine is best given by intramuscular injection at a dose rate of 1–3 mg/kg. Subcutaneous administration is less reliable.

1. Xylazine at a dose rate of 1 mg/kg reliably produces vomiting. This is useful to empty the stomach.

2. For premedication and sedation xylazine will produce a dose-dependent sedation. It has an anaesthetic sparing effect so that the subsequent administration of an anaesthetic for induction requires a reduction of dose by at least one half. At a dose rate of 1 mg/kg xylazine will reduce the muscle tone caused by ketamine anaesthesia. It also reduces the amount of ketamine required.
3. Xylazine can be used in association with pethidine to produce neuroleptanalgesia.

Neuroleptanalgesia

Neuroleptanalgesia involves the administration of a potent narcotic analgesic (often an opiate) together with a neuroleptic (a tranquillizer). This combination produces analgesia and deep sedation without loss of consciousness. In this state the animal will frequently remain sensitive to sound. The combination of the two drugs is often synergistic. The analgesia depends on the opiate drug which is used. The side-effects of the opiate, which include an initial excitement, nausea and vomiting, can be counteracted by the neuroleptic. In veterinary practice the two agents are usually mixed and administered together. The technique is quite good for minor surgery. For more major surgery, potent opiates are required and often produce respiratory depression. The technique is not useful in the cat because opiates have a potent stimulant effect in this species.

Fentanyl + Fluanisone (Hypnorm)

Hypnorm (fentanyl 0.315 mg + fluanisone 10 mg/ml) is given intravenously or subcutaneously to dogs to produce a sedation and analgesia which peaks after 15 minutes. It can be used for premedication and for minor surgery by itself. Fentanyl has a duration of action of about 30 minutes so it is not usually necessary to reverse the action of the opiate using naloxone. The neuroleptic (fluanisone) lasts for some considerable time after the loss of action of fentanyl and maintains a sedation. Hypnorm may produce side-effects including bradycardia which can be controlled using atropine. It may also produce a hypersensitivity to sound, respiratory depression and defaecation. It is contraindicated if there is any respiratory disease, kidney or liver failure (because of prolonged action).

Etorphine + methotrimeprazine (Immobilon)

Small animal Immobilon (etorphine 0.074 mg + methotrimeprazine 10 mg/ml) can be given intravenously or intramuscularly to produce deep sedation and analgesia. The duration of analgesia is about one and a half hours. It can produce severe respiratory depression which is associated with cyanosis, bradycardia and hypotension. In old animals with a depressed liver function the duration of action may be much longer. Etorphine is a particularly potent opiate and is very dangerous to man. It is important to be aware of this. Accidental self-injection may be fatal.

Diprenorphine (Revivon)
This is used to reverse the effects of etorphine and wake the dog. It is prepared in a suitably concentrated solution so that it is given to the same volume as Immobilon. Sedation remains after the administration of diprenorphine because of the remaining effect of the neuroleptic (methotrimeprazine).

Opiate antagonists

These drugs act at the opiate receptor site, essentially as competitive antagonists, to reverse the effect of the opiate agonists. Some antagonists are also known as partial agonists since they have an effect by themselves. The antagonists are useful to counteract the respiratory depression of the opiates and for speeding the return of the animal to consciousness. It is important to realize that the duration of action of the opiate antagonist should match the duration of action of the opiate which has produced the depression. If it is shorter and cleared more quickly there will be a return to unconsciousness as the effects of the opiate return.

Naloxone (Narcan)
This compound is known as a pure opiate antagonist. It has no agonist action on its own so there is little danger of an overdose. Unfortunately it is short acting in dogs and is required in too high a concentration to reverse the effects of etorphine. It is useful in emergency in man at a dose of 0.4 mg which can be repeatedly administered at 2–3 minute intervals.

Diprenorphine
This compound is a partial agonist and is useful for antagonizing the actions of etorphine. It is prepared in a suitably high

concentration and has a sufficiently long duration of action to be useful for countering the effects of the Immobilon.

General anaesthetics

Barbiturates

The barbiturates may be classified according to their duration of action. The classification includes ultrashort-acting (methohexitone), short-acting (thiopentone), medium-acting (pentobarbitone) and long-acting (phenobarbitone) drugs.

Methohexitone (Brietal)

Sodium methohexitone is usually used in a 1–2.5% solution. A fixed dose rate is not recommended because of variation between individuals. Approximately 2–4 mg/kg should be injected quickly (intravenously, taking 5–10 seconds) and then incremental doses given up to 10 mg/kg to induce anaesthesia. Methohexitone is similar to thiopentone in its main effects but can be contrasted in the following ways:

1. It has a shorter duration of action, and a lower dose is required to produce induction of anaesthesia: this is because methohexitone is more rapidly metabolized in the liver and less is deposited in the fat. It therefore shows less accumulative effects.
2. Methohexitone produces greater depression of laryngeal reflexes and allows easier intubation.
3. Methohexitone produces more clonic muscle spasms during induction and recovery. This is usually controlled by premedication and by increasing the rate of injection of methohexitone.

Methohexitone (continuous infusion)

Because methohexitone is relatively rapidly metabolized and does not show accumulative effects, it can be administered as a drip to maintain anaesthesia. Given by infusion of 0.1% methohexitone in 500 ml saline, it allows the depth of anaesthesia to be adjusted by maintaining an appropriate flow rate of the drip. The depth of anaesthesia can be judged from the reflex response and respiratory rate. Approximately 5 drops of a standard drip chamber per kg can be given per minute.

Thiopentone (Intraval)

Sodium thiopentone at a concentration of 2.5–5% is administered intravenously for the induction of anaesthesia. It has an alkaline pH because it is a sodium salt of a weak acid. It is irritant and will cause sloughing if injected perivascularly. It produces the following effects:

1. *Depression of the central nervous system* Barbiturates depress the reticular formation and if given in sufficient dose will produce unconsciousness. It is not a specific analgesic.
2. *Depression of the respiratory system* Barbiturates depress the respiratory centres and sufficient doses will lead to apnoea.
3. *Hypotensive effects* The intravenous injection of thiopentone (and other barbiturates) causes hypotension. It depresses the heart muscle and reduces the heart rate as well as producing dilatation of blood vessels.
4. *Effect on laryngeal reflexes* Thiopentone in normal doses for induction of anaesthesia only just produces sufficient depression of the laryngeal reflexes in the dog to allow intubation. In the cat, the larynx must be anaesthetized by the administration of local anaesthetic to permit intubation.
5. *Depression of the fetus* Barbiturates (including thiopentone) will cross the placenta and depress the central nervous system of the fetus. This means that, following caesarian section, it may be necessary to stimulate respiration in the newborn animal. It is probably better in the parturient animal to avoid intravenous barbiturates or to use very low levels sufficient to produce only narcosis.

Pharmacokinetics

A number of pharmacokinetic factors influence the duration of action and dose of thiopentone required:

1. *Ionization* Barbiturates are weak acids and the proportion of unionized drug which is available for pharmacological effects increases with acidosis. Thus, acidosis will favour the penetration of the barbiturate through the blood–brain barrier. Lower doses of the barbiturate are required in uraemia or other conditions where there is a metabolic acidosis.
2. *Binding to protein* Once again, because barbiturates are acidic drugs, roughly 75% is protein bound to the albumin. The degree of binding depends on the pH of the blood. When there is a metabolic acidosis, less of the barbiturate is protein

bound and so is available for pharmacological effect. Similarly, when there is a hypoproteinaemia due to liver failure or other causes, more barbiturate is available for pharmacological effects.

3. *Fat solubility* Barbiturates with a higher fat solubility will enter the brain and the fat more easily than those barbiturates which have a lower fat solubility. Thiopentone is 16 times more soluble in fat than pentobarbitone.
4. *Distribution, redistribution and elimination* Following intravenous injection, the unassociated thiopentone passes most rapidly into the central nervous system. The drug swiftly produces unconsciousness because of the high lipid solubility of thiopentone and the good supply of the brain. Once it has done this, there is then a process of redistribution of the thiopentone, firstly to the skeletal muscle which has a good blood supply. Redistribution continues to the lipid tissue which has a relatively poor blood supply. In summary, the duration of action of thiopentone is determined by redistribution; metabolism is less important. If thiopentone is repeatedly administered it will lead to saturation of the fat and muscle depots and an increase in the duration of anaesthesia as subsequent doses of thiopentone are administered. Thiopentone is metabolized slowly in the liver as it is gradually released from the fat depots. Inactive products are excreted in the urine. The effect of the redistribution of thiopentone means that small doses given quickly will induce anaesthesia in less than 20 seconds. The animal will then return to consciousness after about five minutes following the redistribution of the barbiturate. If small increments of thiopentone are given, the lipid tissue will gradually become saturated and so each injection will produce anaesthesia which lasts for a longer period of time.

   In animals which have little fat (the greyhound family, the whippet and the Afghan hound) recovery from barbiturate anaesthesia is usually prolonged because of the failure of redistribution. It is better in these breeds to use the ultrashort-acting barbiturate methohexitone which does not rely so much on redistribution for the termination of its action.

Administration

Thiopentone is administered intravenously but the dose required varies dramatically from animal to animal. It is suggested that a dose of 25 mg/kg is prepared initially but that only 5–10 mg/kg is administered intravenously over a period of 5–10 seconds and that this is then followed by a period of approximately 30 seconds to assess the effect of the drug. Subsequently, further increments can be given to produce the depth of anaesthesia required. In animals where the circulation is slow because of cardiac depression, at least 60 seconds should be allowed before the effect is determined.

There is an advantage in using dilute solutions (2.5%, 25 mg/ml) since it allows greater control of the dose. One per cent solutions may also have an advantage. The more dilute the solution injected perivascularly, the less damage will be done to the surrounding tissue. If thiopentone is injected perivascularly it is wise to infiltrate the site with sterile saline, up to 20 ml, to dilute the drug. In addition, 0.5–2 ml of a local anaesthetic (say 5% procaine without adrenaline) can be infiltrated around the site to counteract the alkaline nature of sodium thiopentone. The local anaesthetic solution is acidic. If the perivascular injection is untreated there will be extensive necrosis and possibly sloughing of the overlying skin.

Pentobarbitone (Sagatal)

Pentobarbitone is usually given as a 6% solution (60 mg/ml) sodium salt. It is less irritant than thiopentone sodium and will not produce a perivascular slough. It is less frequently used in practice. Its duration of action is much longer than thiopentone. Although similar in action to thiopentone, it contrasts in the following ways:

1. A greater proportion of pentobarbitone is unbound and undissociated at physiological pH. A greater proportion is available for pharmacological effect.
2. Pentobarbitone is approximately 20 times less soluble in fat than thiopentone and, as a result, will penetrate the brain more slowly and is not effectively redistributed to the fat. The duration of action is much longer.
3. During recovery excitement is more common following pentobarbitone anaesthesia.

Administration

The dose of pentobarbitone can be calculated on a basis of 13 mg/kg (0.5 ml/5 lb.). However, the actual amount given will vary according to the individual and the effect produced. It is suggested that two modes of administration are used:

1. In healthy animals, half of the computed dose is given in ten seconds intravenously to induce unconsciousness. It takes up to two minutes (contrasting with thiopentone) for pentobarbitone to produce its anaesthetic effect following intravenous administration.
2. In unfit or sick animals, one third of the dose should be given intravenously and the remainder injected over a period of four minutes until the depth of anaesthesia is just sufficient for the surgery required.

Euthanasia

Pentobarbitone is most frequently used in small animal practice for euthanasia following an intravenous overdose. It is administered in concentrated solutions for this purpose. It is usually used in a 20% solution. An example is Euthatal. This method provides a humane method of destruction.

Alphaxalone/alphadolone (Saffan)

This is a steroid anaesthetic which is usually used in cats, although it can also be used in rabbits, guinea pigs and primates. The advantage of the steroid anaesthetic is that it has a greater therapeutic ratio and an action which is determined by liver metabolism. Accumulative effects are not seen. Steroids are insoluble in water: alphaxalone has to be solubilized; the agent used is a Cremophor EL (polyoxethylated castor oil). The unfortunate side-effects of the Cremophor EL are that it regularly produces oedema of the paws in cats and sometimes may produce pulmonary oedema. This action is said to be due to histamine release following mast cell degranulation produced by the solubilizing agent. As a result there is often hypotension and tachycardia. The side-effects of the Cremophor makes Saffan by itself unsuitable for use in dogs.

Following intravenous injection, Saffan produces a rapid loss of consciousness which lasts approximately ten minutes. Muscle relaxation is good in most species. Recovery is reasonably rapid following a single injection, although convulsive movements can be seen on recovery in cats. There is little or no tolerance or cumulative effects shown by this compound. The therapeutic index of Saffan is four times that of thiopentone; this compound has little oestrogenic effect. Following intravenous injection it causes a pronounced fall in blood pressure but cardiac output is usually maintained with an increase in heart rate. Normal levels return after two or three minutes. Following the injection, respiration is usually depressed briefly.

Steroids are not exclusively bound to plasma proteins: the duration of action is unaffected by factors which alter the level of plasma proteins. Metabolism is responsible, in the main, for the fall in concentration of the anaesthetic in the plasma. Metabolites are excreted in the bile with some enterohepatic recycling; some metabolites are found in the urine. In cases of reduced hepatic and renal function, the duration of action of Saffan will be prolonged.

Saffan will cross the placenta and produce respiratory depression in the fetus. It would be wise to administer the lowest dose compatible with carrying out a caesarean section in order to minimize the effect on the unborn fetus. Saffan, if injected perivascularly, does not produce slough. In fact it may be injected intramuscularly in the quadriceps group of muscle in front of the femur and can produce anaesthesia/sedation using this method. Higher doses have to be used for this.

Administration

Saffan consists of a mixture of alphaxalone acetate (9 mg/ml) and alphadolone acetate (3 mg/ml) dissolved in a 20% solution of Cremophor EL. Dosages refer to the total amount of 12 mg/ml. A dose of 9 mg/kg is recommended for healthy cats. Normally one should take about ten seconds to administer the anaesthetic intravenously and allow about one minute before the onset of the maximum level of anaesthesia. The duration of anaesthesia following a single injection is usually about ten minutes. One useful approach is to give 5 mg/kg initially and then to administer smaller doses to effect. In sick animals the first dose may be sufficient.

Intramuscular administration in the quadriceps muscle mass is recommended. If the Saffan is injected between the muscle planes, anaesthesia will be delayed. A dose rate of 4 mg/kg is recommended for premedication; a dose of 12 mg/kg is recommended for deep sedation, while 18 mg/kg is recommended for production of anaesthesia.

Contraindications

Saffan is contraindicated in dogs because of the production of histamine release by the solubilizing agent. Saffan must not be given to patients already anaesthetized with other intravenous preparations since extreme hypotension and respiratory arrest are possible. Saffan is not effective in the cat when given subcutaneously or intraperitoneally.

Propofol (Rapinovet)

Propofol is di-isopropylphenol suspended in soya bean oil to form a white emulsion. Its pharmacological properties are very similar to thiopentone but it is non-cumulative. After intravenous injection it is quickly redistributed and metabolized ($T_{1/2}$ 60 min). It may produce a short apnoea if injected too rapidly or overdosed. It is less depressant in the cardiovascular system. Fine muscle tremors may be seen in some dogs.

Uses
Propofol is a 1% emulsion: a dose rate of 6–8 mg/kg in unpremedicated animals and 4–5 mg/kg after acepromazine is used i.v. for induction. There is a rapid return to consciousness and normal behaviour on recovery (useful for day case anaesthesia). It can be used in dogs and cats and does not produce a perivascular slough. It may replace thiopentone and Saffan.

Ketamine (Vetalar)

Ketamine is a dissociative anaesthetic and acts on the dissociative or frontal cortex. It has little action on the reticular formation. It is a rapid onset anaesthetic and is not a barbiturate or a steroid. It produces a state of catalepsy with a loss of consciousness, analgesia but little muscle relaxation. The eyes remain open with pharyngeal and laryngeal reflexes abolished only at higher doses.

Uses
Ketamine can be used alone in cats for restraint or as a sole anaesthetic agent for minor surgical purposes such as castration. Muscle relaxation is not adequate for more major surgery. For restraint a dose of 11–22 mg/kg is used. For minor surgery a higher dose of 22–23 mg/kg of ketamine is required. Ketamine is usually given intramuscularly although the subcutaneous or intravenous route can be used. The duration of the CNS depression lasts about three-quarters of an hour. Complete recovery usually requires about six hours.

Xylazine + ketamine (cats)

The combination of xylazine and ketamine is useful for surgical operations like speying, castration and laparotomy. The following procedure is recommended for the production of surgical anaesthesia:

1. Administer 1.1 mg/kg xylazine by intramuscular injection.
2. Administer immediately 0.04 mg/kg atropine sulphate i.m.
3. After 20 minutes administer a dose of 22 mg/kg ketamine i.m.

The onset of anaesthesia usually occurs within about five minutes of stage 3 and lasts about thirty minutes. Gaseous anaesthetics may be used if required.

Xylazine + ketamine (dogs)

This combination can be used to maintain or induce surgical anaesthesia in the dog. Occasional spontaneous body movements seen after administration of this combination make it unsuitable for delicate orthopaedic or eye surgery.

Dose

The following procedure is recommended for anaesthesia:

1. Administer xylazine intramuscularly at a dose rate of 2 mg/kg.
2. Administer atropine intramuscularly to control salivation (0.04 mg/kg).
3. After 10 minutes administer ketamine at a dose rate of 10 mg/kg by intramuscular injection.

Throughout this period animals should be kept quiet and unnecessary stimulation avoided during the induction period. Anaesthesia is usually induced after 10 minutes and lasts for approximately 30 minutes. It is recommended that in dogs over 25 kg the dosage of xylazine given initially should be reduced to 1.3 mg/kg body weight.

Contraindications

Ketamine is eliminated by the kidney following metabolism by the liver. Thus an impairment in the function of the liver or the kidney will produce a prolongation of anaesthesia. An overdose will produce respiratory depression which is characterized by cyanosis and depressed ventilation. Incubation and ventilation with oxygen is recommended. In dogs and cats myoclonic jerkings and myotonic convulsions have been reported. These are more likely to occur if the animal is stimulated by sound or handling during the recovery period.

The eyes remain open during anaesthesia with xylazine so it is recommended that bland ophthalmic ointments are applied to the cornea if anaesthesia is prolonged. This is to prevent the development of a conjunctivitis and inflammation of the eye.

Gaseous anaesthetics

Nitrous oxide (N_2O)

Nitrous oxide is stored under pressure as a liquid in cylinders which are coloured blue. The high pressure of the nitrous oxide in the cylinder means that a reducing valve is essential for use. Nitrous oxide is a colourless, non-irritant gas which is not inflammable or explosive, although it will support combustion of other agents.

Nitrous oxide is rapidly eliminated from the body through the lungs. It is not a potent anaesthetic but is an analgesic. It does not produce muscle relaxation.

Administration

Nitrous oxide is given with oxygen: it is normally given at a high concentration but the concentration of oxygen should not fall below 30%. At the end of anaesthesia it is essential to ventilate the animal on pure oxygen to avoid the production of diffusion hypoxia. Since nitrous oxide is a weak anaesthetic it is normally given as a supplement with a volatile anaesthetic. It will potentiate the effects of other anaesthetics.

Volatile anaesthetics

Ether (diethyl ether $C_2H_5 \cdot O \cdot C_2H_5$)

Ether is a volatile liquid which is explosive when mixed with air or oxygen. It has a boiling point of 35°C.

Pharmacological properties

Ether is not a potent anaesthetic and is fairly soluble in blood; induction is fairly slow. It has a pungent smell and is irritant to the respiratory tract. A combination of these two factors mean that it is usually unsuitable for induction of anaesthesia. The irritant nature of ether means that it will stimulate salivary and bronchial secretion in all species and may predispose to respiratory infections and aggravate respiratory problems. To counter the effect of these secretions, atropine may be administered for premedication. Good muscle relaxation is one of the features of ether anaesthesia since it has a dual effect on neuromuscular function, depressing it in a curare-like manner, and has a central depressant effect on the spinal cord motor neurones. Ether produces a greater degree of muscle relaxation than other volatile or gaseous anaesthetics. During light levels of anaesthesia, ether may cause a slight hypertension due to a sympathetic stimulatory action. It does not sensitize the heart to the catecholamines and is not arrhythmogenic.

Approximately 90% of the administered ether is recovered from the expired air. Small amounts are retained in the body and metabolized to carbon dioxide and water.

Uses

Ether may be administered by a variety of inhalation methods. It still has a use in cat anaesthesia because of its relative safety. It can be given to the dog by a semi-closed method supplemented by oxygen or nitrous oxide/oxygen.

Halothane ($BrClCHCF_3$; Fluothane)

Halothane (Figure 6.1) is a sweet smelling, potent, volatile anaesthetic sold in amber-coloured bottles to protect against photolytic action. Its stability is further enhanced by the addition of 0.01% thymol. Soda lime does not cause halothane to decompose but long exposure to light turns it brown due to the release of various bromides. These bromides are irritant.

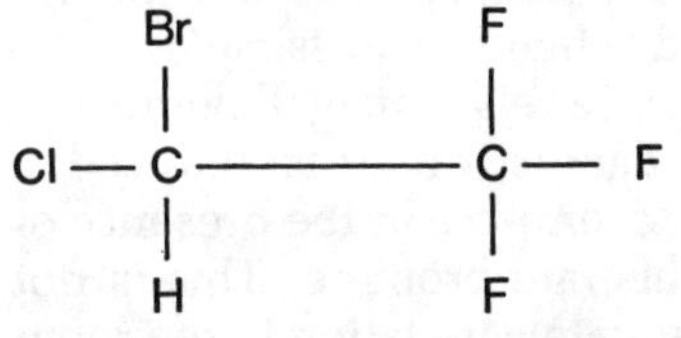

Figure 6.1 The structure of halothane

Mixtures of halothane with air and oxygen are not explosive. Most metals, except nickel and titanium, are corroded by halothane. It interacts with rubber and some plastics and is highly soluble in rubber. This can contribute to slowing of induction and recovery, especially if low flow rates are used in a delivery circuit.

Pharmacological properties

Halothane produces a depression of the central nervous system in a dose-dependent manner. It is more potent than ether and is characterized by a dose-dependent hypotensive effect. Its solubility in blood and the tissues means that a continuous fixed level of administration will give rise to a gradual increasing level of anaesthesia. During long periods of administration the level of halothane administered should be reduced slightly. Ventricular arrhythmias are rare during its administration but may occur in the presence of respiratory acidosis, hypoxia or other causes of sympathetic stimulation. It sensitizes the conducting tissues of the heart to the circulating effects of adrenaline and noradrenaline and therefore predisposes towards arrhythmias. The rest of the cardiovascular system is depressed by halothane; the myocardial muscle is depressed and so is the muscle of the blood vessels. This is the cause of the hypotensive effects produced by halothane.

Approximately 10% of the halothane administered is retained in the body and metabolized. The metabolites include trifluoroacetic acid, bromides and inorganic fluorides.

Uses

Halothane may be used for induction and maintenance of general anaesthesia; it is administered by open, semi-open or closed-circuit methods. Induction is possible using a concentration of halothane of 2–4%. Once the surgical plane of anaesthesia has been achieved it may be maintained by administering a concentration of 0.5–2%.

Contraindications

1. Halothane sensitizes the heart to catecholamines and the use of adrenaline should be avoided whenever possible.
2. It increases the action of the muscle relaxants gallamine and tubocurarine, so doses of these agents should be reduced.
3. It is not inflammable but it will decompose in the presence of oxygen and a naked flame to liberate bromine. This is not normally a hazard if there is adequate ventilation in the room where the anaesthetic is being given.
4. It will cross the placenta and produce depression of the central nervous system of the unborn fetus. This may make respiration difficult in the newborn animal following caesarean section. Minimal concentrations of halothane should be used for caesarean sections.

Methoxyflurane ($CHCl_2CF_2OCH_3$; Metofane)

Methoxyflurane is a clear, volatile, halogenated hydrocarbon. It has a boiling pointof 104°C. It is non-flammable and non-explosive and has a characteristic fruity smell.

Pharmacological properties

Methoxyflurane is a good analgesic and can produce good muscle relaxation. The clinical signs of anaesthesia with methoxyflurane are not as well defined as those with other inhalation agents since the pedal and palpebral reflexes are abolished relatively early and are not reliable signs of anaesthesia. The depth of anaesthesia is best judged by the degree of muscle relaxation and the presence or absence of the swallowing reflex. At deeper levels of anaesthesia methoxyflurane will produce an increasing respiratory depression and a fall in blood pressure. Dysrhythmias are not common with methoxyflurane.

Since methoxyflurane is highly soluble in fat, a substantial proportion (approximately 20%) is retained and ultimately metabolized in the body. The metabolites include various halogenated organic and inorganic substances. One of the main disadvantages of methoxyflurane is the dose-related renal toxicity which is caused by the release of large quantities of inorganic fluoride ion during the biotransformation of the drug in the liver. Signs of kidney damage following methoxyflurane administration include a high output renal failure.

Uses

Although it is possible to induce anaesthesia with methoxyflurane it is not usual to do so. Induction with methoxyflurane is slow and lasts ten minutes or longer. The low vapour pressure does not allow a sufficient concentration to be administered for induction. Maintenance, however, is readily achieved with methoxyflurane. It is customary to use a special delivery system.

Contraindications

1. Methoxyflurane will cross the placental barrier and may produce respiratory depression in the fetus. Possible adverse effects upon fetal development have not yet been assessed.
2. Recovery may be prolonged after long periods of anaesthesia in old or obese animals due to the failure of liver metabolism and storage of the methoxyflurane in the fat.
3. Methoxyflurane is absorbed in rubber and rubber products and the inclusion of it in the material of the anaesthetic circuits may result in prolonged induction and recovery times.

One of the main advantages of methoxyflurane is the good analgesic action it has in subanaesthetic doses. Thus a degree of analgesia will persist following recovery from the anaesthesia.

Local anaesthetics

Local anaesthetics may be used in a variety of ways to produce analgesia:

1. *Surface application* Local anaesthetics which pass through mucous membranes may be applied to surfaces like the cornea, the mucous membranes of the mouth and conjunctiva, as well as for intrasynovial analgesia.
2. *Local infiltration* Local anaesthetics are applied via a needle directly into surgical sites to produce local analgesia.
3. *Regional analgesia* Here the local anaesthetic is applied via injection to nerves to produce a specific nerve block or to produce spinal analgesia or epidural analgesia.
4. *Intravenous regional analgesia* This technique utilizes the intravenous administration of a local anaesthetic during the application of a tourniquet to the limb. The tourniquet must be sufficiently tight to stop the arterial blood flow so that there is back diffusion of the local anaesthetic along the vein to the site required.

Actions of local anaesthetics

Local anaesthetics have systemic and local actions. The local action is to produce a block of nerve conduction in areas supplied by the nerve. As a result there is a loss of pain and sensation as well as vasodilatation and loss of motor function. Pain is the first sensation to disappear and occurs at a much lower concentration of local anaesthetic than that required to produce loss of motor function. The smallest nerve fibres are affected first, probably due to their greater surface area. The effect of the local anaesthetic is to block the sodium currents which give rise to the action potential of the nerve fibre.

The systemic effects which are seen following absorption occur as a result of the 'generalized membrane stabilization' effect of the local anaesthetic and are seen in the cardiovascular and central nervous system. In the heart any dysrhythmias which may be due to hyperexcitability are suppressed as a result of local anaesthetic action. All local anaesthetics except cocaine produce vasodilatation. The effect on the central nervous system if too a high a dose is administered and absorbed is initially to produce a stage of anxiety, restlessness and disorientation. Eventually there is sedation and anaesthesia and, finally, apnoea and cardiovascular collapse due to medullary depression.

Chemical structure of local anaesthetics

Local anaesthetics have the following structure: an aromatic lipophilic group–intermediate chain–hydrophilic group. The intermediate chain may be an ester (-CO-) or an amide (-NH · CO-). Procaine is an example of an ester but lignocaine and most other local anaesthetics are amides. The hydrophilic group is always a quaternary amine. Local anaesthetics are weak bases and can combine with acids to form salts (e.g. lignocaine hydrochloride). The salt can exist in an uncharged form (B) or as a positively charged cation (BH^+). The proportion of uncharged and charged form depends on the pH and the dissociation constant (pK_a).

In acid conditions there will be more cations than free base. In alkaline conditions there will be more free base present. It is the uncharged base form which is free to diffuse and move through the tissues: alkaline conditions favour the diffusion of local anaesthetics. In addition, local anaesthetics with a low pK_a are less highly ionized and more readily diffuse through the tissues. The following local anaesthetics are used commonly in veterinary practice.

Lignocaine

This is an amide (Figure 6.2) and is widely used. It has a moderate potency and duration of action but has superior powers of penetration and a rapid onset. It is effective if applied

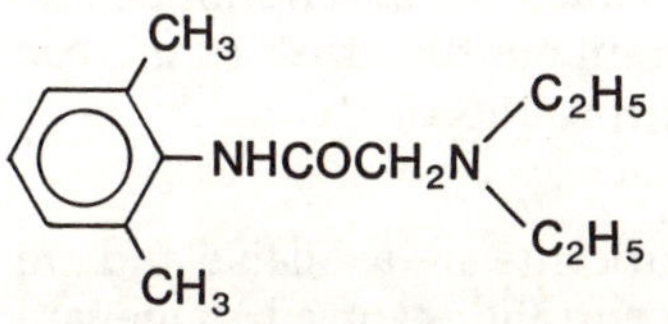

Figure 6.2 The structure of lignocaine

to surfaces for local infiltration or for regional analgesia. It causes relatively little vasodilatation but is often used with adrenaline. Adrenaline with its vasoconstrictor action will counteract the vasodilator effect of lignocaine and limit systemic absorption: there is a decrease in toxicity and increase in the duration of action. Typically, concentrations of 1 in 200 000 adrenaline in the local anaesthetic are used. Frequently adrenaline decomposes and its activity decreases on prolonged storage. The vasoconstriction may sometimes produce ischaemic damage; sometimes hair may change colour after intradermal or subcutaneous administration; ring block around a particular area of limited blood supply may cause serious necrosis. Felypressin is a synthetic polypeptide related to vasopressin which may be used an an adrenaline substitute to delay absorption without having the stimulatory effect on oxygen consumption that adrenaline has. An advantage of lignocaine is that it is stable on autoclaving: this facilitates sterilization.

Lignocaine preparations

1. Solutions for injection in concentrations of 0.5–3%.
2. Cartridges for use intradermal syringes.
3. Aerosols for surface analgesia.
4. Creams and ointments.
5. Gels for lubrication with analgesia.
6. Ophthalmic preparations.

Procaine

Procaine is an ester of short duration of action and it has poor penetration properties. It produces marked vasodilatation and its high pK_a means that it is highly ionized at physiological pHs. It is inactive after topical application to the mucous membranes. Procaine is hydrolysed by plasma pseudocholinesterase and by the liver to para-aminobenzoic acid and diethylaminoethanol. Para-aminobenzoic acid prolongs the action of suxamethonium (a muscle relaxant) and inhibits the effects of sulphonamides. Procaine should not be used at the same time as sulphonamide. Another effect of procaine is to potentiate the effect of digoxin because of the diethylaminoethanol produced.

Uses

Many commercial preparations of procaine are available and are used in veterinary practice. Concentrations of procaine are usually between 1% and 5%. They are used with and without vasoconstrictors. Duration of good analgesia is usually about one hour. Because it has very poor surface analgesic effects and weak powers of tissue penetration, its application is usually limited to nerve block and regional analgesia.

Amethocaine

This compound is also an ester but is more potent and longer acting than procaine. It can be used an an effective surface analgesic. It is incorporated in many skin and oral preparations.

Bupivacaine

This compound is an amide which is 3–4 times as potent as lignocaine and considerably longer lasting. It is useful for many forms of local analgesia especially when long duration is required. If it is used in epidural analgesia its duration of action may be up to four hours. Although bupivacaine does not produce vasodilatation it is often used with adrenaline to produce a longer duration of action. Solutions are often used at a concentration of 0.25–5%.

Proparacaine (proxymetacaine; Ophthaine)

This is an amide local anaesthetic that has superior powers of penetration through mucous membranes. As a 0.5% solution it is applied to the eye for surface analgesia. Thus it is suitable for analgesia for cauterization of corneal ulcers and removal of foreign bodies. It is also useful for the measurement of intraocular pressure (tonometry).

Further reading

Hall, L. W. (1964) A comparison of methoxyflurane and halothane in small animal anaesthesia. *Veterinary Record*, **76**, 650–655

Hall, L. W. and Clarke, K. W. (1983) *Veterinary Anaesthesia*, London, Baillière Tindall

Hall, L. W. and Chambers, J. B. (1987) A clinical trial of propofol infusion anaesthesia in dogs. *Journal of Small Animal Practice*, **28**, 623–637

Chapter 7

Epilepsy

This chapter describes therapeutic aspects of epilepsy. Definitions of epilepsy are considered first, followed by the aims of therapy and a description of the properties of the antiepileptic drugs.

Epilepsy is produced by some imbalance (often due to a localized brain lesion) in the normal pattern and rhythm of the cerebral cortex which gives rise to massive and excessive uncontrolled activity in parts of the cortex. If this is a generalized condition, waves of disturbance spread over the whole of the cerebral cortex. The disturbance can be distributed across the brain to the spinal cord and eventually to the peripheral nerves and muscles. There are a variety of signs and symptoms which include collapse, loss of consciousness and, sometimes, convulsions which vary in duration. Obviously, if the treatment of epilepsy is to be successful after a long period, it is important to select patients which do not have progressive brain lesions (e.g. tumour) producing the epilepsy.

Stages of epilepsy

An epileptic attack has up to five stages which occur in sequence. These comprise:

1. *Aura or prodrome* This stage is characterized by the signs and symptoms (confusion, abnormal motor activity, pacing) which precede an epileptic attack.
2. *Ictus* This stage is the actual seizure and can last from seconds to several minutes. It can be generalized, involving the whole body, or may be partial, involving only one or two limbs. Sometimes no motor activity is involved, in which case the ictus is characterized as non-motor.
3. *Postictus* This stage occurs after the ictus and is characterized by the signs and symptoms of confusion and depression. Sometimes the animal shows signs of confusion, blindness, coma or walking backwards and forwards in a state of anxiety.

4. *The interictal stage* During periods between the ictus there may be no signs or symptoms so that the animal shows no apparent illness. This stage can last very briefly, perhaps 30 seconds, or up to months. During this period the animal may be completely normal in behaviour or occasionally show signs of some apparent psychological disturbance. This disturbance is characterized by abnormal behaviour.
5. *Status epilepticus* If the ictus stage is continuous and runs together without an interictal phase then this condition is known as status epilepticus. The animal remains in a continuous stage of disturbance or convulsion.

Classification of epileptic attacks

Epileptic attacks are classified in a variety of ways based on the neuroanatomical location of the brain lesion and on the symptoms of the seizure. A symptomatic classification is given below:

1. *Major motor epilepsy* This is characterized by tonic–clonic seizures and is the most common. The obvious signs of convulsion make this condition easy to recognize.
2. *Minor motor epilepsy* This condition is not generalized and starts at one part of the brain and gives rise to associated movements of only one part of the body.
3. *Behavioural epilepsy* This is not a motor epilepsy: it is characterized by regular periodic changes in personality or behaviour. Changes in behaviour can include periods of staring, growling, vomiting, fly snapping or occasionally viciousness. It may also be called psychomotor epilepsy.
4. *Sensory epilepsy* This is characterized by hysteria and running. The animal runs continuously and without aim.

Aims of therapy

The general aim of therapy is to control and minimize the frequency of the epileptic attacks. It may not be possible to control the epileptic attacks completely but significant reductions in the severity of attacks can be produced. It may also be possible to increase dramatically the interval between the epileptic attacks: thus, it is often possible to reduce the frequency of the seizures and reduce the severity of them. It is also possible to reduce the postictus stage and prevent the production of status epilepticus. This is usually achieved using CNS depressants specifically chosen for the management of epilepsy. These CNS depressants must not produce unacceptable depression and sleepiness or viciousness in the animal.

Antiepileptic drugs

Table 7.1 shows antiepileptic drugs which are available and the doses at which they are used. The properties of these agents are considered separately below.

Table 7.1 Therapeutic agents for epilepsy

Generic name	*Product*	*Dose*
Phenobarbitone	Phenobarbitone BP	Dog: 1–2 mg/kg 2–3 times daily (initial dose may be increased) Cat: 8–32 mg/cat 2–3 times daily
Primidone	Mysoline 250 mg tab.	Dog: 8–50 mg/kg daily in divided doses Cat: 8–50 mg/cat daily
	Mysoline suspension (oral)	Dog: 1 ml/kg daily Cat: 1 ml/cat daily
Phenytoin sodium	Epanutin 50 mg and 100 mg tabs	Dog: loading dose 8–22 mg/kg; maintenance dose 6.5–11 mg/kg 3 times daily Cat: not recommended
Diazepam	Valium (slow i.v. or i.m. injection)	Dog: 5–35 mg/dog Cat: 2–10 mg/cat

Phenobarbitone

This agent (Figure 7.1) is the most suitable barbiturate for the treatment of epilepsy. It is characterized by selective anticonvulsant properties and possesses a long half-life. The latter features allows administration of doses 3–4 times daily for the control of epilepsy. It does have significant hypnotic (sleep) effects so that at higher doses ataxia, nystagmus and other signs of sedation occur. It is indicated for control of status epilepticus (i.v. or i.m.) in the dog and for all forms of epilepsy in the cat. It is in fact the drug of first choice in the cat. It will reduce the duration of ictus (epileptic seizures) and increase the interval between them. Some animals may become restless and irritable during

Phenobarbitone

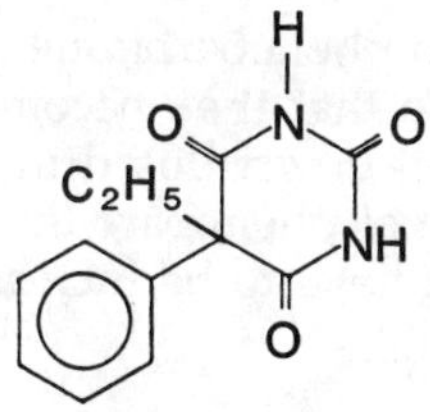

Phenytoin

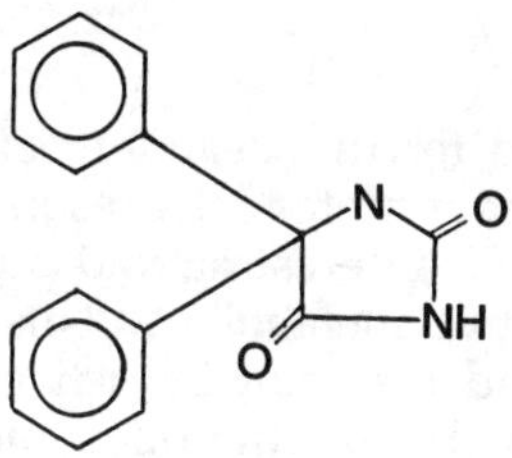

Primidone

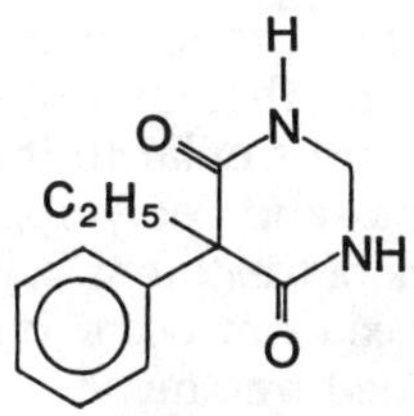

Figure 7.1 The chemical structure of some anticonvulsants

treatment and develop signs of excessive eating and drinking as well as excessive urination.

Phenobarbitone is indicated for the control of generalized major motor seizures, common minor motor seizures and behavioural seizures. It has a serum half-life of some 22–40 hours. If this drug is given at a regular maintenance dose of some 1–2 mg/kg two to three times a day, it will be up to a week before steady plasma concentrations are obtained. This means that dose changes should not be assessed at intervals of less than seven days. Effective plasma concentrations appear to be in the range of 20–40 μg/ml.

Excretion of phenobarbitone is very dependent on the kidney: up to 50% is excreted unchanged in the urine. Since phenobarbitone is a weak acid (pK_a 7.3), increasing the plasma pH will increase the excretion of phenobarbitone. The urine can be made more alkaline by administering sodium bicarbonate orally: this will reduce the half-life of the phenobarbitone.

Continuous exposure to phenobarbitone produces induction of the liver microsomes so that they become more effective at metabolizing and breaking down this drug. Over a period of several weeks the half-life of phenobarbitone will decline. This means that dosages often have to be increased during chronic therapy.

Primidone (Mysoline)

Primidone is indicated for the treatment of generalized major motor seizures and minor motor seizures in the dog. The mode of action of primidone is interesting and probably involves the production of two active metabolites. This means that primidone is a prodrug and may not be active itself. One of the metabolites is phenobarbitone; the other metabolite is phenylethylmalonamide (PEMA). It appears that phenobarbitone and PEMA are the active constituents since the plasma levels of primidone are very low during therapy in the dog.

Side-effects of primidone are similar to those of phenobarbitone and include polyuria and polydipsia, together with polyphagia. In the first week of treatment, when the dose can be increased, sedation and ataxia can occur but these symptoms may disappear after continued treatment.

The liver enzymes show 'induction' so that primidone is metabolized more quickly and doses may have to be increased during chronic therapy. Excretion of the metabolites of primidone will be increased if there is an alkaline urine.

Phenytoin sodium (Epanutin)

This agent is indicated for generalized major motor epilepsy, minor motor epilepsy and behavioural epilepsy. Its use is not recommended in the cat but is restricted to the dog.

The mode of action of phenytoin is unlike phenobarbitone since it has a more marked depressant effect on the motor cortex without significant effect on the sensory cortex; nor is it a general anticonvulsant and it is not used for the treatment of convulsions due to strychnine, or similar clinical syndromes. One advantage of phenytoin sodium is that it has a marked antiepileptic action at therapeutic doses and is not accompanied by a sedative effect. Other advantages include the low frequency of side-effects. Although these are not commonly seen in dogs, observations in humans suggest the following symptoms may occur: lupus erythematosus, various haematological disorders, lymphadenopathy and nystagmus. The presence of nystagmus or ataxia indicates that the dose should be reduced. There is no known specific antidote for toxic overdose. Phenytoin is metabolized in dogs with a half-life of 2–4 hours: at least three daily administrations are required. The minimal plasma concentration for phenytoin appears to be about 10 µg/ml in the dog. Maximal concentrations appear to be in the region of 20 µg/ml. When the drug is metabolized it is converted to 5-(*p*-hydroxyphenyl)-5-5-phenylhydantoin. This metabolite does not have antiepileptic actions of its own and is removed from the body by conjugation with glucuronic acid in the liver. The cat does not possess glucuronyl transferase (an enzyme required for the formation of the glucuronate) so that the half-life of phenytoin sodium in the cat is very long. The use of phenytoin sodium in the cat is therefore restricted: it also produces sedation in this species.

Phenytoin sodium is particularly well bound to plasma proteins: if there is a hypoalbuminaemia it will give rise to much higher free plasma concentrations and the half-life of phenytoin will be reduced.

Diazepam (Valium)

This agent is a benzodiazepine and is the drug of choice for the treatment of status epilepticus. Intravenous doses of 5–35 mg/dog or 2–10 mg/cat are recommended. Half-life is in the region of 6–8 hours. Diazepam is more effectively administered intravenously since absorption following intramuscular injection is poor. The drug has not been evaluated as an oral anticonvulsant in the dog. The use of diazepam in cats may be considered if they do not respond favourably to phenobarbitone.

Containers of plastic should not be used for the storage of diazepam since diazepam is adsorbed by plastic.

Medroxyprogesterone acetate

Medroxyprogesterone acetate, a potent progestogen (Perlutex), is indicated in dogs for the treatment of epileptiform convulsions, particularly if they are associated with oestrus. An initial dose of 20 mg/kg, repeated 14 days later, is suggested. A third dose of 20 mg/kg can be given 4–6 months later. If this is found to be effective, any subsequent treatment may be given at the first signs of epileptic fits returning.

Not to be used

Phenothiazines like acepromazine should not be used for the treatment of epilepsy. These compounds, which interfere with the extrapyramidal motor system, may precipitate and aggravate epileptic seizures.

Convulsions

Convulsions can be produced by a variety of poisons including lead, metaldehyde, organophosphorus compounds, strychnine or antifreeze. Other causes of convulsions include sequelae of canine distemper, neoplasia or trauma. Tetanus, encephalitis, eclampsia, rabies, toxoplasmosis, hypoglycaemia, uraemia and liver encephalopathy are also causes of convulsions. Like epilepsy they can give rise to tremor, twitching, rigidity, ataxia and violent muscle spasms. It is therefore important to distinguish these conditions from epilepsy. Treatment may be very similar, with the use of phenobarbitone and primidone to control the convulsions while appropriate steps are taken to correct the underlying causes.

Further reading

Averill, D. R. (1970) Treatment of Status Epilepticus with diazepam sodium. *Journal of the American Veterinary Medical Association*, **156**, 432

Baggot, J. D. and Davis, L. E. (1973) Comparative study of plasma protein binding of diphenyl hydantoin. *Comp. Gen. Pharmacol.*, **4**, 399

Bogan, J. and Smith, M. (1968) The relation between primidone and phenobarbitone blood levels. *Journal of Pharmacy and Pharmacology*, **20**, 64

Croft, P. G. (1977) Treatment of epilepsy in the working dog. *Veterinary Record*, **101**, 394

Higgins, G. (1977) Treatment of epilepsy in the working dog. *Veterinary Record*, **101**, 335

Kay, W. J. (1975) Epilepsy in cats. *J. Amer. Amin. Hosp. Assoc.* **11**, 77

Nash, A. S., Thomson, H. and Bogan, J. A. (1977) Phenytoin toxicity: A fatal case in a dog with hepatitis and jaundice. *Veterinary Record*, **100**, 280

Turner, T. (1967) Treatment of convulsion in dogs. *Veterinary Record*, **81**, 386

Chapter 8

Endoparasite Therapeutics

Internal parasites are a common problem in small animal practice: eradication is not practicable. The veterinary practitioner must continue to recognize and treat parasite infestations in an appropriate way for the foreseeable future. This chapter describes the properties of the therapeutic agents available and the treatment of endoparasite infections.

Therapeutic agents

There are comparatively few effective anthelmintics used for the treatment of parasites in small animals: this contrasts with the large number of products available for the treatment of ruminant animals. Because the market is small, it is likely that newer anthelmintics for the dog and cat will be developed from compounds originally used for ruminants or human medicine. The main agents currently available and their spectra of action are shown in Table 8.1.

Table 8.1 Anthelmintics: spectrum of action

Compound	*Nematodes*			*Tapeworms*		
	Ascarids	*Hookworm*	*Whipworm*	*Dipylidium*	*Taenia*	*Echinococcus*
Piperazine	+	+	–	–	–	–
Pyrantel	++	++	–	–	–	–
Mebendazole	++	++	++	–	++	+
Fenbendazole	++	++	++	–	++	–
Febantel	++	++	++	–	–	–
Nitroscanate	++	++	–	+	++	+
Praziquantel	–	–	–	++	++	+
Bunamidine	–	–	–	++	++	+
Niclosamide	–	–	–	++	++	–

–, Not effective; +, moderately effective; ++, effective.

Piperazine

This drug was originally used for the treatment of ascariasis in man. It has been used for a considerable period of time and appears to be reasonably safe. It has a limited spectrum of action, being effective against ascarids in the dog and cat and hookworm in the dog but has limited effect against whipworm and no action against tapeworm. Piperazine can be given by mouth as the adipate, citrate or phosphate. It is readily absorbed from the gut; 40% is excreted in the urine within the first twenty-four hours. Since piperazine mimics the action of a normal inhibitory transmitter found in the parasitic worn, it paralyses the worm so that it cannot maintain its position in the intestine. The parasite is then expelled by the peristaltic movements of the gut.

Multiple dosing is often required to control toxocariasis since piperazine does not remove the migrating larvae. A practical regime is to use fortnightly dosing from four weeks of age up to three months of age, with further treatments at six months and then annually. Hookworm, although affected by piperazine, is less sensitive. Up to three times the therapeutic dose for ascarids may be used for the treatment of hookworm.

Piperazine has produced signs of CNS depression (ataxia, etc.) in cats when given in overdose; careful attention to proper dosage is advised. Sometimes damage to the gut by the parasite has led to too rapid absorption of piperazine and CNS disturbances in man.

Mebendazole (Telmin)

This drug is a benzimidazole anthelmintic. Its mode of action is to inhibit microtubule polymerization in the parasite. Microtubules act like intracellular muscles, moving small particles within the cell. Mebendazole causes degenerative changes in the intestinal cells of the parasite as a result of its interaction with the cytoplasmic microtubules. It is very poorly soluble and very little is absorbed through the gut; most of it is excreted unchanged in the faeces. Lower doses are effective against ascarids but higher doses are required for the treatment of hookworm and whipworm. Although it has an action against *Taenia* and *Echinococcus* spp. it is not effective against *Dipylidium* spp.

Fenbendazole (Panacur)

Fenbendazole is also a benzimidazole anthelmintic, presumably acting in the same way as mebendazole by interfering with microtubule synthesis in the parasite. It is available in a variety of preparations, including 2.5% and 10% suspensions, powder, granules and paste preparations. It is effective against ascarids, hookworm, whipworm and *Taenia* species but has little effect against *Dipylidium* and *Echinococcus* species. A particularly useful indication for this drug is in the control of pre- and postnatal transfer of helminth infection to puppies. This is carried out by dosing the pregnant bitch with 50 mg/kg daily, from 21 days prewhelping to 14 days postwhelping, to control the transfer of the larvae.

Pyrantel (Strongid)

This drug acts rapidly as an excitatory transmitter (like acetylcholine) to produce contraction of most nematode muscle. If this drug were to gain access to the muscarinic and nicotinic receptors of the host animal, it would produce vomiting, diarrhoea, muscle tremors, etc. It is therefore presented in a highly ionized form for oral administration so that its distribution is confined to the gut. It will therefore only act on gut-dwelling nematodes. These include *Toxocara canis, Toxascaris leonina, Uncinaria stenocephala* and *Ancylostoma* spp. It is reasonably safe because of limited distribution and can be given to dogs of all ages, including young puppies and pregnant and lactating bitches. It is available as a paste or as a suspension. The suspension should be used with particular care since accidental inspiration produces severe cardiovascular disturbances. Its use is not recommended for cats.

Febantel (Bayverm)

This drug is a prodrug and is activated by a metabolism to fenbendazole and oxyfendazole. Its use is not recommended for cats. It has an indication for the treatment for ascarids, hookworm and whipworm in dogs. It must *not* be used in the dog during the first 4 weeks of pregnancy because of possible teratogenic effects. It is administered in granules (10%).

Nitroscanate (Lopatol)

This is a broad spectrum anthelmintic for use in dogs but not cats. It has an action against tapeworms as well as nematodes. It is effective against ascarids, hookworm (but not whipworm), as well as *Dipylidium, Taenia* and *Echinococcus* spp. For best effects, nitroscanate should be given with a small quantity of food on an empty stomach and food should be withheld for a further eight hours. Because nitroscanate is slightly irritant it is given as film-coated tablets which should not be divided. Side-effects include vomiting after administration.

Praziquantel (Droncit)

Praziquantel is effective against both immature and mature forms of cestodes, but not roundworms, in dogs and cats. It is effective against *Taenia* and *Dipylidium* spp. but less effective against *Echinococcus* spp. It can be given either intramuscularly or subcutaneously by injection or orally in tablet form. Praziquantel is quickly absorbed and metabolized by the liver. Praziquantel impairs the normal tegument function of the tapeworm, making it permeable to excessive glucose loss and more easily attacked by proteolytic enzymes. Because of this, the whole tapeworm disintegrates so that it is rarely passed in the faeces after administration of the drug. If echinococcus infestation is suspected, intramuscular injection is preferred. Few toxic actions of praziquantel are recorded so it may be administered to pregnant females: it is safe to the pregnant female herself as well as the unborn fetus. It is well tolerated by both dogs and cats so that withholding food is not necessary. Vomiting is not usually seen after oral administration of praziquantel.

Bunamidine (Scolaban)

Bunamidine has been shown to be effective against *Dipylidium* and *Echinococcus* species, as well as various *Taenia* species, in the dog. It is given in tablets of 100 or 200 mg. Since the powder is irritant, dust particles may irritate the eyes or the buccal mucous membranes. Toxic effects so far described include vomiting and diarrhoea in certain dogs and, on occasion, deaths have been reported due to ventricular fibrillation since bunamidine sensitizes the heart to adrenaline and noradrenaline.

Niclosamide (Yomesan)

Niclosamide is effective against *Taenia* as well as *Dipylidium* in dogs and cats. However, it has limited effect against *Echinococcus* species. Infections of *Echinoccus* could be treated with up to four times the dose required against *Taenia* and *Dipylidium*. Niclosamide is apparently safe but is not recommended in cases of intestinal atony or acute diarrhoea.

Ivermectin

Ivermectin is not yet available for small animals in the UK but is used in the USA.

Common endoparasite infections

Toxocariasis

This condition is seen in dogs, usually due to *Toxocara canis*, and in cats, due to *Toxascaris leonina*. Toxocariasis is a common problem in dogs, particularly when the animal is under the age of six months. A variety of symptoms are seen which include general illthrift, a poor coat colour, vomiting and diarrhoea, occasionally alternating diarrhoea and constipation, anaemia, a distended abdomen ('pot belly') and, very rarely, a ruptured bowel. These symptoms occur as a result of the mature parasite being located in the intestine. A variety of other symptoms may be seen when the immature larvae are migrating. For example, migrating larvae may produce a peritonitis, septicaemia, liver damage, or even pneumonia as a result of their presence in the lungs. Coughing is frequently commented on by owners of young pups heavily infested with worms.

In cats toxascariasis is usually less severe than in the dog. *Toxascaris leonina* does not show a tracheal migration. In general, severe symptoms, if seen, are similar to those in the dog.

Diagnosis is usually on the basis of history (age and symptoms), which can be confirmed on the basis of faecal examination, and the history of the kennel or cattery. Occasionally worms may be passed in the faeces. Table 8.1 shows that a variety of compounds may be used for the treatment of toxascariasis. Agents suitable for use include piperazine, mebendazole, fenbendazole, febantel and nitroscanate. Table 8.2 shows a list of appropriate doses which may be used. Since infection is from ingestion of infected larvae or by direct infection of the embryo *in utero* from the bitch after the 42nd day of pregnancy, prevention is by an improvement of hygiene or treatment of the bitch to remove the encysted larvae in the muscle.

Table 8.2 Treatment of roundworm in dog and cat

Generic and trade names	*Oral dose in dog and cat*	*Comment*
Piperazine (Coopane) as phosphate, adipate or citrate	100 mg/kg for ascarids; up to 300 mg/kg for hookworm. A second dose may be required in 10 days	Effective against ascarids, hookworm at higher doses but not whipworm
Pyrantel (Strongid, paste or suspension)	Dose: 5 mg/kg pyrantel. Puppies: from birth dose at 10, 20 and 30 days and at 8 and 12 weeks. Bitches: pregnant – dose at 30 and 50 days. During lactation at 1, 4 and 7 weeks postwhelping. Otherwise: every 3 months starting at 6 months	For dogs only
Mebendazole (Telmin KH)	Ascarids: 50 mg twice daily for 2 days (under 2 kg body weight) or 100 mg twice daily (if over 2 kg body weight) for 2 days. Other helminths: same daily dose (50 mg below 2 kg, 100 mg above 2 kg) but increase to 5 consecutive days treatment; heavy dogs over 30 kg, 200 mg twice daily for 5 days	Lower dose effective against ascarids, higher dose required for hookworm, whipworm, taenia and echinococcus. Not very effective against Dipylidium
Fenbendazole (Panacur)	Preparations available including 2.5%, 10% suspensions, powder, granules and paste. Dose 20 mg/kg body weight daily for 5 days	To control pre- and postnatal transfer of toxocara larvae in pups, dose pregnant bitches with 50 mg/kg daily from day 40 to 14 days postwhelping
Febantel (Bayverm granules 10%)	Adults 10 mg/kg three times at 8–24 hour intervals, puppies 30 mg/kg three times at 8 hour intervals – *dogs only*	Do not use during first four weeks of pregnancy
Nitroscanate (Lopatol)	100 or 500 mg tablets available. *Not recommended in cats*. In dogs, dose: 1 × 100 mg tab per 2 kg or 1 × 500 mg tab per 10 kg	Give whole on empty stomach, do not divide tablet. Also effective against some cestodes

Hookworm

This condition is caused by *Uncinaria stenocephala* or, less commonly, *Ancyclostoma caninum*. It is usually seen in kennel dogs housed under unhygienic conditions. The signs of infestation include general debility, as a result of the parasite in the gut taking massive quantities of blood, or lesions that affect the surface of the feet and abdomen which may come in contact with the ground. The signs are erythematous skin, produced by penetation of the parasites, pruritus and possibly secondary bacterial infection. Similar symptoms can occur in the cat. Diagnosis can be based on the history, which shows an anaemia, black tarry faeces and an enteritis, together with a parasitological examination of the faeces.

Treatment is summarized in Tables 8.1 and 8.2. To prevent the condition, improvements in hygiene with prompt removal of faeces should be encouraged.

Whipworm

In dogs this condition is caused by *Trichuris vulpis*. In general it does not cause severe symptoms; however, in severe infections there may be an enteritis with a secondary bacterial infection, as well as an anaemia, weight loss and general unthriftness. Diagnosis is usually made on the basis of the history and a parasitological examination of the faeces. Tables 8.1 and 8.2 show appropriate treatments. Prevention is by an improvement in hygiene and removal of the contaminated faeces. Periodic treatment will also facilitate prevention.

Tapeworm

In dogs two main types of tapeworm infection occur. These are *Echinoccus granulosus* and *Dipylidium caninum*. In the cat a variety of *Taenia* species are found. The clinical symptoms produced by these infestations in the dog and cat are most often not obvious. However, in severe cases of infection there may be vague clinical signs which include chronic diarrhoea and some abdominal discomfort, together with poor weight gain and possibly anal pruritus. Diagnosis is usually based on a demonstration of proglottids in the perianal region or in the faeces. Tables 8.1 and 8.3 describe appropriate treatments. In general, *Echinococcus* is more difficult to remove than *Dipylidium*. It should also be remembered that the intermediate stage of the

Table 8.3 Treatment of tapeworm in dogs and cats

Generic and trade names	*Dose*	*Comment*
Nitroscanate (Lopatol)	As in Table 8.2	Limited action against echinococcus
Niclosamide (Yomesan)	Dogs: 500 mg/4 kg body weight. Cats: up to 2 kg, 250 mg; over 2 kg, 500 mg	Fast for 12 hours before treatment. 4 × recommended dose is required for echinococcus
Praziquantel (Droncit Tablets)	Dogs: 50 mg per 10 kg. Kittens: 12.5 mg. Cats: 25 mg	Droncit Injectable is also available. Dogs: 56.8 mg/10 kg up to 12 kg body weight; thereafter 45.4 mg/kg. Subcutaneous or i.m. Cats same dose but maximum of 34 mg
Bunamidine (Scolaban)	100 and 200 mg tabs available. Dogs: 5–10 mg/kg up to a maximum of 600 mg. Cats: 100 mg	Give whole after fasting. Feed 3 hours later. Not to be given to unweaned puppies or kittens. For echinococcus repeat after 48 hours and again in 3–6 weeks for immatures
Mebendazole (Telmin KH)	Ascarids: 50 mg twice daily for 2 days (under 2 kg body weight) or 100 mg twice daily (if over 2 kg body weight) for 2 days. Other helminths: same daily dose (50 mg below 2 kg, 100 mg above 2 kg) but increase to 5 consecutive days treatment; heavy dogs over 30 kg, 200 mg twice daily for 5 days	Lower dose effective against ascarids, higher dose required for hookworm, whipworm, taenia and echinococcus. Not very effective against *Dipylidium*
Fenbendazole (Panacur)	Preparations available including 2.5%, 10% suspensions, powder, granules and paste. Dose 20 mg/kg body weight daily for 5 days	To control pre- and postnatal transfer of toxocara larvae in pups, dose pregnant bitches with 50 mg/kg daily from day 40 to 14 days postwhelping

parasite of *Dipylidium caninum* is found in fleas. Therefore to complete the treatment against *Dipylidium* it is necessary to treat the animal against fleas as well.

Prevention is achieved by avoiding contact with the intermediate host. This means that raw meat and viscera should not be fed to dogs or cats. Fleas should be eliminated to prevent *Dipylidium caninum*. Animals should not be allowed to roam or hunt since this may permit access to uncooked food. However, despite these precautions periodic treatment may be the only course of action.

Treatment of rare endoparasite infestations

Filaroides osleri

This nematode parasite is found in the dog; it is diagnosed on faecal examination and can produce lesions in the trachea or bronchi. It can produce a chronic dry cough, dyspnoea and wasting. Although no products have been licensed for the treatment of this nematode parasite, albendazole (Valbazen), fenbendazole (Panacur), ivermectin (Ivomec), levamisole (Nilverm) and thiabendazole (Thibenzole) have been used with differing levels of success.

Aelurostrongylus abstrusus

Again no product has been licensed for the treatment of this nematode parasite of the cat which can cause respiratory difficulties but is often asymptomatic. Diagnosis is on the basis of faecal examination. Levamisole (Nilverm) at a dose of 30–40 mg/kg every second day for three treatments has been used successfully.

Coccidiosis

A variety of species of coccidia including *Levincia, Hammondia* and *Sarcocystis* may infect the dog. If the infection is severe, diarrhoea occurs as a result of an intermediate stage of the parasite multiplying in the intestine. Diagnosis is usually based on a history which shows an outbreak in young animals closely housed. Treatment involves the use of a sulphonamide (e.g. sulphadimidine, at a dose rate of 100–200 mg/kg body weight). Potentiated sulphonamides have also been used. The disease may be prevented by improving hygiene and avoiding close housing of young animals.

Babesiosis

This disease is not endemic in the United Kingdom but can occur in quarantine kennels. It is caused by *Babesia canis* which is transmitted by ticks (*Rhipicephalus sanguineus*). The disease produces pyrexia, anaemia, jaundice and sometimes death. Diagnosis is confirmed using Giemsa-stained blood smears which show intraerythrocytic pyriform bodies. Quinuronium sulphate (Ludobal) has been used for treatment at a dose of 0.5 mg/2 kg diluted 1:9 with water s.c. Side-effects of quinuronium include a fall in blood pressure, intestinal contractions and salivation; dogs are particularly susceptible. These effects of quinuronium are due to its potent anti-cholinesterase activity and may be prevented by a large dose of atropine before its administration.

Toxoplasmosis

This disease is caused by *Toxoplasma gondii*. The signs of the disease are varied and can include weight loss, pyrexia, respiratory symptoms, abortion and neonatal disease. Specific immunofluroescent tests are required for diagnosis. A variety of sulphonamides may be used to treat the condition, although none have been specifically licensed. Pyrimethamine (Daraprim) is a human preparation which may be useful in conjunction with the sulphonamides. It is important to point out that the zoonotic aspects of this disease should not be overlooked. The oocysts shed in cat faeces may contaminate pregnant women and give rise to abortion. Serological tests for suspected toxoplasmosis would be sensible where pregnant women are in contact with cats which may be infected.

Further reading

Arundel, J. H. (1970) Control of helminth parasites of dogs and cats. *Australian Veterinary Journal*, **46**, 164

Jacobs, D. E., Pegg, E. J. and Stevenson, P. (1977) Helminths of British dogs: *Toxocara canis* — a veterinary prospective. *Journal of Small Animal Practice*, **18**, 79

Rew, R. S. (1978) Mode of action of common anthelmintics. *Journal of Veterinary Pharmacology and Therapeutics*, **1**, 95

Van den Bosche, H. (1976) In *Biochemistry of Parasites and Host–Parasite Relationships*, p 553. North Holland, Amsterdam

Chapter 9

Ectoparasite Therapeutics

A variety of external parasites attack dogs and cats which are then frequently presented for treatment in small animal practice. This chapter considers firstly the therapeutic agents which are available for the treatment of these conditions and, secondly, the specific conditions produced by each parasite.

Selective toxicity

Many chemical substances may be used to kill ectoparasites but their usefulness is limited by toxicity to the animal and to man. In general, the selective toxicity of the antiparasitic agent depends on selective uptake by the parasite. The chitinous cuticle of the ectoparasite allows a greater rate of absorption of the antiparasitic agent than does the skin of the animal. In addition, there is a much greater ratio of surface area to body weight in the parasite compared to the host animal.

Most antiparasitic agents act on the parasite by disrupting nerve function. Since the nerves of the ectoparasites are usually located just beneath the cuticle, the relatively quick absorption of the antiparasitic agent produces a selective toxic effect on the parasite. However, it should be pointed out that large amounts of an antiparasitic agent, when administered either orally or intravenously to the host animal, will also produce toxic effects, usually of neural type.

Resistance

Resistance to antiparasitic agents has been recognized for some time. This resistance appears as a result of the selection pressure produced by the continuous use of one type of antiparasitic agent. Over a considerable period this selection pressure results in the appearance of new genes in the parasite, conferring resistance. The resistance of the population of parasites is slowly lost if the antiparasitic agent is not used for a considerable

Table 9.1 Ectoparasite preparations

Drug	*Product*	*Presentation*	*Dog*	*Cat*	*Recommended for treatment against*									
					Flies	*Fleas*	*Ticks*	*Lice*	*Otodectics*	*Cheyletiella*	*Sarcoptes*	*Notoedres*	*Demodex*	*Trombicula*
Sulphur compounds														
Monosulfiram	Tetmosol	5% soap; 25% solution	√	√	–	√	√	√	√	–	√	√	√	–
Selenium sulphide	Seleen	1%	√	√	–	√	–	√	–	–	–	–	√	–
Sulphur	Skin Dressing Sulphur 22%	22% wettable powder	√	–	–	–	–	–	–	–	√	–	–	–
Naturally occurring compounds														
Benzyl benzoate	Benzyl Benzoate BP	25% applic. (liquid)	√	–	–	–	–	–	–	–	√	–	√	–
Derris	Skin Dressing Derris 2%	2% wettable powder	√	–	–	√	√	√	–	–	–	–	–	–
Rotenone	Demodectic Mange Dressing (concentrate)	3% conc. liquid	√	–	–	–	–	–	–	–	–	–	√	–
Chlorinated hydrocarbons														
γ-Benzene hexachloride (lindane)	Lorexane, Kilsect Dogwash, Skin Dressing BHC. Skin Dressing Nos 2 and 3, also in Clendrol, GAC and Otoryl ear drops	Emulsions, liquids, powders and drops	√	Limited use in cat (ears)	–	√	√	√	√	√	√	√	√	√

Bromyocyclen	Alugan	0.8% aerosol spray; 42.5% wettable powder; 4.25% dusting powder	√	√	–	√	–	√	√	√	√	√	–	√
Pyrethroids														
Pyrethrins + piperonyl butoxide	Pybuthrin dusting powder	0.1% dusting powder; 1.1% dusting powder	√	√	–	√	√	√	–	–	–	–	–	–
Permethrin	Coopers head to tail veterinary flea powders, spray, shampoo	1% powder; spray and shampoo	√	√	–	√	–	–	–	–	–	–	–	–
Neopynamin + sumithrin	Willothrin	Aerosol spray	√	√	–	√	–	–	–	–	–	–	–	–
Organophosphorus compounds														
Diazinon	Canovel collars	15% collars	√ Dog collar	√ Cat collar	–	√	√	–	–	–	–	–	–	–
Cythioate	Cyflee	30 mg tablets	√	√	–	√	√	–	–	–	–	–	–	√
Ronnel	Ectoral	250 mg, 500 mg and 1 g tablets; 33% and 56% emulsion	√	√	–	√	–	√	–	–	–	–	√	√
Dichlorvos + fenitrothion	Nuvan Top, Zeprox	0.2% aerosol; 0.8% spray	√	√	–	√	√	√	√	–	√	√	√	√
Carbamates														
Carbaryl	Derasect	Shampoo	√	√	–	√	√	√	–	–	–	–	–	–
Propoxur	Belfo Collar and Flea Spray (also in Negasunt)	Collar; aerosol; (powder)	√	√	√	√	–	–	–	–	–	–	–	–
Amitraz	Taktic	Liquid	√	–	–	–	–	–	–	–	–	–	–	√

period of time. If a parasite develops a resistance to a particular type of antiparasitic agent, say organophosphorous compounds, it means that resistance to other compounds in the same group is also likely. Should resistance appear, it is logical to use compounds which are believed to have a differing mode of action.

Therapeutic agents (Table 9.1)

Sulphur compounds

Lotions of sulphur are still used occasionally in small animal practice for the treatment of sarcoptic mange in the dog. However, it is not suitable for use in the cat which will lick its coat and so ingest the irritant oxides of the sulphur which may be formed. The mode of action of sulphur is believed to involve the blocking of the oxidative phosphorylation in the parasite by the oxides of the sulphur which are formed.

Selenium sulphide (Seleen)

This is used as a 1% w/v suspension in a mild detergent base in the control of various ectoparasites and dermatoses (Table 9.1). It is applied topically but care should be taken to prevent the animal from licking the suspension since it is an irritant. Care should also be taken to avoid the eyes. Treatment should be repeated at intervals of one week if necessary.

Monosulphiram (Tetmosol)

This is a yellowish powder which is made up with a wetting agent in a 25% solution or as a soap at a concentration of 5% (w/v). This preparation can be used to eliminate fleas, ticks, lice and has been suggested for use against demodex, notoedres and sarcoptes. For the treatment of sarcoptic mange in the dog, the animal is first cleaned with soap and then an alcoholic solution of monosulphiram (diluted 1/10 with water) is scrubbed into the skin. Like the other sulphur compounds, monosulphiram is irritant if it gets into the eyes or if it is consumed orally.

Naturally occurring compounds

Benzyl benzoate

This is an oily liquid toxic to mites. It can be used for the treatment of sarcoptic or demodectic mange. Again, like the sulphur compounds, benzyl benzoate is contraindicated in cats because of the likelihood of cats licking the substance applied to its fur. If consumed in sufficient quantities, benzyl benzoate will cause gastroenteritis and, if sufficient is absorbed, stimulation of the central nervous system. Contact with the eyes should be avoided since the compound is an irritant.

Derris

This drug is obtained from the dried rhizome of *Derris elliptica*. The most important and active constituent is rotenone which is insoluble in water. It is therefore prepared as a 2% wettable powder and can be used on dogs for the treatment of fleas, ticks and lice.

Rotenone

As a concentrated liquid rotenone is used for the treatment of demodectic mange in the dog. It acts by inhibiting the electron transport chain in the mitochondria, so depressing respiration in both vertebrates and the parasite. The selective action of rotenone is a result of its selective uptake. Rotenone is more rapid in onset of action when compared with γ-BHC but is lower and more prolonged than the pyrethroids. Contact of mucous membranes with rotenone may lead to irritation of the eyes and some numbness of the lips. It is not well absorbed through the skin or intestines since it is inactivated in the alkaline intestine. Since it is unstable in the environment it is not very persistent. One specific recommendation for rotenone is the treatment of demodectic mange. Here it can be used as an alcoholic solution (0.75% w/v). It is applied to one-third of the animal's skin daily for a week. This particular approach is effective in about 90% of cases and this compares favourably with many alternative antidemodectic treatments. Probably the reason for the effectiveness of this approach is that this application method ensures contact of the rotenone with the demodectic parasite.

Chlorinated hydrocarbons

γ-Benzene hexachloride (Lorexane)

γ-Benzene hexachloride is a white crystalline powder with a characteristic musty smell. It is soluble in alcohol and organic solvents, but not water. The γ isomer is used since this is less toxic than the β isomer which is selectively absorbed from the intestine and slowly cleared from the body. γ-Benzene hexachloride has a quicker action than DDT but is less persistent. It is used in a variety of preparations which include powders, drops, liquids, soaps and emulsions (Table 9.1). Its mode of action involves an increase in neuronal excitability by acting as a sodium channel stimulator. It has an action against fleas, ticks, lice and a wide variety of mange. In the cat it is of limited use because of the likelihood of licking of the coat. If sufficient quantities are consumed it may produce excitability and CNS stimulation which can be treated with calcium borogluconate or pentobarbitone sodium.

Bromocyclen (Alugan)

Like γ-benzene hexachloride, bromocyclen is a chlorinated hydrocarbon. It is available in a variety of preparations including an aerosol, a wettable powder and dusting powder; thus, washes, dips or sprays can be used. It has a similar mode of action to γ-benzene hexachloride and affects neuronal excitability of the parasite. Its selective effect is on the basis of the greater uptake by the parasite compared with the host. It can be used for the treatment of fleas, lice, sarcoptes, notoedres, otodectes, chorioptes and cheyletiella but is not recommended for the treatment of demodectic mange.

A 0.07% suspension of bromocyclen concentrate powder is suitable for the treatment of flea infestations, with a repeat treatment one or two weeks later. For generalized sarcoptic mange animals should be bathed in a 0.07% suspension but localized lesions may be treated by painting or rinsing the affected areas with a 0.2% suspension. For the treatment of fleas and lice, the aerosol spray or dusting powder may also be used. Cats may be treated with bromocyclen powder or the spray, rather than the suspension of concentrate powder, in order to minimize the risks which ensue from licking of the coat. The dusting powder and aerosol preparations are usually effective for feline mange but severe lesions may require the concentrate powder, using a suspension of 0.07%. Toxic symptoms due to an increase in neuronal excitability of the host animal may occur, particularly in cats if the amount of this compound consumed is too great. Calcium borogluconate may be used to counteract the increased neuronal excitability.

Pyrethroids

Pyrethrins + piperonyl butoxide

Pyrethrum is prepared from the flower heads of *Chrysanthemum cinerariaefolium*. This plant was cultivated for its insecticidal esters, now called the pyrethrins. These substances can be used to control fleas, ticks, lice and, in appropriate preparations, flies. One slight problem with the use of these substances is that they are unstable in the atmosphere and have to be protected from the light. Despite this problem they are useful as antiparasitic agents since they are much safer than the other insecticides. The reason for this increase in safety is the poor absorption of these substances from the alimentary tract of the host animal. They are also rapidly metabolized in the liver. They have a selective effect on the parasite, being preferentially taken up through the cuticle to act on the neuronal tissue lying underneath. The increase in neuronal excitability is again the result of increasing the influx of sodium ions.

The pyrethrins are inactivated by hydroxylation, a process which occurs rapidly in the host animal but more slowly in the parasite. It is possible to inhibit this hydroxylation using piperonyl butoxide. Piperonyl butoxide also has a weak insecticidal action of its own but, in the main, acts as a synergist to the pyrethrins. Preparations containing synergized pyrethrins are therefore useful. They are safer than most other insecticides.

Permethrin

This is a synthetic ester and has the general pyrethroid structure. Because it is an ester it is rapidly hydrolysed in the tissues of the host, so decreasing its half-life. Permethrin is used as a 1% w/w insecticidal powder or spray. It can be used for the control of fleas on dogs and cats of all ages and may produce protection against reinfestation for up to two weeks. The powder is administered evenly over the whole body by dusting it in while stroking the hair against the direction of lie. A medium-sized dog will require 8–15 g of powder, while a cat will require 6–9 g and a kitten 3–5 g. Repeat treatments every 2 to 3 weeks may be necessary.

The preparation is for external use only so that contact with eyes and inhalation should be avoided. It is also known that this substance, like many of the other insecticides, is dangerous to fish in aquaria so that it is important to avoid contamination.

The aerosol spray may also be used in a similar way but particular care with kittens is required. Kittens must not be sprayed for more than 2–3 seconds at the most. An overdose with this substance is seen as hyperaesthesia which may be countered with calcium borogluconate or barbiturates. Keeping the animal quiet in a darkened cage has proved effective even in the most severe cases of overdose.

Neopynamin + sumithrin (Willothrin)

These two compounds are used in combination as an aerosol spray against fleas in dogs and cats. The synthetic pyrethroids are used in a similar way to permethrin. However, the contraindications are that they should not be used on puppies or kittens less than one month of age. Treatment of any animal should not exceed once per week. Thus it appears that the combination of these two substances given as an aerosol is associated with very slightly increased toxic hazards. These hazards are similar to those of permethrin.

Organophosphorus compounds

The first organophosphorus compounds were produced as a result of the development of nerve gases for chemical warfare. Their toxic effects and therapeutic effects arise as a result of antagonizing the enzyme cholinesterase. As a result of inhibiting this enzyme, the neurotransmitter acetylcholine increases in concentration at the neuroeffector junctions. The blocking of this enzyme and the subsequent rise in concentration of acetylcholine at these junctions may occur in either the host animal or, preferably, in the parasite.

The safest organophosphorus compounds are precursors of active metabolites. Activation produces a delay in toxicity and so provides an opportunity for other enzymes to degrade the active metabolites. The enzymes degrading the organophosphorus compounds are more active in the mammal hosts than the ectoparasite; this helps to produce the selective toxicity of the organophorphorus compound. The ratio of activation to inactivation is very important in these antiparasitic agents. The organophosphorus compounds are very fat soluble and are quickly absorbed through the cuticle of the parasite where they inhibit the cholinesterase of its nervous system. A consequence of the accumulation of acetylcholine in the parasite is a loss of function, and death ensues.

Oral preparations of organophosphorus compounds are available. Following digestion they are distributed throughout the body to reach the skin in sufficient quantities to kill off mange-mites and fleas digesting plasma. Resistance to the various organophosphorus compounds in the parasite (fleas particularly) is increasing. There appear to be many mechanisms for this resistance, including possession of a cholinesterase which is insensitive to organophosphorus compounds.

Side-effects of the organophosphorus compounds are uncommon when used as recommended. However, incidences of overdose have been known to occur. The symptoms are of cholinergic poisoning and include constriction of the pupil, salivation, colic, diarrhoea, muscular tremors and respiratory failure. Atropine sulphate (0.1–0.2 mg/kg) is repeatedly injected to reverse the muscarinic actions of acetylcholine. Effective treatment of organophosphorus poisoning with atropine may be judged by the appearance of a dilated pupil, decreased salivation and a speeding of the heart rate. The effect of the organophosphorus compounds may persist for several days but atropine is cleared from the body within a period of a few hours so that subsequent treatments with atropine may be necessary. Pralidoxime (Protopam 20 mg/kg) has been suggested for reactivating the cholinesterase at neuromuscular junctions.

Diazinon (Canovel collars)

This is available as an insecticidal collar for dogs and cats. The collar is manufactured from a strip of polyvinyl chloride impregnated with diazinon (50%) which is released gradually over a period of up to 120 days. The diazinon is deposited on the animal's neck hair and becomes available for contact with the fleas. These collars are very useful in dogs and cats but care must be taken to recognize any irritation around the neck which may occur. The limited period of duration of action must also be recognized.

Cythioate (Cyflee)

This compound is available in 30 mg tablets. It is indicated for repeated oral administration to dogs of all ages for the control of fleas, mange (demodex) and ticks. It is also specifically indicated for repeated oral administration to cats of all ages for the control of fleas.

In dogs, 1 tablet per 10 kg bodyweight is the recommended oral dose, given every third day or twice weekly for four weeks and thereafter every second week, to control flea reinfestation. To control demodectic mange the recommended dose should be given every third day or twice weekly for at least six weeks. Should it prove necessary it is safe to repeat the treatment for up to six months. In cats, one quarter tablet per 5 kg bodyweight is recommended as an oral dose, given once a week for the first four weeks and thereafter every second week, to control flea infestation.

Cythioate is rapidly absorbed from the gastrointestinal tract within two or three hours and is well distributed throughout the body. Fleas and other ectoparasites which ingest body fluids are therefore vulnerable. The drug appears to persist for a maximum of eight hours after administration. It then appears that the compound is rapidly eliminated from the body. The therapeutic index of cythioate has been suggested to be ten-fold in the dog and twenty-fold in the cat. It is pointed out that this ratio may be considerably lower in susceptible animals, particularly those animals exposed to other anticholinesterase drugs.

Ronnel (Ectoral)

Ronnel is a systemic insecticide for oral and topical administration to dogs and cats. It is used for the treatment of demodectic mange in dogs as well as the control of flea infestation in cats and dogs.

To control demodectic mange in dogs a combined oral and topical treatment appears to be most effective. A solution of 1% ronnel is applied over the entire body every four days, together with the administration of 25 mg ronnel per pound bodyweight every day. It is preferable to administer the tablets in divided doses throughout the day. For very severe conditions the dose may be increased to 35 mg/lb/day. It is important to monitor the course of this treatment by periodic microscopic examination of skin scrapings to look at the demodectic mange-mite and to continue treatment until the parasite appears dead.

Fleas in dogs and cats or lice in dogs can be treated by giving ronnel at a dose rate of 25 mg/lb every other day in single or divided doses. In order to continue the control, a decreased dosage of 12.5 mg/lb every other day may be given. A 0.25% solution of ronnel may be given over the entire body by sponging or dipping for the treatment of fleas in dogs or cats.

Dichlorvos + fenitrothion (Nuvan Top; Zeprox)

These two organophosphorus compounds are prepared in an aerosol for the control of fleas, lice and flies on dogs and cats. They can also be used for the control of ticks and mange in dogs and cats. They are sprayed on the affected areas after raising the animal's hair and applying the aerosol at a distance of 6–8 inches from the lie of the coat. The eyes and the mouth should be avoided. For mange, treatment should be applied every seven days; for lice, the treatment should be applied every ten to twelve days; for the control of fleas the spray should be applied every seven to fourteen days; to kill ticks the spray should be applied every seven days. Two to three treatments normally kill off existing populations of lice and fleas. Mange-mites are sometimes more resistant and treatment may be repeated for several weeks. When there is repeated infestation it is advisable to spray the area of the animal's resting place (baskets, carpets, skirting boards, etc.).

Dichlorvos and fenitrothion are cholinesterase inhibitors: they should not be used in conjunction with the flea collars containing other organophosphorus compounds (diazinon). A period of at least one week should be allowed after removal of the flea collar and before treatment with the organophosphorus aerosol mixture.

Carbamates

Carbamates also antagonize the action of cholinesterase and act in a similar manner to the organophosphorus compounds. However, the inhibition is reversible so that it is of a different nature. Carbamates are inactivated in the liver by the mixed function oxidases.

Carbaryl (Derasect)

This is an ester of methyl carbamic acid and is sparingly soluble in water. Because it is fat soluble it is rapidly absorbed through the cuticle of the parasite. Once in the parasite it inhibits the cholinesterase, leading to the death of the parasite. In the host animal, carbaryl may produce toxic symptoms in very high doses but the signs do not last very long since the carbaryl is removed within a period of three to four hours and its symptoms are readily abolished by atropine. Unlike the organophosphorus compounds, pralidoxime is ineffective as an antidote since it does not reactivate the carbamylated cholinesterases.

Carbaryl is used in an insecticidal shampoo in dogs and cats for the control of fleas, mange mites, lice and ticks. The eyes should be avoided. For the best results it should be left on for five minutes before rinsing. Repeat shampooing at seven-day intervals is advised if there is heavy infestation. It should not be used on puppies or kittens under one month of age, nor should it be used on pregnant animals. In order to minimize risk to the owner of the animal, shampooing should take place using rubber gloves.

Propoxur (Bolfo)

This carbamate is found in wound powders and is also used in flea collars which contain propoxur 9.4% w/w in a plastic strip. A flea collar is used as a long-term control for flea infestation in dogs and should be replaced after five months. It is not suitable for use on a sick or convalescent dog. Irritation of the neck is possible with this preparation. A 0.25% w/w presentation of propoxur as an aerosol spray is also used. This is useful for the control of fleas in dogs and cats.

Amitraz (Taktic)

Amitraz is the active constituent of Taktic liquid concentrate. Recent reports have suggested that this compound is useful for the treatment of demodectic mange in dogs. It is used at a concentration of 0.025% w/v applied to the whole body of affected animals at 14-day intervals for a total of 4–8 applications. In approximately 86% of treated animals recovery from demodectic mange has been seen. In the remainder (14%) maintenance treatment is able to keep the condition under control.

The mode of action of amitraz is unknown but toxic symptoms may be seen in about 10% of dogs and present themselves as sleepiness which lasts from a few hours up to two days.

Ivermectin (Ivomec)

This antibiotic is useful for the treatment of demodex, cheyletiella and heartworm, but is not currently licensed in the UK. It is available in the USA as Heartguard.

Specific conditions

Flea infestation

This is a very common problem of dogs and cats. It is caused by *Ctenocephalides felis* in the cat and *Ctenocephalides canis* in the dog. Occasionally infestation may be due to the flea of the hedgehog, rabbit or human. Signs include itching (pruritus), small scabs or papules (especially along the back), flea dirt in the coat, self-inflicted damage and occasionally anaemia. The differential diagnosis includes the presence of other ectoparasites, hypersensitivity due to other allergens, contact irritants, bacterial or fungal infection, or anal gland disease. Specific diagnostic tests include the wet paper test on flea dirt (the application of small quantities of water to flea dirt producing a red coloration) or the identification of fleas in the coat. The presence of *Dipylidium caninum* proglottids are also of diagnostic value.

Treatment

Numerous insecticidal preparations are available to control and kill fleas on pet animals (Table 9.1). In general it is important to remember that cats tend to be more sensitive to the insecticides than dogs, so that a product should not be used on a cat unless it is specifically recommended for that species. It is also important to remember that the concurrent use of flea medications and certain organophosphorus anthelmintic compounds may result in poisoning. The pyrethrins have the advantage that they are the least toxic and that they are contact poisons with rapid action. They can also be used on kittens. Carbamates are less toxic than the organophosphorus compounds and can be used on cats. The organophosphorus compounds have been widely used and should be used with caution in cats. Some resistant flea populations have developed.

There are a variety of ways of administering the parasiticide. Flea collars may be used and are useful for the control of the flea population but are not adequate or sufficient treatment for the complete prevention and control of an animal allergic to flea saliva. They can also irritate the skin. Shampoos and sprays have good knock-down effects but usually have little residual action. Sprays can be alarming to the animal because of the noise. Powders usually have a residual action lasting at least seven days but they must be worked well into the coat. Dips appear to be the most effective and best at producing a residual action lasting seven days.

Prevention is an important part of treatment. The environment of the animal, including the bedding, carpets and cushions on which it lies, must be vacuum cleaned or sprayed effectively with an antiparasitic agent.

Flies

Fly strike is caused by fly larvae invading dirty or damaged flesh. The clinical symptoms include a very depressed animal, a pungent smell and the presence of fly larvae. Many antiparasitic agents are effective for the treatment of this condition, including dichlorvos and fenitrothion. However, propoxur in a mixture with coumaphos and sulphanilamide (Negasunt) is specifically recommended for the treatment of this condition.

Ticks

In the UK, tick infestation with *Ixodes* is seen during spring or autumn in dogs or cats that have access to long grass and bush. The ticks are usually found on the ears, head and toes but may also be found on the body. At the site of the attachment there may be some irritation and possibly infection. In severely infected animals, particularly the young, anaemia is possible. The ticks may serve as carriers of bacterial, viral, protozoal or rickettsial diseases.

Successful treatment uses a variety of approaches. Sometimes only one tick is present on the animal. This may be removed manually after an appropriate anaesthetic solution (chloroform, ether) has been applied to the tick. Care must be taken to avoid leaving the head parts of the tick in the skin. These may remain and cause irritation. Large numbers of ticks can be treated by an appropriate antiparasitic agent (Table 9.1).

Lice

This is a contagious condition which is usually associated with poor sanitary arrangements, neglect and debility. The lice are frequently found on the ears, neck and shoulders and cause marked irritation (pruritus), inflammation of the skin, hair loss and restlessness. Symptoms are the same in both the dog and the cat.

Diagnosis is on the basis of the clinical symptoms together with the presence of eggs (nits) attached to the hair follicles, or the presence of the lice themselves. Treatment is relatively simple and involves isolation of the animal so that the infection may not spread. It also involves the application of a suitable antiparasitic agent (Table 9.1) which should be applied weekly for a period of 2–4 weeks. Further spread of the infection to other animals can be avoided by treating all the animals on the premises.

Otodectes (ear mite infestation)

In the dog and cat this condition is caused by *Otodectes cynotis*. This condition is more frequently seen in cats than dogs. It is a highly contagious condition and occurs as a result of mites in the ear canal. These mites give rise to pruritus, head shaking, possibly oral haematomas, scratching of the ears, thick black-brown exudate in the ear canal and secondary bacterial infections of the outer ear. Diagnosis can be made on the basis of the history and a physical examination of the ear revealing the presence of the mites in the canal.

Treatment includes the cleansing of the ear canal and the application of ear drops containing a suitable insecticidal agent (Table 9.1). If there is a secondary bacterial infection the application of suitable antibiotics is indicated. Since this condition is contagious it is appropriate to treat all animals in the immediate environment which are likely to be in contact with the affected animal.

Notoedric mange (feline scabies)

This condition is caused by *Notoedres cati* and presents as crusting around the borders of the ear which quickly spreads to the face, neck, elbows and feet. There is intense pruritus which produces self-trauma.

Diagnosis is made on a basis of microscopic observation of the parasite or its eggs in skin scrapings. Differential diagnosis includes otodectic infestations, cheyletiella infestations, lice, dermatomycosis, allergies, systemic lupus erythematosus and bullous autoimmune diseases. The condition is rare in the UK.

Sarcoptic mange (canine scabies)

This condition is caused by *Sarcoptes scabiei* var. *canis*. The condition is a contagious one giving rise to reddening, scaling and papule formation of the skin, initially around the ear borders, hocks, elbows and sternum. It can become generalized later. It causes severe pruritus, particularly when the animal is near heat. It is also associated with a peculiar mousey odour.

Diagnosis is on a basis of a strong positive scratch reflex from the pinna and microscopic observation of the parasite or its eggs in skin scrapings. Differential diagnosis includes allergy, primary seborrhoea, dermatomycosis and cheyletiella infestation.

Treatment should include isolation of infected animals together with the application of an appropriate insecticide (Table 9.1). Since this condition is contagious, all animals on the premises should be treated. In long-haired animals it may be an advantage to gently clip and cleanse the affected areas to remove the hair and crusts. Glucocorticoids may help to relieve the pruritus and self-trauma.

Demodectic mange

This condition in dogs is caused by *Demodex canis* (a follicular mite). The condition is usually seen in a young animal where there are localized or generalized skin lesions not associated with pruritus. If pustules and hair loss are seen, the condition is referred to as pustular demodex.

Diagnosis is usually made on the basis of the history which is confirmed by the presence of mites seen after a microscopic examination of the pustules. The differential diagnosis includes other skin parasites, ringworm, bacterial infections and hypersensitivity.

Treatment is usually more difficult than for the other parasite infections since demodex is localized deep in the skin and access is difficult. Specific treatments are recommended (Table 9.1). Also recommended is Alphosyl lotion for use after an initial treatment with Dermisol, as an aid to insecticidal therapy. In addition, amitraz (Taktic) has been used successfully in the treatment of demodex but is not licensed in the UK.

Since this condition is sometimes seen in litters, wih young animals being infected, it appears that the condition may be handed on from the parents. Animals with generalized demodex should not be used for breeding. Although not licensed, ivermectin (Ivomec) has been found very useful for this condition.

Trombiculiasis (harvest mites or berry bugs)

This condition is caused by *Trombicula autumnale* and is seen in July to October. It shows a variety of symptoms including pustules, papules, crusts and irritation of the areas that come into contact with the ground (feet, ventrum, etc.). Pruritus may be absent or intense.

Diagnosis is usually made on the basis of the identification of orange mites which are seen macroscopically or microscopically. Treatment involves washing the infected animal in an appropriate insecticide (Table 9.1) and avoiding areas which contain these mites (usually grasses).

Cheyletiella infestations

This condition is more commonly recognized and caused by the trombiculid thermite of the rabbit *Cheyletiella parasitovorax*, the dog-adapted *Cheyletiella yasguri* and the cat-adapted *Cheyletiella blakei*. Infestation with cheyletiella produces pruritus and self-inflicted damage. The owners of the animals may also show characteristic lesions and pruritus. The skin of the infected animal shows dry scaling, especially along the back. Mites are just visible to the eye and appear like 'walking dandruff'. Diagnosis is usually on the basis of microscopical identification: differential diagnosis includes lice, demodectic mange, scabies, otodectic mange and nutritional alopecia. Treatment is with a suitable ectoparasiticide (Table 9.1).

Further reading

Brown, A. W. and Pal, R. (1971) *Insecticides*, No. 38, World Health Organization, Geneva

Campbell, W. C., Fisher, M. H., Stapley, E. O., Albers-Schonberg, G. and Jacob, T. A. (1983) Ivermectin: A potent new antiparasitic agent. *Science*, **221**, 823–827

Silver, A. (1974) The biology of cholinesterases. In *Frontiers of Biology*, Vol. 36. North Holand, Amsterdam

Chapter 10

Fluid Therapy

Fluid therapy is now an important aspect of small animal practice. This chapter describes the solutions suitable for, and an approach to fluid therapy.

Substances available for fluid replacement

There are two main types of fluid used for therapy: the first are crystalloid solutions which are based on extracellular fluids; the second type of solution are the plasma expanders.

Crystalloid solutions

Mild water or electrolyte deficits may be corrected by oral or intravenous administration of crystalloid solutions. The solutions must be sterile and pyrogen free; they should have a pH close to that of plasma and match the osmotic pressure. Table 10.1 illustrates the composition of the crystalloid solutions commonly used. They comprise sodium chloride BP and sodium bicarbonate BP solutions, glucose solutions and Hartmann's solution.

In animals with moderate fluid deficits the most important function of fluid therapy is to provide an adequate volume expansion of extracellular fluid so that normal renal function will be restored: this allows the animal to carry out self-regulation of electrolyte levels.

Dextrose injection BP

This is a 5% solution of glucose which is approximately isotonic with plasma. In normal animals, glucose administered intravenously is rapidly metabolized unless the rate of intravenous injection is so high that it saturates renal absorption. If this occurs, and glucose appears in the urine, the effect of the dextrose injection may be to provoke diuresis. Obviously it is important to inject the dextrose saline slowly to avoid this effect.

Table 10.1 Composition of extracellular fluid and fluid replacement solutions

	Concentration (mmol/litre)						
	Na^+	*K^+*	*Cl^-*	*HCO_3*	*Lactate*	*Glucose*	*Ca^{2+}*
Extracellular fluid	140	4	100	28	2	5	–
Sodium bicarbonate injection BP	150	–	–	150	–	–	–
Dextrose injection	–	–	–	–	–	280	–
Hartmann's solution	130	5	110	–	30	–	2
Sodium chloride injection BP	150	–	150	–	–	–	–

Higher concentrations of glucose (10% or 50%) may be administered with caution if the intention is for glucose to act as an energy source.

Hartmann's solution

This contains sodium lactate and closely resembles extracellular fluid. It may be used to replace extracellular fluid loss. The lactate which is in the solution is metabolized in normal animals in a period of 1–2 hours following administration. The combination of the lactate with H^+ to form lactic acid prior to its uptake by the liver reverses acidosis. Lactate is more stable than bicarbonate and shows fewer incompatibilities with the other components used for fluid therapy. Its slow metabolism in the body helps protect the animal against overdosage. It is pointed out, however, that Hartmann's solutions are contraindicated if lactic acidosis is present or if there is severe liver damage. In these cases, sodium bicarbonate solutions are more appropriate.

Plasma expanders

These substances are administered intravenously and are not intended to cross capillary membranes. They are indicated when the fluid deficit has occurred from the vascular compartment. Severe haemorrhage or plasma loss due to burns or peritoneal effusions are indications.

Plasma expanders should be easy to obtain and store. They should not interfere with the viscosity or ability of the blood to clot and they should persist in the circulation for a reasonable length of time before removal by excretion or metabolism. It is obvious that they should not cause toxicity or provoke an allergic response (histamine release). Most commercially available preparations are designed to minimize the possibility of an allergic response. Despite this, such responses are still known to occur, with the consequent release of histamine and other autocoids (5-HT, prostaglandin, etc.).

Dextrans

Dextran 70 or dextran 40 solutions are most often used. The '70' or '40' indicates the average dextran molecular weight (in daltons), for example dextran 70 contains molecular weights in the range of 25 000 to 110 000 daltons. The 6% solutions which are usually supplied often cause movement of water from the interstitial fluid to the vascular compartment as well as producing plasma expansion. The increase in plasma volume normally lasts six to seven hours. After this, 25–35% of the dose of the original dextran comprising the smaller molecules is excreted in the urine. The larger molecules of dextran are taken up by the reticuloendothelial cells or slowly metabolized to carbon dioxide and water. Some of the dextran may last in the circulation for up to two days.

The dextrans improve the circulation in other ways than by plasma expansion: they line capillary endothelium and prevent aggregation of red blood cells. However, one problem which may occur with the dextrans is that of the lower molecular weights being found in the renal tubule shortly after intravenous injection. Here, they raise the luminal viscosity and cause the renal failure which is sometimes seen in cats. Since the effect on renal tubules and the effect on microcirculation is due to lower molecular weight dextrans, these two effects are more likely to occur with dextran 40 than with dextran 70.

Polygeline (Haemaccel)

Gelatine has been used to produce a number of plasma expanders. One of the commonly used derivatives is a urea–gelatine polymer called polygeline. In this compound molecules have an average molecular weight of 35 000 daltons but their range is from 4300 daltons to 280 000 daltons. At the concentration of 3.5%, the osmotic pressure and viscosity are very similar to that of plasma. The half-life of polygeline is about 4.5 hours which results in a clinically useful effect lasting about 2 hours. However, it is known that in animals suffering from hypovolaemic shock this compound persists for twice as long. Most of the compound is excreted in the urine after two days.

Polygeline does not interfere with the microcirculation or affect blood coagulation. It does have a tendency to release histamine; an effect which varies with different batches of polygeline and is known to occur in dogs after rapid infusion.

Selection of fluid

The fluid selected for treatment will depend upon the kind of losses that have been incurred. The aim of the treatment is to replace those constituents that are missing. A knowledge of the type of deficit which occurs with various disease states indicates

Table 10.2 Fluid disorders and treatment

History	*Disorder*	*Treatment*
Neglect/unable to drink; diabetes insipidus; pyrexia and panting; polyuric renal failure	Primary water depletion	N/5 (0.18%) saline + 4.3% dextrose
Severe vomiting	Gastric vomiting, loss of H_2O, H^+, Cl^-, K^+ – mixed depletion + metabolic alkalosis	Normal saline (0.9%)
	Bile stained vomiting, loss of H_2O, Cl^-, HCO_3, Na^+ – mixed depletion +/– metabolic acidosis	Normal saline (0.9%)
Diarrhoea	Loss of H_2O, Na^+, HCO_3, Cl^- (chronic also K^+) – mixed depletion + metabolic acidosis	Hartmann's solution, KCl and HCO_3 may be added
Bowel obstruction	Loss of H_2O, Na^+, Cl^-, HCO_3 – mixed depletion +/– metabolic acidosis	Colloid solution + Hartmann's solution + HCO_3 2 mmol/kg may be added
Ruptured bladder; urethral obstruction	K^+, H^+ accumulation – hyperkalaemia + metabolic acidosis	N/5 saline (0.18%) + 4.3% dextrose or 0.9% saline. HCO_3 (2.3 mmol/kg) may be added
Haemorrhage	Loss of blood	Whole blood of PCV below 0.25 litre/litre or dextrans or Haemaccel
Burns; peritonitis; pancreatitis	Loss of plasma + extracellular fluid – hypovolaemic shock	Dextrans or Haemaccel + Hartmann's solution
Prolonged anorexia	Loss of calories and protein	10% glucose added to infusions. If over 4 days add 30 ml/kg lipid emulsion (Intralipid) + 30 ml/kg 5% amino acids (Aminoplex)

the composition of the fluid to be used (Table 10.2). Most patients respond favourably to standard normal saline or Hartmann's solution provided that sufficient quantity is given.

Estimation of fluid requirements

The estimation of the fluid requirements is based on the history, clinical examination and laboratory testing of the animal.

History

In the history it is important to gather information on the presence or absence of diarrhoea, vomiting, polyuria, polydipsia, panting and anorexia. This information will indicate the type of deficiency present (Table 10.2). It will also be important to assess the duration of these signs and their frequency, when appropriate. For example, it would be important to determine how long any urinary losses have been occurring and to determine the frequency and the duration of vomiting.

Clinical examination

An estimation of the level of dehydration may be based on the texture and elasticity of the skin, together with the appearance of the mucous membranes. As an approximate guide, losses less than 5% of the body weight are undetectable clinically. Losses exceeding 15% of the body weight, however, are usually associated with a moribund animal. The assessment of the level of dehydration between 5% and 15% is subjective and depends on the degree of loss of elasticity when a skin fold is lifted. In addition to these signs, the dryness of the mucous membranes of the mouth may also indicate primary water depletion. This may be complicated by dryness associated with panting and is not, therefore, an exclusive indication of dehydration. Capillary refill time is a useful indicator since the normal pink colour of the gum should return within two seconds of compression. A time longer than two seconds suggests a degree of hypovolaemia (7–10% deficient). If the capillary refill time exceeds three seconds and is associated with a tachycardia and cold limbs it indicates a hypovolaemic shock which, if caused by dehydration, shows a high percentage deficiency (12–15%).

Pulse

Palpation of peripheral pulses at the paw or tongue to obtain information about changes in pulse rate, volume and rhythm will give an indication of the degree of peripheral tissue perfusion and will indicate severe hypovolaemia, which will be associated with intense vasoconstriction.

Temperature

Animals suffering from hypovolaemic shock respond by showing intense peripheral vasoconstriction. This leads to marked temperature differences between the peripheral tissues, like the skin and the toes, and the core tissues as measured by the rectal temperature. Under normal conditions, temperature gradients of 3–4°C between the peripheral and the core temperatures are seen. In hypovolaemic shock the gradient can increase up to 10°C. A temperature difference between the ambient air and peripheral tissues of less than 2°C indicates very poor peripheral perfusion and a poor prognosis.

Respiration

Metabolic acidosis and hypovolaemic animals will hyperventilate. A marked improvement and a reduction in respiratory rate associated with treatment is a favourable indication that the treatment is successful. Pulmonary oedema as a result of a failing heart or overhydration may be detected by auscultation which will show an increase in the respiratory sounds.

Central venous pressure

The central venous pressure may be measured (Figure 10.1) during fluid infusion to indicate the success with which the heart can cope with the volume of blood returning to it. A low central venous pressure shows that there is a hypovolaemia and a need for more fluids. A raised central venous pressure indicates that there is either a fluid overload or a right sided heart failure. An indication of the central venous pressure can be obtained by examining the peripheral veins such as the jugular or carpal veins.

ECG

The ECG may be used to detect arrhythmias associated with severe raised serum K^+. This can show itself as a widening of

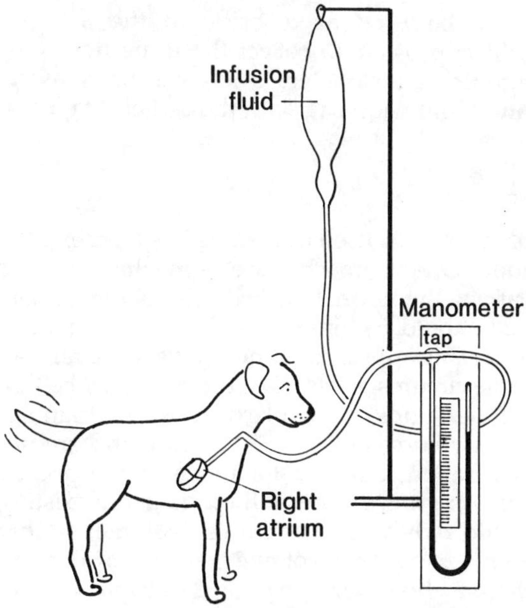

Figure 10.1 Measurement of central venous pressure. The jugular vein is cannulated and pressure measured with the manometer

the QRS complex; with a peaking of the T wave so that the ECG appears to have an abnormal pattern.

Urine

The production of urine is a useful guide to the performance of the cardiovascular system. A decrease in urine production will occur if there is decreased glomerular filtration associated with a reduced renal perfusion and a reduction in systemic arterial blood pressure. The glomerular filtration rate will fall dramatically if the systemic arterial pressure falls below 60 mmHg. A reduction in the rate of urine production can, therefore, indicate severe hypovolaemic shock. The normal rate of urine production is 1–2 ml/kg body weight per hour. A flow of less than 0.5 ml/kg body weight per hour may be considered significant and constituting oliguria. Urine with a high specific gravity (therefore concentrated) often indicates that the kidneys are responding well to dehydration although protein or glucose, which are abnormal constituents of urine, can also increase specific gravity. The pH of the urine in the absence of any urinary infection can be used as a guide to the animal's acid–base balance. It is possible to collect the urine hourly by continuous drainage using a catheter. One particularly useful method is to use an old infusion bag with the catheter taped or sutured in place.

Packed cell volume

The packed cell volume can be used as a guide in estimating the degree of dehydration. One approach is to assume that for every 0.01 litre/litre rise above the normal packed cell volume of 0.45 litre/litre, the animal should be given 10 ml/kg body weight of fluid for replacement. This approach, although very useful, can be misleading in some circumstances. One problem may be that certain dogs like greyhounds, particularly those in training, have high packed cell volumes over 0.55 litre/litre and are not suffering from dehydration. Single estimations of the packed cell volume may also be misleading if there is a pre-existing anaemia, which would reduce the packed cell volume, so that during dehydration the packed cell volume may appear normal. Despite these limitations, however, the packed cell volume is an invaluable guide for indicating the success of any fluid therapy.

Acid–base balance

There are four types of acid–base imbalance: respiratory acidosis, respiratory alkalosis, metabolic acidosis and metabolic alkalosis.

The pH of the blood may be considered to be governed by the ratio of the carbon dioxide tension and the bicarbonate concentration. An increase in the partial pressure of CO_2 leads to a respiratory acidosis; a reduction in the normal CO_2 partial pressure of the blood leads to a respiratory alkalosis. A loss of bicarbonate ions or the accumulation of hydrogen ions produces metabolic acidosis; the abnormal loss of hydrogen ions or the excessive administration of bicarbonate will lead to a metabolic alkalosis.

In severe diarrhoea, where there is a loss of bicarbonate leading to a metabolic acidosis, CO_2 will be blown off during hyperventilation so that the $P\text{CO}_2$ is reduced in an attempt to compensate for the metabolic acidosis. During vomiting, when hydrogen ions are lost, there is a metabolic alkalosis which results in a rise in the pH of the blood: CO_2 is retained within the body in an attempt to compensate for the blood pH changes. The $P\text{CO}_2$ therefore rises during a metabolic alkalosis.

Although in practice is it not often possible to measure the venous pH, bicarbonate ion concentration and CO_2 tension using a blood gas analyser, it is possible to predict on the basis of the history and severity of the clinical signs presented whether or not an acid–base disturbance is likely to have occurred.

Correction of fluid imbalance

There are four main aims of fluid therapy:

1. The correction of plasma fluid deficit (hypovolaemia).
2. The correction of the fluid deficit and the acid–base and electrolyte disturbances.
3. The administration of adequate amounts of fluid and electrolytes to match continuing daily losses.
4. The administration of fluids and nutrients to match normal daily requirements.

Correction of hypovolaemia

Hypovolaemia is the first deficit to correct since it is life threatening and the most common abnormality in severely ill animals. The amount of fluid required depends on the size of the deficit and may be estimated by the method advocated by Hall (1967) (Table 10.3) as one-twelfth of the total fluid deficit. It is important to give this volume as quickly as possible in the form of a colloid infusion such as dextran 40 or 70 or polygeline (Haemaccel).

Correction of the fluid deficit and acid–base and electrolyte disturbances

This usually takes place at a slower rate: for example, one half may be given in the first eight hours while the rest may be spread over the following twenty-four hours (Table 10.3).

Electrolyte and acid–base imbalances should be corrected early in treatment to enhance the success rate. Correction of acid–base imbalances in, for example, a metabolic acidosis occurring from diarrhoea requires the administration of bicarbonate or one of its precursors (Hartmann's solution). The quantity of bicarbonate required for the correction of acidosis may be estimated by the following formula:

one-third body weight (kg) × body deficit
= mmol bicarbonate required.

Table 10.3 Examples of fluid therapy requirement estimation

History
A 7-year-old 20 kg female labrador has been anorexic for 3 days and has vomited 5 times daily for 2 days. The vomit is bile stained. The animal has not urinated for 2 days. X-ray shows a foreign body in the small intestine. Laboratory examination gives a PCV of 0.45 litres/litre.

Estimation from history
1. 3 day inevitable water loss at 20 ml/kg/day (20 × 20 × 3) = 1200 ml.
2. 1 day urinary loss (before urination ceased) at 20 ml/kg/day (20 × 20 × 1) = 400 ml.
3. Vomiting losses at 4 ml/kg/vomit (4 × 20 × 5 × 2) = 800 ml.

Total water deficit = 2400 ml; this is 12% of the total body weight and serious.

Extracellular loss = 1/3 × total deficit = 800 ml.
Plasma deficit = 1/12 × total deficit = 200 ml.

Estimation from packed cell volume
PCV assumed when normal = 0.45 litres/litre.
Percentage increase = 0.56 − 0.45 = 0.11 or 11%.

Total water deficit at 10 ml/%/kg (10 × 20 × 11) = 2200 ml.

Treatment
200 ml colloid (dextran or Haemaccel) immediately before surgery; 2000 ml crystalloid, 1000 ml being given within 8 hours, the remainder over 24 hours.

The base deficit is estimated by the difference between the normal 25 mmol/litre bicarbonate which is usually observed in the plasma and the actual plasma bicarbonate concentration observed in the patient. The formula given for the correction of the bicarbonate imbalance should avoid over-correction since only one-third of the total deficit is given. It is important where the plasma bicarbonate levels are not known that treatment should avoid excessive bicarbonate administration, producing a metabolic alkalosis which may be more damaging than the original acidosis. Since the estimation of the plasma bicarbonate often involves equipment not available in general practice, it may be difficult to estimate accurately the amount of bicarbonate to be given under these conditions.

An animal known to have a raised potassium concentration above 6.0 mmol/litre is regarded as being hyperkalaemic. Hyperkalaemia is likely to occur in association with a ruptured bladder or a complete urinary obstruction. It may also be indicated from the ECG which shows the characteristic reduction in the P wave, peaked T waves and increase in P–R intervals. Mild cases of hyperkalaemia (6.0–8.0 mmol/litre) may be treated by administration of potassium-free fluids together with sodium bicarbonate (1 mmol/kg if the bicarbonate plasma concentrations are unknown). This is usually all that is needed. In severe cases of hyperkalaemia with potassium concentrations above 8.0 mmol/litre, and in association with severe cardiac irregularities, more specific action will be required. Calcium gluconate (1 ml 10% solution per kg) administered i.v. over ten minutes will directly counter the effects of the high potassium on the heart. Unfortunately, this approach is short lived since the calcium is quickly returned to resting levels. It is therefore important to encourage the movement of the potassium back into the intracellular environment by the administration of glucose with soluble insulin (1 g glucose/kg as a 10% solution with 0.5 IU insulin/g glucose).

Although under practice conditions estimation of the bicarbonate and potassium concentration may be difficult, it should be appreciated that most patients respond well to the infusion of standard isotonic or normal saline or Hartmann's solution if given in sufficient quantity.

Correction of continuing losses each day and the normal daily requirements

It is possible to correct for the continuing losses and to estimate the amount of the solutions required in the same way as that used for the original deficit. The normal daily requirements may be met by administering crystalloid solutions (40 ml/kg body weight) to meet the inevitable water losses and the normal urinary losses. This should continue until the animal is able to drink voluntarily.

Infusion rates

If there is a severe shock, with a fluid deficit of up to 15% of the total body weight, then the rate of replacement needs to be very rapid; up to 5 ml/kg per minute for the first 15 minutes until the animal's condition improves. In less severe conditions the total replacement requirements may be given over 24 hours, perhaps with half being given within the first eight hours. The rate of administration under these conditions need not exceed 10 ml/kg per hour. It may not be practicable to administer the fluid at this slow rate since it requires continuous supervision of the animal. Under these conditions, the faster infusion rate of about 20 ml/kg per hour may be employed. A useful guide in estimating the flow rates is to remember that most infusion sets deliver 15–20 drops/ml. This may be checked over a longer period of time (say 30 minutes) by the change in volume of the infusion bag.

Administration routes

In most conditions where fluid therapy is necessary, patients will receive intravenous fluid administration. This allows direct access to the circulation. Occasionally subcutaneous routes may be employed in animals where peripheral perfusion is adequate. Usually, however, in hypervolaemic shock where there is peripheral vasoconstriction, this mode of administration will be precluded. Intraperitoneal injection may be used to give large volumes of fluid. This approach is likely to be more successful than the subcutaneous route of administration but suffers from the disadvantage that absorption will be delayed in severe hypovolaemic states. The oral route, by means of a pharyngostomy tube, is a useful method of administering fluid to animals unable to drink because of head and neck injuries. Cases of severe diarrhoea may be managed by means of oral administration.

It is usual to administer the fluids by means of the cephalic vein, which is the most accessible route. Other veins, including the saphenous vein or the jugular, can be used. Although it would seem most convenient to use needles for intravenous administration, these are only suitable for the short-term administration of fluid because movement of the needle within the vein tends to cause damage. Catheters made of Teflon are the preferred method if fluids are going to be given over a longer period of time. There are two types of catheter. Over-the-needle catheters are short and designed for percutaneous introduction. Through-the-needle units consist of a plastic sleeve, a needle guard, a catheter and needle: the catheter is long and only suitable for insertion into the jugular vein. Unfortunately, since the needle has to remain attached despite being withdrawn from the skin there is a chance of the sharp edge of the needle tearing off the catheter. Over-the-needle catheters are probably easier to use.

Further reading

Hall, L. W. (1967) *Fluid Balance in Canine Surgery – An Introduction*, London, Baillière Tindall

Watermann, A. (1984) Practical fluid therapy for small animals. *In Practice*. **September,** 143

Chapter 11

The Gastrointestinal Tract

This chapter discusses the therapeutics of the gastrointestinal tract. The physiological control of vomiting is described and followed by an account of drugs which are commonly used for the control of vomiting. Purgatives and the treatment of constipation and diarrhoea are also described. The symptomatic treatment of other disorders of the GI tract are considered.

Vomiting

The physiological control of vomiting

Vomiting in the dog and cat is a natural physiological defence mechanism and is necessary since these animals frequently consume food which is slightly 'off'. In fact, manufacturers add substances to make pet food smell attractive to dogs and cats; these include substances which make the food smell like slightly decaying flesh. An account of the physiological control of vomiting is now given.

Figure 11.1 illustrates the control mechanisms involved in the production of vomiting. Vomiting (emesis) is brought about by a number of reflex mechanisms:

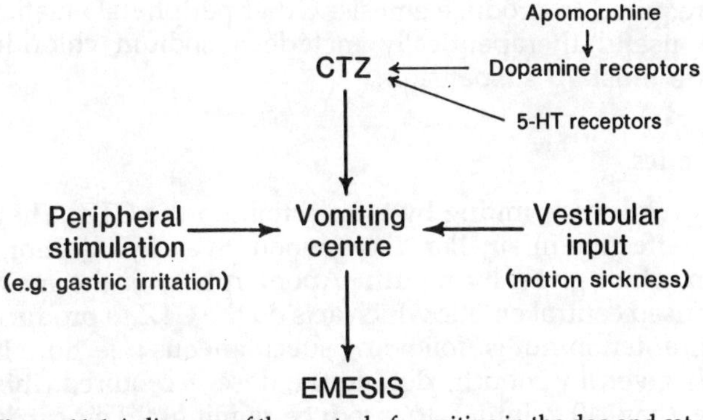

Figure 11.1 A diagram of the control of vomiting in the dog and cat. CTZ, chemoreceptor trigger zone

1. The stimulation of the chemoreceptor trigger zone (CTZ) which is found in the area postrema of the medulla. It can be stimulated by a variety of drugs which activate dopamine receptors or 5-HT receptors. Apomorphine acts centrally on the CTZ to stimulate these dopamine receptors. Hydergene also acts on the CTZ but stimulates emesis by activation of 5-HT receptors.
2. Peripheral stimulation. Various irritants acting to stimulate sensory nerves in the stomach and duodenum will stimulate the peripheral pathway which acts on the vomiting centre to induce emesis. Drugs which act in this way include ipecac, copper or zinc sulphate, and tartar emetic. Other substances which irritate the stomach may also produce vomiting in this way.
3. Disturbances of the labyrinth act via the vestibular nerve to stimulate the vomiting centre. A disturbance of the labyrinth is usually regarded as the cause of motion sickness.
4. Disturbances in the activity of the vomiting centre.

Peripheral emetics

A variety of substances which can stimulate sensory nerve endings in the stomach and duodenum will act as peripheral emetics. These include the salts of a variety of metals and various irritant organic compounds. Some of these are considered in Table 20.1. Examples of these compounds include ipecacuanha which contains the alkaloids emetine and cephaline which irritate the mucous membranes of the gastrointestinal tract and will usually produce vomiting about 30 minutes after consumption. This drug is not given parenterally since large doses are required to produce emesis. Other peripheral emetics which are useful therapeutically include a sodium chloride solution or a mustard suspension.

Central emetics

These drugs induce vomiting by their action on the CTZ. They are usually effective in smaller doses when given by injection, rather than when given by mouth. Apomorphine is the most commonly used central emetic which acts on the CTZ to produce vomiting after ten minutes, following subcutaneous injection. If this drug is given by mouth, double the dose is required: this takes more than 40 minutes to produce vomiting. The cat is much less sensitive than the dog to the actions of apomorphine and may require over a hundred times the dose. Because apomorphine at this high dose has a depressant action it is not useful for therapeutic purposes in the cat.

Other central emetics like hydergene also action the CTZ but, instead of acting on dopamine receptors, they act on a separate class of 5-HT receptors.

Motion sickness

Travel sickness occurs frequently in small animals. It is also a common condition in human medicine. Dogs have been used as experimental animals to study this condition but it turns out that drugs effective in the human are not as effective in the dog, and vice versa. In man, drugs which can depress motion sickness include:

1. *Antiacetylcholine drugs* These compounds include atropine and alkaloids of hyoscine.
2. *Antihistamines* This group of drugs includes acepromazine and chlorpromazine. Although there are antihistamines such as cyclizine and meclozine which do not depress the central nervous system, it has been found in the dog and the cat that central depression for the control of motion sickness is an advantage.

Drugs used for the suppression of vomiting

Acepromazine

This is a powerful sedative and antiemetic. It has an antidopaminergic action and depresses the CTZ. It is of particular value in treating vomiting associated with uraemia or motion sickness.

Chlorpromazine

This compound is similar in its action to acepromazine.

Metoclopramide (Emequell)

This compound is chemically related to procainamide and acts on the CTZ by antagonizing 5-HT and dopamine receptors. Since its action in the central nervous system is limited to the sites of the CTZ, it does not produce sedation. The drug also has an action on the gastrointestinal musculature and promotes peristalsis, encouraging gastric emptying into the small intestine. It therefore has a central action depressing the CTZ and a peripheral action reducing nausea and vomiting. Metoclopramide can be given by intravenous or intramuscular injection; tablets are also available. The most important side-effects include an extrapyramidal syndrome affecting motor activity similar to that seen with the other phenothiazines. This complication disappears when the drug is withdrawn.

Drugs which affect intestinal movements

The intestines are in a state of constant activity: their function is to mix the digesta with the secretions of the intestine and associated glands. There are two types of activity: a mixing movement and a propulsive movement. The propulsive movement normally conveys the contents of the intestine aborally: it is controlled by the intrinsic nerve plexus which produces coordinated contraction of the gut, preceded by a relaxation aborally. The rhythm of contraction decreases in rate from the duodenum aborally. The movements of the intestines are influenced by the autonomic nervous system: the vagus stimulates gastrointestinal secretion and movement; the sympathetic nervous system, which includes the splanchnic nerves, stimulates a reduction in secretion and a reduction in gastrointestinal movement.

Drugs with muscarinic actions will increase intestinal motility: such drugs include carbachol, pilocarpine and bethanechol. An antagonism of the muscarinic receptors with atropine will diminish the propulsive movements of the intestine. Clinical cases of diarrhoea, however, are often exacerbated by atropine because it increases the faecal excretion of water and electrolytes. Gastrointestinal activity is also influenced by painful stimuli or irritants of the peritoneum which reflexly produce splanchnic inhibition. The pyloric and ileocaecal sphincters are relaxed under the influence of muscarinic stimulation but contracted by adrenergic stimulation. In the dog and cat considerable digestion takes place in the stomach. The contents of the small intestine consist of a soup-like chyme; this becomes firmer in consistency in the colon following the reabsorption of water. The transit time from the mouth to the anus is less than 24 hours. Drugs can influence the gastrointestinal movement by acting on the intrinsic or extrinsic nerves of the bowel or by direct action on the plain muscle. Sympathomimetic drugs (adrenaline, ephedrine) in general will decrease gut activity while the parasympathomimetic drugs (carbachol) will increase that activity. Barium, histamine, salts of lead, nitrate and opium alkaloids will act directly on the intestinal muscle and generally increase tone.

Bulk purgatives

Purgatives are drugs which are used to promote the evacuation of faeces. Those which increase the bulk or water content of the faeces and facilitate passage are described as bulk purgatives. The character of the faeces is determined in the main by the content of indigestible cellulose and fibre. A high cellulose content will increase the faecal bulk; water is retained within the faecal mass, softening the stool and promoting passage. Compounds which mimic the effect of cellulose and fibre can be added to the diet to stimulate passage of the gut contents.

Methylcellulose (Celevac)

This absorbs water and swells to form a gel with the result that the faecal bulk is increased. It acts to promote purgation.

Sterculia (Peridale)

This agent is a bulk purgative and acts in a similar way to methylcellulose. The sterculia takes up as much as sixty times its own volume of water and forms a gelatinous mass to increase the bulk of the intestinal contents. Again, this promotes peristalsis and helps ensure an easy passage of a soft stool. Sterculia is inert: it is not absorbed and does not produce systemic effects. It is useful for the control of constipation and the management of infected anal sacs. In all cases it is necessary to ensure an adequate supply of drinking water for this substance to be effective. Contraindications include impactions where there is a need for an enterotomy.

Ispaghula husks BP (Vi-Siblin)

These husks are obtained from the plant *Plantago ovata*. Like the previous bulk purgatives, they assist peristalsis. It is not advisable to use bulk laxatives when there is abdominal pain, nausea and if vomiting is present.

Agar

This is derived from seaweed and has a similar action to the substances mentioned above. Typical dose is between 1 and 3 g/day for the dog.

Dietary modifications

An increase in the fibre content of the diet with the inclusion of bran and similar substances will help as a means of controlling the consistency of the faeces.

Osmotic purgatives

A number of inorganic salts which are not well absorbed from the small intestine will retain water and act as purgatives because of their osmotic effect within the colonic lumen.

Magnesium sulphate (Epsom salts)

This compound is a potent osmotic purgative. The magnesium and sulphate ions are not absorbed from the small intestine; they provide a means of producing nearly complete evacuation of the small and large intestine.

Magnesium hydroxide (milk of magnesia)

This has a similar action to Epsom salts but is less potent. It also has a gastric antacid effect.

Anthraquinone purgatives

This group of compounds includes senna, cascara, rhubarb and aloes. The active component of these substances is liberated on hydrolysis of the parent glycoside in the small intestine. They are all chemically related to anthraquinone. They are absorbed and subsequently re-excreted into the colon where they are thought to stimulate the myenteric plexus. As a result they induce contraction of the colonic muscle. There is some delay between their consumption and their onset of action. Senokot is the best known.

Castor oil

Castor oil acts in a similar way to the authraquinone purgatives and is hydrolysed in the small intestine, liberating ricinoleic acid. This is a mild irritant to the small intestine and causes peristalsis. The absorption of ricinoleic acid probably modifies the motility of the colonic muscle. Castor oil is an old remedy and has little place in modern veterinary practice.

Lubricant purgatives

These substances are not absorbed from the gastrointestinal tract. They remain in the lumen and mix with the stool so that it becomes soft and oily. They have no action on the bowel. Although these substances have been used for many years they appear to be no more effective than the bulk purgatives and also inhibit the absorption of fat-soluble drugs and vitamins.

Liquid paraffin BP

This is frequently used in cats at a dose of 2–6 ml daily for the control of megacolon.

Soft white paraffin (Katalax)

This preparation is a soft brown paste with soft white paraffin as the active ingredient. It is used as a palatable laxative for cats as an aid for the treatment and elimination of hair balls. It is only given orally. It is made in a palatable base and may be given to a fussy animal by placing a small amount on the paw and allowing the animal to lick and become accustomed to the taste.

Dioctyl sodium sulphosuccinate (Dioctyl)

This is a surface activating agent (a wetting agent) which softens the faeces and increases the water content. It is safe and effective and is useful for the treatment of painful anal conditions such as fissures and anal sac conditions. It is available in tablet or syrup form and is used in doses of 8–40 ml three times daily in dogs.

Glycerin

This can be used by introducing it into the rectum as a suppository and acts to initiate defaecation within 30 minutes.

Constipation

In dogs and cats constipation is characterized by straining on defaecation, irregular and painful defaecation, the absence of defaecation or, when there is an enlarged prostate gland in the male dog, the faeces may be hard and flattened ('ribbon like'). There are a variety of causes of constipation in the dog and cat. One cause is a highly refined diet with little fibre. Examples include animals which are fed on meat-only diets without the addition of any meal. A bony diet can also lead to constipation with the spicules of bone impacting in the large colon. In cats, hair balls may lead to difficulty in defaecation. Other causes of constipation include megacolon, neoplasia, an enlarged prostate, various strictures and pelvic deformities, rectal diverticula and perineal hernias. Table 11.1 summarizes some of the products which are available for the treatment of constipation.

Table 11.1 Agents for the treatment of constipation

Generic name	*Product*	*Dose*
Liquid paraffin	Liquid paraffin BP	5–30 ml in dogs 2–6 ml in cats
Soft white paraffin	Katalax	0.5″–1″ in cats
Senna	Senna BP	1–8 g in dogs 0.1–0.3 g in cats
Castor oil	–	5–25 ml in dogs 3–10 ml in cats
Magnesium sulphate	Epsom salts	5–25 g in dogs 2–5 g in cats
Magnesium hydroxide	Milk of magnesia	5–10 ml in dogs 2–6 ml in cats
Methylcellulose	Celevac	0.5–5 g in dogs 0.5–1 g in cats
Isphaghula husk	Vi-Siblin	0.5 tsp/10 lb Not recommended for cats
Dioctyl sodium	Dioctyl-Medo syrup	8–40 mg dogs three times daily
Glycerin	–	Administered as a rectal suppository

Enemas

Enemas may be given to evacuate the faeces from the large colon. Traditionally, slightly soapy water is used. Alternatively, a buffered phosphate solution may be preferred. A large volume of solution (20–100 ml) is instilled into the rectum and evacuation of the bowel generally occurs within a few minutes. The large water content of the enema allows the sometimes solid faecal mass to be broken down. Mini-enemas like Micralax can be used but are less effective.

Antidiarrhoeal drugs

There are a number of drugs that are used for the symptomatic treatment of diarrhoea. They have a variety of mechanisms of action. Diarrhoea is usually described as an excessively liquid faeces; the action of many diarrhoeal compounds is to diminish the free water content of the faeces. This may be achieved by

Table 11.2 Agents for the prevention/treatment of diarrhoea

Generic name	*Product*	*Dose*
Atropine	Atropine Sulphate	30–100 μg/kg
Aminoacetic acid, citric acid, potassium citrate, potassium dihydrogen phosphate, sodium chloride and dextrose	Lectade	See data sheets
Wood charcoal, light kaolin, calcium phosphate and bismuth subnitrate	BCK granules	1 tsp/10 lb for dogs and cats
Bismuth nitrate, heavy kaolin and charcoal	Carsub granules	3–10 g once or divided into 3 doses given daily
Light kaolin and pectin	Kaogel suspension	1 ml/kg daily in divided doses
Kaolin	Kaopectate V suspension	0.5–1 ml/kg daily in divided doses
Sterculia	Peridale granules Peridale paste Peridale capsules	0.5 tsp/10 lb daily for dogs 120 mg/cat daily 120 mg/cat daily
Methylcellulose	Celevac	0.5–5 g in dogs; 0.5–1 g in cats
Isphaghula husk	Vi-Siblin	0.5 tsp daily in dogs
Diphenoxylate (+ atropine)	Lomotil	0.06 mg/kg daily for dogs
Loperamide	Imodium	See data sheets

enhancing water reabsorption from the gastrointestinal tract or by the administration of non-absorbable agents which act by absorbing the excess water and rendering the faeces more solid. Contrary to original belief, diarrhoea is not usually associated with an increase in the contractility of the gastrointestinal tract. In fact, the reverse is usually the case: pathological causes give rise to a depression of gastrointestinal movement but a decrease in the water absorption. The symptomatic treatment of diarrhoea is really only permissible when appropriate specific treatment of the cause of the diarrhoea has been initiated. Table 11.2 summarizes the drugs used for the treatment of diarrhoea.

Atropine

Atropine will inhibit contractions of the gut by its muscarinic antagonistic action and is useful for treating some types of colic. When it acts in this way it relieves the spasm of the intestinal muscle; it can also exacerbate diarrhoea by increasing the faecal water content. Atropine is the active principle of belladonna.

Kaolin

This is naturally occurring aluminum silicate. It is the most commonly used absorbent in veterinary practice. Since it is insoluble it acts, when given by mouth, to form a protective layer on the bowel wall. It also absorbs certain toxins which are produced during enterotoxaemias.

Charcoal

Charcoal is incorporated into a number of proprietary preparations which are used for the treatment of diarrhoea. It acts to absorb extra and excessive water, so firming up the faeces. In addition, its particular characteristic is to absorb certain toxins in a similar way to kaolin.

Methylcellulose, sterculia and isphaghula husks BP

Methylcellulose and the other water absorbing agents will help in many cases of diarrhoea by reducing the amount of free water and firming up the faeces. It is interesting that they are used for the treatment of both constipation and diarrhoea. The reason for their effectiveness in both these conditions is based on their hydrophilic nature.

Astringents

These compounds precipitate proteins which form an insoluble layer over the surface of the mucous membrane of the gut. This then protects the gut from further irritation and irritant substances present in the faeces. It will inhibit further exudation and small haemorrhages. An example of a vegetable astringent which acts by liberating tannic acid to precipitate protein is catechu. Examples of other types of astringents which are also used in small animal practice are bismuth and pectin. Both of these substances tend to act to precipitate protein and lead to a protective effect on the surface of the gut mucosa.

Opiates

Many opiates have a spasmogenic action. Morphine, for example, will increase the tone of the intestinal muscle and delay the movement of digesta along the alimentary tract. This may be an appropriate symptomatic treatment in the treatment of diarrhoea. Preparations which contain crude opium, such as tincture of opium or powdered opium, may be used for this. Related substances are more commonly used. These include loperamide (Imodium) and diphenoxylate (Lomotil). These substances are related to pethidine in structure and are used for the treatment of diarrhoea. Although they have an opiate-like action they are insoluble in water and almost totally unabsorbed from the gut.

The symptomatic treatment of diarrhoea should also include the administration of appropriate fluids. This is considered in Chapter 10.

Colitis

Colitis is often characterized by straining (tenesmus) and sometimes by blood in the faeces, frequent evacuation and watery faeces. It appears to be caused by a variety of agents. A particular type of colitis (histiocytic ulcerative colitis) is only seen in Boxers. This causes an inflammatory condition of the rectal and colonic mucosa which gives rise to diarrhoea. It may be treated by the administration of prednisolone which is effective in acute attacks. One preparation which may be useful for the treatment of this condition is Predsol which contains prednisolone (20 mg as the disodium phosphate/100 ml). It may be administered once or twice daily.

Sulphasalazine (Salazopyrin)

This compound is formed by the combination of sulphapyridine and 5-aminosalicylic acid. It has a specific indication in the treatment of ulcerative colitis. Although the mechanism of its action is unknown, it is believed that the drug is broken down into its two components in the alimentary tract. In man, sulphasalazine reduces the relapse rate of ulcerative colitis but the efficacy in the treatment of acute attacks is uncertain. Side-effects in man include vomiting and nausea.

Hepatic/bile disorders

Acute hepatitis is characterized by vomiting and pain, together with loss of appetite, dehydration and sometimes jaundice. Chronic hepatitis is sometimes more difficult to detect and is characterized by lethargy, selective feeding and weight loss. Very occasionally there is jaundice, associated with hepatic encephalopathy. Once a diagnosis has been confirmed, appropriate specific treatments should be initiated. These might include the use of antibiotics, together with symptomatic treatments to control the build up of fluid (diuretics) or the administration of electrolytes to treat dehydration. Vitamins and anabolic steroids may also be indicated. Other substances which may be indicated are described below.

Menbutone (Genebile)

In dogs and cats this is indicated for the treatment of a variety of conditions including constipation, toxaemia, septicaemia and hepatitis. It is also indicated for digestive disturbances due to impaired hepatic and pancreatic function. Menbutone appears to act by stimulating the secretion of the glands of the stomach, liver and pancreas. Bile secretion can be increased in volume and content. Menbutone acts as a choleretic and acts for 2–5 hours. It increases the flow of the pancreatic secretions by up to four times the normal level. It increases the level of trypsin and pepsin secretion by up to five times the control levels. It is used at a dose rate of 10 mg/kg body weight and is administered by deep intramuscular administration or slow intravenous injection because of its irritant nature. It is precipitated by solutions which contain calcium salt, procaine penicillin and the vitamin B complex. It should not be administered in cases which are associated with serious cardiac disease.

In addition to using therapeutic agents, diets for the treatment of hepatitis should contain protein and be of high biological value with adequate carbohydrate. It is important to avoid foods which have a high fat and nucleic acid content.

Cholestyramine (Questran)
This is an ion-exchange resin which absorbs bile salts. It is taken orally to prevent the reabsorption of the bile salt pool by the distal ileum. It is particularly useful for clinical syndromes where the normal secretion of bile salts into the bile is imparied. Cholestyramine will cause serum concentrations of bile acids to fall and will relieve the associated itching when there are high serum concentrations present (jaundice).

Lactulose (Duphalac)

Lactulose is a disaccharide which is not hydrolysed by the enzymes of the pancreas and intestine. Once it has been taken orally it passes unchanged into the alimentary tract and is hydrolysed by the bacteria present in the gut. It causes the growth of particular organisms in the gut, favours a fall in the faecal pH and has a mild laxative action. It is of particular value in the treatment of hepatencephalopathy. The beneficial effects of lactulose probably occur as an indirect result of the lowering of the faecal pH which inhibits the growth of bacteria producing ammonia or other nitrogenous substances thought to be the cause of the encephalopathy. Lactulose is available as a 50% w/w solution (Duphalac). Doses of 5–10 ml may be given 2–4 times daily to the dog. In addition to the administration of lactulose, antibiotics, particularly neomycin, are indicated for the control of the ammonia-producing bacteria in the gut. Low-protein diets containing readily digestible low-residue foods are also particularly helpful.

Pancreatic insufficiency

This condition is seen rarely in the cat but occurs in the dog, typically the German shepherd. It is characterized by weight loss, sometimes emaciation, with voracious appetite. In extreme conditions the faeces appear like undigested food. There is often a steatorrhoeic faeces; usually there is flatus and the animal looks in poor condition. The most common cause is a degenerative atrophy of the pancreas. Sometimes the pancreas fails to develop properly. To confirm the diagnosis, enzyme tests on the gastrointestinal contents are used. Faecal trypsin and the presence of starch or fat in the faeces are useful indicators. PABA absorption tests, serum trypsinogen and trypsin-like immunoreactivity tests are useful to confirm the diagnosis. Table 11.3 summarizes the preparations which are available for the treatment of this condition.

Table 11.3 Agents for the treatment of pancreatic insufficiency

Generic name	*Product*	*Dose*
Trypsin, amylase, lipase	Tryplase capsules	2–5 capsules/day in dogs (5 capsules for 1 lb tin of dog food) 1–2 capsules/day in cats (2 capsules are enough for 1 tin of standard cat food)
Protease, lipase, amylase	Pancrex Veterinary Tablets, Granules or Powder	2–4 tabs for 100 g of food or 400–800 g powder or 2–4 g granules for the same dose of food
Pancreatin	Pancrin	2–4 tabs with 100 g food
Pancreatin, sodium tauroglycocholate	Panteric Compound Tablets	1–2 tabs/3 oz of food
Cimetidine	Tagamet	5–10 mg/kg orally 1 hour before feeding

Pancreatin (Pancrin)

This preparation contains pancreatic enzymes, mostly trypsin and lipases, and is used for replacement therapy in cases of pancreatic exocrine insufficiency. The steatorrhoea is reduced and the animal's nutritional state is usually improved.

A variety of pancreatic enzyme replacement formulations are available. These include powders, tablets, enteric-coated tablets and tablets which include bile salts. The powders have the advantage that they may be added to moistened food 10–15 minutes before ingestion and permit preincubation. This effect appears to be superior to that of tableted products. Enteric-coated tablets designed to diminish the gastric acid hydrolytic activation appear to be less effective than intended. A variety of methods have been used to limit the hydrolysis of the administered enzymes. It appears that the most effective way is to use preincubation, although neutralization of the gastric acid and the use of enteric-coated tablets have been attempted. A more recent method of reducing the acid secretion is the administration of the H_2 antagonist cimetidine at a dose rate of 10 mg/kg by mouth about half an hour before the ingestion of the food containing the pancreatin. General experience suggests that the dose rate recommended by the manufacturers should be followed initially but, if this proves inadequate, an increase in dose may be required to alleviate clinical symptoms.

Malabsorption syndrome

This condition is characterized by the presence of diarrhoea, which may be steatorrhoeic. Usually there is polyphagia associated with weight loss. The condition may arise as a sequel to a severe enteritis which results in a villous atrophy and sometimes an excessive infiltration of the gut with inflammatory cells. Diagnosis can be confirmed using specific tests which include absorption of D-xylose and serum B_{12} and folate levels.

This condition may be treated by using appropriate systemic corticosteroids and endoparasiticides or antibiotics. Diets containing fairly easily digestible foods, for example chicken and lamb with potatoes or rice, have been useful. In addition, preparations containing medium chain triglycerides may also be beneficial. The medium chain triglycerides consist of esters which are 8–12 carbon atoms long. Their absorption by the intestine occurs through the portal venous system, in contrast to fatty acids which have a longer chain length and are largely resynthesized to triglycerides within the mucosa and transported to the systemic circulation by the lymphatic system. The greater solubility in water of the medium chain fatty acids means that they are less dependent on bile salts. In conditions where there is an intestinal disease which can give rise to an inadequate amount of bile salt production, leading to a reduction in the absorption of dietary fatty acids, medium chain triglycerides are more likely to be well absorbed. Adequate nutrition can be achieved by using a diet low in normal fat, with the administration of 3–10 ml medium chain triglyceride three times daily. The preparation can be added to other fluids or to the food.

Acute pancreatitis

This condition is characterized by anorexia, malaise and abdominal pain. Sometimes there is pyrexia, vomiting and diarrhoea, together with fluid in the abdomen. Diagnosis is confirmed using blood biochemistry to assay serum amylase and lipase. Treatment includes the administration, as indicated, of electrolytes, analgesics, glucocorticoids and antibiotics. In addition, anticholinergic drugs such as atropine can be useful in reducing pancreatic secretion. Pethidine is the analgesic of choice; morphine is contraindicated because it will stimulate secretion from the pancreas.

Canine parvovirus infection

This condition is caused by a parvovirus. It produces sudden death in young pups, often of several pups within the litter. In some there is dyspnoea, collapse and cyanosis. In others there may be difficulty in exercise and rapid breathing with dyspnoea. Sometimes there is ascites.

Older pups and adults usually show a depression with vomiting and diarrhoea, which is often haemorrhagic with a characteristic unpleasant smell and can give rise to dehydration and eventually death. Very occasionally there are respiratory signs, including tachypnoea and dyspnoea.

Diagnosis may be made on the basis of the heart lesions, particularly in young animals, which are characterized using radiography and the ECG or at post-mortem histology of the cardiac muscle. When there is gastroenteritis, faecal matter can be used for a haemagglutinin assay. The blood can be used for HA inhibition and SN tests. Treatment, once diagnosis has been made, is with the antiserum (Maxagloban P) which is administered at three-day intervals until the clinical signs have subsided. Other supportive treatment includes the administration of antiemetics, antidiarrhoeals and antibiotics, together with appropriate fluid replacement.

Feline infectious enteritis (panleucopenia)

This condition is also produced by a parvovirus. It causes abortion and fetal resorption in the queens. The kittens which are born can suffer from cerebellar ataxia. Normally the condition is very infectious and the mortality rate is high, especially in young animals. The young kittens show a sudden onset of vomiting and severe depression with abdominal pain and may have a profuse watery or bloody diarrhoea with threads of mucous lining. The diagnosis is confirmed using white cell counts and histology of the small intestine on post-mortem material. Supportive treatment includes the use of anabolic steroids, antiemetics and antidiarrhoeal compounds. Fluids are necessary to combat dehydration. Administration of atropine may be helpful in reducing the severe fluid loss in the intestine.

Key-Gaskell syndrome (feline dysautonomia)

This condition is seen in cats and is characterized by dilated pupils which fail to respond to light. The third eyelid may be protruded, there may be a dry mucous membrane, inappetence and dehydration. The animal may also fail to defaecate properly so there is constipation. Urine may be retained or there may be incontinence as a result of the loss of the control of the bladder. The cause of this condition is not known. Treatment is usually symptomatic and consists of fluid replacement to combat the dehydration, and the use of lubricant purgatives. Pilocarpine or physostigmine eyedrops may be used to contract the pupil. This may also lead to an increase in saliva flow and sometimes to an increase in parasympathetic activity. Bethanechol (Myotonine) has also been used to try and increase the level of parasympathetic activity. Generally, prognosis is poor. Occasionally some animals will recover if supportive treatment is given.

Flatulence

This condition occurs with particular types of diet which contain low fibre. Treatment may best be carried out by attending to the diet. BCK granules or Carsub can be used since they both contain wood charcoal and act to absorb the offensive gases.

Further reading

Burder, H. J. (1977) Pharmacology of laxatives. *Annual Review of Pharmacology and Toxicology*, **17**, 355

Steway, J. J., Gaginella, T. S., Olsen, U. A. and Bass, P. (1975) Intubitory action of laxatives. *Journal of Pharmacology*, **192**, 458

Chapter 12

The Cardiovascular System

This chapter considers therapeutic aspects of congestive heart failure and the treatment of arrhythmias. The pharmacological properties of the agents used (diuretics, glycosides, xanthines and antiarrhythmics) are described first, followed by an account of the treatment of specific conditions.

Diuretics

Diuretics act by directly or indirectly inhibiting tubular reabsorption of sodium. A result of this inhibition is that water reabsorption is inhibited in the kidney. Responses to modern diuretics are rapid, even in the presence of congestive heart failure.

Frusemide (Lasix)

This diuretic is commonly used in practice. It acts by inhibiting chloride uptake and, therefore, indirectly affects sodium reabsorption in the ascending loop of Henle. The drug has a half-life of about 15 minutes so that, after intravenous injection, the duration of action is about two hours. The dose given orally can be varied according to the severity of the condition. A dose given once every three days may be a minimal course but administration of tablets every six hours or the administration of an intravenous dose once every hour is possible. Although it is usually considered that frusemide produces an increased loss of sodium and water without a loss of potassium, it is recognized that overdose can result in a hypokalaemia and poor tissue perfusion.

Hydrochlorothiazide (Vetidrex)

The major action of hydrochlorothiazide is the inhibition of chloride absorption in the cortical portion of the thick ascending limb of the loop of Henle. Because of the way in which hydrochlorothiazide acts, it leads to an increase in the luminal sodium content which results in a compensatory aldosterone secretion. The compensatory aldosterone secretion in turn leads to sodium resorption and potassium loss in the distal tubule of the kidney. The potential long-term hazard of this effect is that there is an increased potassium loss which can lead to a hypokalaemia. A reduced plasma potassium concentration will increase the toxic effects of the cardiac glycosides. To reduce this danger, it is possible to use potassium-sparing diuretics like spironolactone.

Bendrofluazide (Berkozide)

This compound is also a thiazide diuretic like hydrochlorothiazide. It is approximately ten times as potent as hydrochlorothiazide but is approximately half as potent in its ability to act as a diuretic when compared with frusemide. Bendrofluazide or hydrochlorothiazide may be administered together with frusemide to promote additional sodium loss in animals which are refractory to the action of a single diuretic.

Spironolactone (Aldactone)

Spironolactone is a potassium-sparing diuretic that is not frequently used in veterinary practice. It is an analogue of aldosterone and therefore acts as a competitive antagonist at the receptor site for aldosterone. The potential advantage of using spironolactone is to prevent an excessive loss of potassium caused by other diuretics. It is, therefore, best used in conjunction with other diuretics to promote water and sodium loss in animals refractory to one diuretic. A suggested dose is 1.25–2.5 mg/kg t.i.d. It takes two to three days to become effective.

Captopril (Capoten)

This drug acts by inhibiting the enzyme responsible for the production of angiotensin. The net effect is a reduction in the secretion of aldosterone. Although its diuretic effects are very weak it is often used to enhance the action of other diuretics which cause sodium loss; it reduces potassium loss.

Agents used primarily to treat congestive heart failure

Cardiac glycosides

Glycosides are frequently used in practice for treatment of congestive heart failure and certain types of arrhythmia. Glycoside preparations available for therapeutic use include digitalis BVetC, digoxin, digitoxin and ouabain. These are prepared from the leaves of the plant *Digitalis purpurea* and *Digitalis lanata*. Ouabain is infrequently used in veterinary practice; it is destroyed by intestinal enzymes and has to be administered intravenously to produce a rapid effect. Digoxin (Lanoxin) and digitoxin (Table 12.1) are more frequently used than digitalis BVetC which contains a mixture of glycosides.

Actions of cardiac glycosides

Glycosides act directly on the heart and via the vagus nerve. The direct effect on the heart is to increase the force of contraction, the excitability of the heart and the refractory period of specialized conducting systems (Purkinje fibres). These effects are best seen in a congestive heart failure uncomplicated by valve defects. Glycosides increase cardiac output despite a reduction in heart rate. The reduction in heart rate allows a better filling of the heart and an improvement in circulation. The consequent reduction in venous blood pressure allows a relief of oedema. Higher doses of glycoside can give rise to conduction block between S–A and A–V nodes, due to depression of A–V nodes and Purkinje fibres, together with increased vagal activity. Since glycosides have an effect on muscle excitability they will decrease the refractory period of atrial muscle in flutter and convert it to atrial fibrillation. However, electrical coupling between the fibrillating atrium and ventricles is reduced because of the longer refractory period of the A–V node. In cases of atrial fibrillation with a high ventricular rate, there is a beneficial slowing of ventricular rate allowing an increase in filling and consequent cardiac output. The effect of glycosides on the ECG is to prolong the P–R interval due to depression of the conducting system; there is a shortening of the Q–T interval and a reduction or inversion of the T-wave because of the direct excitatory action on the cardiac muscle. Because of increased excitability of the heart muscle (in contrast to the depression of the conducting system within the heart) there is a characteristic double beat in toxic overdose, known as the 'pulsus bigeminus'.

Table 12.1 Agents used during cardiac therapy

			Dose		
Active principle	*Product*	*Presentation*	*10 lb dog*	*40 lb dog*	*Cat*
Cardiac glycosides					
Digitoxin	Cardio-Tabs	Chewable tabs	1–2	4–6	Not to be used
Digitoxin	Digitoxin Tablets BP	100 μg tabs	1–10		Not to be used
		30 mg tabs	1–8		
		60 mg tabs	0.5–4		
Glyceryl trinitrate Belladonna dog ext.	Heart tonic and stimulant		No specific dose advised		Not to be used
Digoxin	Lanoxin	Tabs	0.125 mg	0.5 mg	0.06 mg/cat
Diuretics					
Frusemide	Lasix	Injectable 50 mg/ml	0.25–0.5 ml	1–2 ml	0.25 ml
		Tabs 40 mg	0.5	2	0.25–0.5
Hydrochlorothiazide	Vetidrex	Injectable 50 mg/ml	0.25 ml	0.5 ml	0.25 ml
		Tabs 25 mg	0.25–0.5	1–2	0.25
Bendrofluazide	Berkozide	Tabs 2.5 mg	0.25	0.5	0.25
		5.0 mg	–	0.25	–
Captopril	Capoten	Tabs	1–2 mg t.i.d.		
Xanthine derivatives					
Etamiphylline camsylate	Millophyline-V	Injectable 140 mg/ml	1–2 ml	2–3 ml	1–2 ml
		Tabs 100 mg	1	2	1
Diprophylline	Theocardin	Tabs 200 mg	1	1–2	1
		Injectable 250 mg/ml	0.5–2 ml	2–4 ml	0.5 ml
Quinidine	Quinidine BP	Tabs	8–24 mg/kg every 2 h or 6–8 hrs		
Procainamide	Pronestyl	Injectable or tabs	Daily dose not exceeding 50 mg/kg. May also be given to cats. Divide dose into four equal quantities		
Propranolol	Inderal	Injectable or tabs	1–2 mg slow i.v. or 5–6 mg every 6 hrs for maintenance		
Lignocaine	Lignocaine Injection; Xylocard	Injectable 20 mg/ml (adrenaline must *not* be present)	1–2 mg/kg as a bolus or 4–8 mg/kg over a few minutes		

Factors modifying the action of the glycosides

1. *Potassium* A reduction in plasma potassium concentration will sensitize the heart to cardiac glycosides. Thus, diuretics like the thiazides which can cause a potassium loss may potentiate and increase the toxic hazards of cardiac glycosides. It is important to consider the use of potassium-sparing diuretics in conjunction with glycosides.
2. *Calcium and magnesium* A low magnesium and a high calcium plasma concentration will increase the sensitivity of the heart to the glycosides.
3. *Thyroid function* Hypothyroid patients require lower levels of the cardiac glycosides for maintenance.
4. *Propranolol* Propranolol will interact with the glycosides and produce a slowing of the heart rate.

Absorption and metabolism of the glycosides

The chemical structure of the glycosides affects the absorption and distribution of these compounds and so, in the end, influence their therapeutic use. Figure 12.1 shows the structure of ouabain, digoxin and digitoxin. The important difference between the compounds is the addition of the -OH groups. It can be seen that the difference between digitoxin and digoxin is the addition of the -OH group at the C-12 position. This change, although it appears small, significantly alters the degree of plasma protein binding (digitoxin most bound) and increases the polarity of the molecule, which in turn reduces the absorption of the drug through lipid cell membranes of the

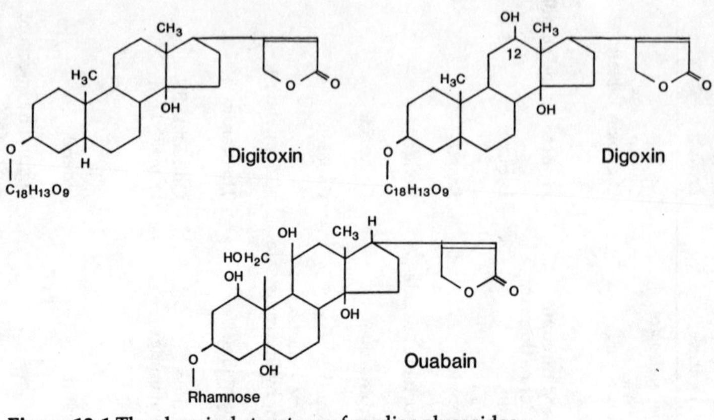

Figure 12.1 The chemical structure of cardiac glycosides

gastrointestinal tract. The most polar compound, the compound with the most -OH groups, is ouabain; it is so polar that it is not absorbed through the gastrointestinal tract and can only be given intravenously.

Digitoxin and digoxin are absorbed from the small intestine after oral administration. It has already been pointed out that the main factor which governs absorption is the degree of ionization of the compound. This means that the more nonpolar and nonionized compound (digitoxin) is more readily taken up across the intestinal mucosa. Digoxin, a slightly more polar glycoside, is less well absorbed. Finely divided or micronized preparations of digoxin, however, allow nearly 70% absorption. Liquid preparations or tinctures are also well absorbed. Once the glycosides have been absorbed across the intestinal mucosa they are transported in the plasma. These drugs are then eliminated in the urine or metabolized in the liver. The route of excretion and also their half-lives depend upon the nature of the glycoside, as well as the species to which the drug has been given. Digoxin and ouabain are excreted through the kidney; this is possible since they are highly ionized and are the least protein bound. Digitoxin, the least ionized glycoside, is metabolized in the liver and then excreted in the bile, conjugated to glucuronide. The conjugating system is deficient in the cat so that digitoxin is metabolized slowly in this species.

In summary, digoxin is eliminated via the kidney and has a half-life in the dog of 24–26 hours and in the cat it has a half-life of 24–48 hours; digitoxin is mainly removed via the liver and has a half-life of 8–12 hours in the dog and greater than 100 hours in the cat. The very long half-life of digitoxin in the cat prohibits its use in this species. A high percentage of digitoxin bound to the plasma protein means that a relatively high dose of digitoxin compared to digoxin is needed to obtain a therapeutic serum concentration. Usually 100% of digitoxin, compared with only 60–75% of digoxin, is absorbed from the gastrointestinal tract.

Dosage: general guidelines

There are a number of factors which influence the dose necessary.

Ouabain

This is used for emergencies and given by the intravenous route. A dose of 0.04 mg/kg is given intravenously (25–50% initially) and then 25% every hour until the desired effect is achieved.

Digoxin

1. 0.05 mg/kg intravenously (25–50% initially) then 25% every hour for the desired effect.
2. 0.025 mg/kg per day orally divided into two doses for the dog and 0.01 mg/kg/day orally for the cat.

Digitoxin

A dose rate of 0.05–0.1 mg/kg per day orally divided in equal doses.

Digitoxin may be used as a second choice agent but is suitable for use in dogs where there is a decreased glomerular filtration rate associated with kidney disease. Under these conditions it might be expected that digoxin has an increased half-life; digitoxin would not be expected to be affected since it is mainly eliminated by the liver. Digitoxin may also be used where digoxin produces excessive vomiting as it is supposed to produce less vomiting than the latter.

Other factors influencing dose include the loss of skeletal muscle; in affected animals smaller doses are required because the skeletal muscle is a large storage depot for glycosides. Digoxin is not soluble in fat so that the lean body weight should really be used to calculate the dose of digoxin required for fat dogs.

Digoxin has possible advantages in being more efficient at relieving congestive heart failure when compared with digitoxin. It has the added advantage that it can be used in the cat where digitoxin has too long a half-life.

The slow oral digitalization method

This regime consists of administering a maintenance dose of digoxin 0.0125 mg/kg per day twice daily to the dog. The plasma concentration rises over 10 days to a plateau. The dose of digoxin under this schedule may be reduced as the patient improves.

The rapid oral digitalization method

Using this dose regime, a loading dose of 0.066 mg/kg of digoxin is given the first day in divided doses. It is then followed by the administration of the maintenance dose (0.0125 mg/kg twice daily). This is given from day two onwards. This approach allows more rapid digitalization but is more likely to produce digitalis toxicity.

The rapid parenteral digitalization method

This method consists of intravenous administration of ouabain or digoxin (doses given above) to obtain immediate high plasma concentration of the cardiac glycoside. The intramuscular administration of the glycoside should be avoided since it causes pain at the injection site. Since the intravenous dose of the cardiac glycoside produces a rapid rise in the concentration of the agent, toxic symptoms as well as therapeutic effects may occur rapidly. It is therefore important to monitor the heart, using an ECG. In addition to the use of the cardiac glycosides, it is also appropriate to use an intravenous diuretic (frusemide 5–10 mg/kg every two hours). Morphine may also be given to reduce the dyspnoea produced by the pulmonary oedema; it may also provide a necessary and useful sedation as well as promoting the pooling of blood in the splanchnic vessels and reducing the pulmonary blood pressure. Rapid digitalization should not be attempted in the cat since this species is particularly sensitive to the toxic effects of the glycosides.

Glycoside toxicity

Because of the tremendous variations in dosages, toxicity is likely to be seen on a regular basis. Mild symptoms of toxicity include loss of appetite, vomiting and occasionally diarrhoea. This is sometimes associated with a weakness and general lethargy. More severe signs of toxicity will produce cardiac dysrhythmias (coupled beats or 'pulsus bigeminus'). The commonest cause of A–V heart block in small animal practice is toxicity due to the cardiac glycosides. Ventricular dysrhythmias are the most serious and require immediate therapy. Suitable therapy includes the use of the local anaesthetic lignocaine (lidocaine) or the use of the β-adrenergic blocking agent propranolol. Obviously, during the treatment of the cardiac glycoside toxicity, therapy with the glycosides must be discontinued.

Xanthine derivatives

This group of agents includes etamiphylline (Millophyline) and diprophylline (Theocardin). Xanthines have a variety of beneficial effects including a powerful inotrophic and chronotrophic action on the heart. There is also a relaxation of the bronchial smooth muscle and the smooth muscle surrounding the coronary artery. There is a central stimulatory action which increases the respiratory rate and volume. The effect on the heart gives rise to an increase in the heart rate and an increase in the cardiac output which leads to an increase in the glomerular filtration rate and causes a mild diuresis.

Uses

Xanthines can be used for the treatment of mild congestive heart failure, or for the treatment of more severe congestive heart failure, in association with cardiac glycosides. Oral preparations can be given at intervals of 4–8 hours in adequate dosage. Signs of xanthine toxicity include CNS stimulation, which can be readily countered with the use of a suitable hypnotic. This is not likely to occur at usual therapeutic doses.

Milrinone

This is an orally active agent still under experimental development which appears to act by potentiating the effects of adrenaline and noradrenaline. At a cellular level it appears to act in a similar way to the xanthines by increasing the intracellular levels of cyclic-AMP. It has a brief half-life of two hours in the dog and may be given at a dose rate of 0.5 or 1.0 mg/kg orally twice or four times per day. It has been suggested that this agent is useful for the treatment of congestive heart failure and is effective in about 70% of dogs with severe heart failure. This compares with about 50% success with digoxin. This agent acts by increasing heart contractility as well as acting as a moderate arterial dilator. One potential disadvantage is that desensitization to the action of this drug is frequently seen. It remains to be evaluated under practice conditions.

The use of vasodilators

A number of dogs and cats do not respond to the glycosides or milrinone: they usually have a poor prognosis. Under these conditions vasodilators may provide a useful means of improving the clinical signs together with the quality of life but they may not significantly prolong survival time. The vasodilators act to reduce the peripheral resistance, so relieving load on the failing heart in an attempt to improve cardiac output. They may consist of drugs which are arterial dilators or dilators of the veins; some drugs act at both sites.

Hydralazine (Apresoline)

This agent is described as being a pure arterial dilator. Its action is to decrease the peripheral vascular resistance and so lead to a reduction in the systemic arterial blood pressure. This permits an increase in cardiac output. A dose of 1 mg/kg twice daily is suggested; this may be increased up to a maximum of 3 mg/kg every twelve hours.

Prazosin (Hypovase; Sinetens)

This agent is a selective α_1-adrenergic receptor blocker. Its action is described as dilating arteries and veins. It increases the cardiac output by reducing the peripheral resistance, so decreasing congestion and oedema. A dose rate of 1 mg three times daily for dogs less than 15 kg has been suggested. Larger dogs may respond to 2 mg given three times daily. Because prazosin dilates the peripheral vasculature, hypotension is a possible side-effect. To minimize this effect, low doses should be given initially and gradually increased until a response is seen.

Low-salt diets

Low-salt diets with less than 250 mg sodium chloride per 100 g dry food weight should be used to reduce sodium retention. By reducing sodium retention, water retention is also expected to be reduced. Thus, whenever diuretics are used low-salt diets should be prescribed. Salt substitutes using KCl can be used to increase the palatability of low-salt diets and may also be used to add potassium to the diet.

Vitamin E

Vitamin E is claimed to be useful if given in therapeutic doses. It may act in a nonspecific way by allowing the normal integrity of the cardiac muscle. This is likely to be impaired during congestive heart failure.

The treatment of progressive left-sided heart failure

Progressive left-sided heart failure in the dog is most frequently seen as a result of mitral valve incompetence. The condition can be divided into four stages which describe increasing severity of symptoms and are associated with the requirement of more rigorous therapy.

Stage I is not associated with fatigue, dyspnoea or coughing.

The appearance of a systolic murmur indicating mitral incompetence may be an incidental finding on auscultation. At this stage the pulse is normal in character with the heart rate being in the normal range.

Treatment of Stage I is not strictly necessary. It would be advisable to reduce the weight of obese dogs. Weekly monitoring may be a useful aid to achieving weight loss.

Stage II is marked by some intolerance to exercise associated with some breathlessness. Coughing is the most likely sign. This coughing or dyspnoea is usually worse following exercise.

Treatment may involve the limiting of exercise to that which causes no distress. Obese dogs must be dieted strictly to reduce the load on the heart. Low-sodium diets may facilitate and reduce the load on the heart. Xanthine derivatives may be used to dilate the bronchi and so alleviate coughing.

Stage III At this stage any exercise produces dyspnoea, coughing and pronounced fatigue. The heart rate is high, even at rest. There may be dysrhythmias. Auscultation reveals a systolic cardiac murmur that is heard over large areas of the chest. A generalized enlargement of the heart is detectable on X-ray. There is also congestion in the pulmonary vasculature together with evidence of systemic venous congestion.

Treatment allows only minimal exercise. A low-sodium diet and xanthine derivatives may be beneficial. Digitalization may be advised, together with diuretics.

Stage IV marks the onset of congestive heart failure with the appearance of dyspnoea and coughing even when the dog is at rest. These signs are exaggerated after any physical exertion. The mucous membranes are either slightly pale or cyanosed. The heart rate is rapid and jerky but may become very irregular and weak in advanced disease. X-ray may demonstrate the possibility of pulmonary oedema together with hydrothorax and gross enlargement of the heart. Cardiac arrhythmias can include atrial and ventricular ectopic beats which may be heard on auscultation or revealed on ECG. Atrial fibrillation can be seen in larger dogs.

Treatment involves the same management as described for Stages II and III, together with the vigorous use of diuretics and cardiac glycosides.

Drugs for cardiac arrhythmias

Cardiac arrhythmias are seen less frequently than congestive heart failure. Diagnosis is made on the basis of the signs and symptoms together with an ECG. The properties of drugs used for the treatment of arrhythmias are considered first. Second, an account of the treatment of various types of arrhythmia is considered.

Quinidine sulphate

Quinidine has a depressant action on the heart muscle. It depresses contractility, conduction and automaticity. It also prolongs the refractory period of the heart muscle and the Purkinje fibres. It has vagolytic effects which block or reduce the input of the vagus so reducing the chances of conduction block at the A–V node. It has an additional action on the peripheral vasculature in that it produces a degree of dilatation. All these features combine to reduce the arterial blood pressure and depress the heart rate at therapeutic doses. There is also an inhibition of ectopic activity.

Dose

Doses of 8–20 mg/kg, starting at the 8 mg/kg dose, should be used and repeated every two hours in severe cases and every 8 hours in established cases of arrhythmia. Therapy should continue until conversion is achieved or until the toxic symptoms prevent further therapy. The quinidine may be administered orally if it is being used for the treatment of established conditions; quinidine given intramuscularly may be used for the treatment of acute cases. If quinidine is given orally, its maximal effect starts about two hours after administration and lasts for about six hours. If it is given intramuscularly its peak effect occurs one hour after administration. Long-acting quinidine preparations are available; these may be given every twelve hours.

Therapeutic uses

Quinidine has had a limited use for the control of atrial and junctional arrhythmias in dogs. It appears more useful for the treatment of ventricular premature contractions and tachycardia. Quinidine can be used to depress the ectopic ventricular beats and can be used in conjunction with digitoxin or digoxin to improve the performance of a failing heart. If quinidine proves effective for the control of ventricular premature contractions and tachycardia, it can be used for periods of up to five weeks to achieve long-term control. A severe and persistent tachycardia should be controlled with lignocaine or procainamide.

Toxicity

Quinidine frequently gives rise to toxic symptoms. These include loss of appetite, sickness, diarrhoea and incoordination. The incoordination stems in part from the effect of quinidine on the cardiovascular system. High doses can lead to hypotension and excessive depression of the heart musculature. This can be seen as an atrioventricular block or ventricular tachycardia. Quinidine is not safe for use in cats. It is contraindicated when there is sinoatrial, atrioventricular or intraventricular block. It is also contraindicated in cases of known hypersensitivity. Some animals show a peculiar idiosyncratic hypersensitivity to quinidine.

Procainamide (Pronestyl)

This drug acts in many ways like quinidine and depresses conduction and automaticity in atria and ventricles. It prolongs the effective refractory period of the heart and gives rise to an increase in the duration of the QRS complex and the P–R and Q–T intervals.

Dose

Doses up to 6 mg/kg every three hours may be given if necessary. Intravenous injections of 6–8 mg/kg can be used if an immediate situation arises. Intramuscular dose ranges are 8–10 mg/kg every three to six hours.

Therapeutic uses

Procainamide, with its depressant action on the heart, is used for the treatment of ventricular arrhythmias (ventricular premature contractions and unifocal and multifocal ventricular tachycardia). It seems that quinidine is less effective than procainamide for treating these conditions when they arise as a result of the disease process *per se* but lignocaine or propranolol are preferred when the arrhythmias arise as a result of toxic symptoms of the cardiac glycosides. Procainamide has only a limited effect on atrial tachycardias.

Toxicity

Like quinidine, procainamide can produce toxic symptoms which arise as a result of excessive pharmacological action. Thus, hypotension and a severely depressed cardiac contractility can arise as a result. This is seen as anorexia, vomiting and occasionally CNS depression. Chronic administration may lead to agranulocytosis. The only effective treatment for toxicity with procainamide is to withdraw therapy.

Lignocaine (lidocaine; Xylocard)

Lignocaine at normal therapeutic doses has little effect on the arterial blood pressure or myocardial contractility. It does, however, depress ventricular excitability and automaticity. It increases the effective refractory period of the heart and as a result it has been used widely for the treatment of ventricular arrhythmias.

Dose

Lignocaine can be used at doses of 1–2 mg/kg given intravenously as an acute bolus or used at a higher dose rate of 4–8 mg/kg given slowly over a period of a few minutes. The duration of action is about 15 minutes and repeat doses can be given at 20-minute intervals. Lignocaine is not usually administered orally since quinidine or procainamide are preferred when this mode of administration is required.

Therapeutic uses

Lignocaine must be used without adrenaline and its prime indication is for the control of serious and acute ventricular arrhythmias arising during the induction of anaesthesia with halothane or as a result of cardiac glycoside intoxication. It is, therefore, useful for the treatment of ventricular premature contractions or ventricular tachycardia. It may also be used for the treatment of ventricular fibrillation.

Propranolol (Inderal)

Propranolol is known as a β-blocking agent. It will block the β_1-adrenoreceptors that are found on the heart, and so reduce heart rate, and will lead to an increase in the effective refractory period of the heart muscle. Propranolol also has a local anaesthetic action and will depress heart muscle in a way independent of its β_1-blocking actions. It is therefore useful for the treatment of various cardiac arrhythmias.

Dose

A dose of 1–3 mg may be given slowly by intravenous injection and stopped when the desired effect has been achieved; 0.2–1.0 mg/kg may be given orally at 6-hour intervals for maintenance.

Therapeutic uses

Propranolol is used for atrial arrhythmias and arrhythmias that are produced by the cardiac glycosides. It can also be used to reduce the ventricular rate when there is an atrial fibrillation. It is particularly useful when the arrhythmias are thought to arise as a result of excessive sympathetic activity. Propranolol may be one of the safest antiarrhythmic drugs to use in the cat. It is contraindicated when there is a sinus bradycardia and in severe and intractable heart failure.

Toxicity

Propranolol toxicity may show itself as cardiac depression, bradycardia and hypotension. During heart failure there may be a retention of water and sodium as a result of the diminished cardiac output.

Cardiac arrhythmias

Atrial fibrillation

Atrial fibrillation usually produces the signs associated with congestive heart failure; it is due to the absence of any synchronized atrial contraction and conduction. The normal P-wave is replaced by undulating F-waves on the ECG. Since atrial fibrillation in the dog and cat is usually associated with a general failure of the heart it is not usually treated in isolation. During the treatment of atrial fibrillation the prime objective is to decrease the ventricular rate. Cardiac glycosides are indicated in the treatment of atrial fibrillation to reduce the ventricular rate through the vagal action and the direct depressant action the glycosides have on the conducting system of the heart. Usually there is a slowing of the ventricular contraction rate as a result of therapy.

If use of the glycosides fails, it is usual to try propranolol. This agent has negative inotrophic effects due to its β_1-adrenergic blocking action. Diuretics should also be given with atrial fibrillation in the dog or cat: this will help the general condition and the symptoms of congestive heart failure.

Atrioventricular block

Atrioventricular block is divided into three conditions or degrees depending on the severity or the completeness of the block.

1. *First degree* The P–R interval is greater than 0.13 seconds and each P-wave is followed by the QRS complex.
2. *Second degree* The P–R interval increases progressively until the QRS complex is missed or the P–R interval remains unchanged and is associated with occasional dropping of the QRS complex.
3. *Third degree* At this degree the atrial rate is rapid and not associated with QRS complexes.

The treatment will depend on the severity of the clinical signs. (Check it is not due to cardiac glycoside toxicity.) First degree A–V block is not usually associated with clinical symptoms unless it is caused by cardiac glycoside toxicity. Second degree A–V block may be associated with some weakness or syncopy but usually it is only third degree A–V block that is associated with listlessness and poor exercise tolerance. Treatment may involve the use of an anticholinergic (atropine). This is particularly indicated if the animal is to be anaesthetized. Alternatively, the animal may be treated using a β_1-adrenergic agent such as isoprenaline (Saventrine) given intravenously at a sufficient dose to increase the heart rate up to 80–100 beats per minute.

Ventricular premature contractions

Premature contractions arising from an ectopic focus distal to the bundle of His can give rise to ventricular premature contractions. The ECG appearance may show normal QRS complexes without an associated P-wave or can show a wide variety of more exotic complexes. This condition may result from glycoside toxicity or be associated with other cardiovascular diseases. The clinical signs will depend on the severity of the condition; single and isolated ventricular premature contractions will not result in clinical signs. Multiple ventricular premature contractions will result in fainting and weakness. Treatment will involve the removal of any known cause. Clearly, if glycosides are responsible for this condition they must be stopped. Lignocaine (Xylocard) is considered the drug of first choice. Premature ventricular contractions resistant to lignocaine may be treated with procainamide or propranolol. Preparations containing the cardiac glycosides may be useful if a patient is suffering from congestive heart failure.

Ventricular tachycardia

This condition is somewhat similar to ventricular premature contractions but arises as a result of an ectopic focus within the ventricular myocardium which produces an impulse at a greater rate than the existing sinus node pacemaker. The QRS complex may vary from fairly normal to a wide variety of odd patterns. P-waves may or may not be detectable. Ventricular tachycardia is serious and may herald the onset of ventricular fibrillation. The clinical signs will depend on the severity of the condition. When it is sufficiently severe, weakness and collapse are signs. There is usually a pulse deficit and poor peripheral perfusion.

The cause of ventricular tachycardia is varied. It can include advanced congestive heart failure, myocarditis or electrolyte disturbances (particularly low serum potassium). The treatment is directed towards correcting any possible underlying cause. For example, if there is a low serum potassium it is appropriate to correct this by the administration of potassium chloride (at a rate not exceeding 0.5 mEq/kg/h). Ventricular tachycardias may benefit from the digitalization if they are associated with congestive heart failure. Obviously it is important to monitor the heart with an ECG to make sure that cardiac irritability is not increased. Antidysrhythmic drugs may be used. Lignocaine, procainamide and quinidine are considered to be the drugs of choice. Lignocaine is preferable for short-term therapy, followed by procainamide and quinidine.

Congestive cardiomyopathy in cats

This condition produces dilatation of all cardiac chambers and leads to dyspnoea and accumulation of thoracic fluid. Severely dyspnoeic cats should be given cage rest and diuretics (frusemide 4 mg/kg every 8 hours) initially. Use of cardiac glycosides is controversial. Aspirin at a dose rate of 100 mg three times weekly will minimize thromboembolism. Prognosis is extremely poor.

Hypertrophic cardiomyopathy in cats

This is characterized by bouts of tachypnoea associated with stress. Radiographs show cardiomegaly involving the left ventricle. Treatment involves cage rest and diuretics (frusemide). Propranolol (5 mg thrice daily) is indicated to control the tachydysrhythmias and stress-induced tachycardia. Aspirin is also indicated to minimize thromboembolism. Prognosis is reasonable.

Further reading

Detweiler, D. K. and Knight, D. H. (1977) Congestive heart failure in dogs. Therapeutic concepts. *Journal of the American Veterinary Medical Association*, **171**, 106

Hamlin, R. L., Dutta, S. and Smitti, C. R. (1971) Effects of digoxin and digitoxin on ventricular function in normal dogs and dogs with heart failure. *American Journal of Veterinary Research*, **32**, 1391

Jenkins, W. L. and Clark, D. R. (1977) A review of drugs affecting the heart. *Journal of the American Veterinary Medical Association*, **171**, 85

Tilley, L. P. and Weitz, J. (1977) Pharmacologic and other forms of medical therapy in feline cardiac disease. *Veterinary Clinics of North America*, **72**, 415

Chapter 13

The Respiratory Tract

This chapter discusses therapeutic aspects of the respiratory tract. Expectorants, mucolytics, cough suppressants, bronchodilators and respiratory stimulants are described. The treatment of cat influenza (flu), kennel cough, pneumonia and pulmonary oedema are also described.

Expectorants

Stagnant viscid mucus produced in the respiratory tract as a result of inflammation can remain and lead to bronchiectasis. Normally mucus in the terminal bronchi is very viscous. It is carried upwards to the trachea by the action of the ciliated epithelium which lines the respiratory tract. As the mucus progresses upwards, it is usually diluted, becoming less viscous. Sometimes, during inflammation of the respiratory tract, this is not the case and it is necessary to stimulate the secretion of mucus in order to dilute it and to protect and reduce inflammation in the respiratory tract. Expectorants serve this purpose.

Salt expectorants

These expectorants include salts of ammonium, typically ammonium chloride, and are believed to act reflexly following stimulation of receptors in the stomach. In toxic doses, ammonium chloride can produce pulmonary oedema. A commonly used preparation is Benylin (Table 13.1).

Benylin expectorant

This is a clear syrup which contains diphenhydramine, ammonium chloride and menthol. The diphenhydramine is used as an antihistaminic agent to relieve histamine-induced bronchoconstriction. The other agents included have expectorant and demulcent actions.

Table 13.1 Therapeutic agents for the respiratory tract

Generic name	*Preparation*	*Dose*
Expectorants		
Ammonium chloride, menthol and diphenyhydramine	Benylin syrup	Dogs 5–10 ml every 2–3 hours. Cats, not recommended
Camphor, morphine sulphate, Ipecacuanha, squill syrup and tolu syrup	Linct. Morphine Co	1 ml/kg 2–3 times daily. Dogs only
Mucolytic		
Bromhexine	Bisolvon injection 3 mg/ml	i.m. 0.25–0.5 ml/kg in dogs and cats daily for 5–7 days
	1% Bisolvon powder	2 mg/kg twice daily for dogs; cats, 1 mg/kg twice daily
Cough suppressants		
Butorphanol	Torbutol injection 0.5 mg/ml	0.05 mg/kg (1 ml/20 lb) in dogs only
	Torbutol tablets 1 mg, 5 mg and 10 mg	2.5 mg/10 lb dogs only
Dextromethorphan	Cosylan	1–2 mg/kg 3–4 times daily
Codeine	Codeine Sulphate	1–2 mg/kg 3–4 times daily
Bronchodilators		
Etamiphylline camsylate	Millophyline-V injection 140 mg/ml	1–2 ml/10 lb in dogs; 1–2 ml in cats
	Millophyline-V tablets 100 mg	0.5–1 tablet per 10 lb in dogs. Cats, one tablet
Diprophylline	Theocardin ampoules containing 500 mg in 2 ml	0.5–2 ml in dogs and cats
	Theocardin tablets 200 mg	1–2 tablets every 4–8 hours
Atropine	Atropine sulphate BP 600 μg/ml injection	Dogs and cats 30–100 μg/kg
Adrenaline	Adrenaline 1–1000 1 mg/ml	0.05–0.15 ml/10 kg in dogs
Salbutamol	Ventolin syrup and inhaler	
Respiratory stimulants		
Doxapram	Dopram-V injection and drops	Complex. See data sheets
Crotethamide and cropropramide	Respirot syrup	10 drops/10 lb on tongue

Demulcent expectorants

These expectorants consist of syrups which are thick and sweet and are believed to reduce the irritation of the pharynx. Although this action is not particularly marked, they are often used as a vehicle for administering other expectorants.

Nauseant expectorants

These expectorants act by producing a very slight feeling of nausea and this gives rise to reflex secretions in the respiratory tract. An example of a nauseant expectorant is ipecacuanha.

Irritant expectorants

Many volatile organic compounds are excreted in the respiratory tract where they induce a hyperaemia and increase the secretion of mucus. Examples of this sort of expectorant are oil of lemon and oil of eucalyptus.

Steam (water vapour)

Steam or water vapour has an expectorant action and when inhaled will help to break down and liquify secretions present in the respiratory tract. Nebulizers and vaporizers have a similar action.

Mucolytics

Bromhexine (Bisolvon) (Table 13.1) is used as a bronchial mucolytic in dogs and cats. It acts in some ways like an expectorant by reducing the viscosity of the secretions. An added effect of bromhexine is an increase in the level of antibiotic (oxytetracycline; Bisolvomycin) secreted into the bronchial mucus during simultaneous administration of these agents.

Cough suppressants (antitussives)

The function of a cough suppressant is to decrease the frequency and severity of the cough without a reduction of the evacuation of the bronchial and pulmonary secretions. Narcotic (opiate) antitussives are used because of their depressant action on the cough centre in the brainstem. Morphine and codeine are used for this purpose. Non-narcotic opiates like butorphanol and dextromethorphan are also used. These latter agents have fewer side-effects than the narcotics but have a similar cough suppressant action.

Butorphanol (Torbutol)

This agent (Table 13.1) is used in dogs for the relief of acute and chronic non-productive cough associated with tracheobronchitis and similar conditions. General experience suggests that treatment with this agent should last for three to four days. It is recognized that cough suppression is accompanied with mild, dose-dependent sedation. High doses may produce a transient ataxia, anorexia and, very occasionally, diarrhoea. As with other cough suppressants it should not be used to suppress coughing which is associated with copious mucus production. Since this compound is an opiate it can produce excessive respiratory depression which may be reversed with naloxone. It should not be used in cats or in dogs with a history of liver disease.

Dextromethorphan (Cosylan)

This agent is very similar in action to butorphanol. It may also produce CNS depression in high doses.

Bronchial dilatation

Figure 13.1 illustrates the control of bronchial diameter. The vagus nerve (X) innervates the mucous glands and smooth muscle of the bronchial tract. Stimulation of the vagus nerve releases acetylcholine which brings about stimulation of muscarinic receptors, constriction of the bronchial tract and secretion of bronchial mucus. Stimulation of the sympathetic nerves gives rise to the release of noradrenaline and dilatation of the bronchi, together with a reduction in bronchial secretion. The diameter of the bronchial tract is controlled by the tone of the smooth muscle which encircles the bronchial tubes. The smooth muscle may be relaxed using muscarinic blockers to block the effect of acetylcholine; it may be relaxed by using sympathomimetics to stimulate the β_2-receptors on the smooth muscle; it may also be relaxed by other smooth muscle relaxants like the xanthine derivatives.

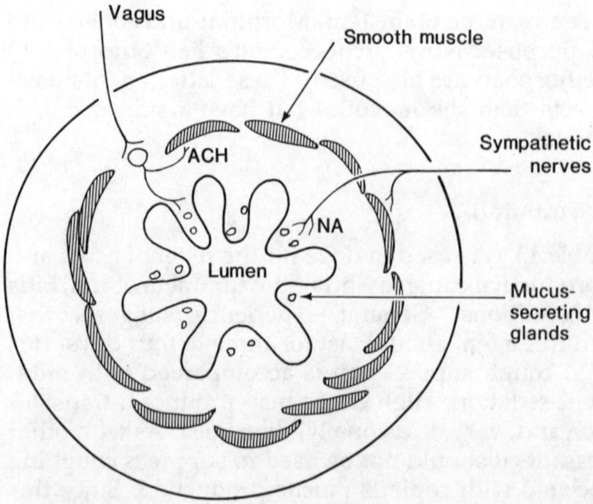

Figure 13.1 Control of bronchial diameter. ACH, acetylcholine; NA, noradrenaline

Atropine

Atropine sulphate at a dose rate of 30–100 μg/kg is used in dogs and cats to produce dilatation of the respiratory tract and an inhibition of bronchial secretion. This may be advantageous during anaesthesia with ether, for example, but it is not usually considered advantageous during the treatment of respiratory tract inflammation. The antiexpectorant action of atropine may be deleterious. Muscarinic antagonists like atropine are not usually used for the treatment of asthmatic type conditions.

Adrenaline

Adrenaline acts on α-, β_1- and β_2-receptors and, at a dose rate of 50–150 μg/10 kg, is sometimes used to produce a short-lasting bronchial dilatation. Its brief action and the fact that it may also act on the heart and other receptors of the body are usually considered as reasons for using other agents, like the selective β_2-agonists.

Salbutamol (Ventolin)

This agent is a selective β_2-agonist and will produce dilatation of the respiratory tract without having an effect on the heart. It may be administered by inhalation or as a syrup.

Xanthine derivatives

These compounds act to produce dilatation. The two xanthine derivatives commonly used in practice are etamiphylline (Millophyline) and diprophylline (Theocardin) (Table 13.1).

Etamiphylline camsylate (Millophyline)

This preparation is available for injection or administration in tablet form. Like xanthines it has a CNS stimulant effect, a diuretic action, a cardiac stimulant action and a bronchial dilatory effect. It is therefore useful for the treatment of bronchitis, cardiovascular and respiratory failure and collapse. It may also be used for pleurisy, pulmonary oedema and syncope.

Diprophylline (Theocardin)

This preparation is another xanthine derivative and is available for injection and in tablet form. Because it is freely soluble it is rapidly absorbed and produces adequate blood levels which last for a period of six to eight hours. It is not irritant so it does not give rise to any pain at the injection site. It is useful for the treatment of heart failure (left- or right-sided) or for the treatment of bronchospasm and congestion of the lungs. It can be used for chronic bronchitis as well as pulmonary oedema. Its use is recognized for the treatment of lung congestion in breeds like pugs and Pekingese where there is an inbred impediment; prolonged administration may be required because of cardiac insufficiency.

Respiratory stimulants

Doxapram (Dopram-V)

This preparation (Table 13.1) is available for injection or from a dropper. Its prime use is as a respiratory stimulant in dogs and cats. It can be used to stimulate respiration after a general anaesthetic and to facilitate return of the reflexes after anaesthesia. It can also be used in the neonate to stimulate respiration following dystocia or caesarean section. Its action is rapid in onset; the intensity of the response depends on the dose. A repeated dose should not be given until effects of the first dose have passed and the condition of the animal requires it. If an overdose is given, hyperventilation will result in a loss of carbon dioxide which can produce a cerebral vascular constriction, hypoxia and possible brain damage. Excessive doses may produce cardiac arrhythmias when administered with halothane or methoxyflurane (halogenated hydrocarbons).

Doxapram is contraindicated if the dog has been sedated with morphine. Since the drug is prepared as the hydrochloride, it is incompatible with alkaline solutions such as frusemide and thiopentone.

Crotethamide + cropropamide (Respirot)

This is available as a syrup: it is administered from a dropper and deposited on one side of the tongue so that it can stimulate respiration in neonatal animals. It should act fairly quickly, within 30 seconds of application, and can be used in repeat doses at intervals of about 30 seconds until a response appears. It should not be repeated more than twice.

Some respiratory conditions

Kennel cough

A variety of pathogens are believed to cause this condition. Canine distemper virus may be one of these agents and canine parainfluenza virus, canine adenovirus type 2, canine herpesvirus and reoviruses have also been isolated. *Bordetella bronchiseptica* is known to multiply and colonize the trachea and bronchial tract following the primary viral infection. The condition of kennel cough is characterized by exhaustive paroxysmal coughing which is usually non-productive. There is sometimes a fever, tonsillitis, pharyngitis and rhinitis. This cough is easily initiated following tracheal palpation. The animal may be suffering from a mild, uncomplicated tracheobronchitis and is usually bright and alert, or it may be suffering from a more severe, complicated tracheobronchitis where it shows a temperature and is mildly or moderately depressed.

Treatment

The most distinctive sign of kennel cough is the paroxysmal coughing due to the tracheobronchitis. It is useful to use an antitussive to decrease the frequency and severity of the cough, especially if it is non-productive. A variety of antitussive agents can be used (Table 13.1). If the kennel cough is more severe and there are signs of severe, complicated tracheobronchitis with a temperature and a productive cough with frequent gagging associated with a nasal discharge, antibiotic treatment may be required. Susceptibility patterns of *Bordetella bronchiseptica* isolates suggest that the most suitable antibiotic agents are oxytetracycline, gentamicin or kanamycin. Ampicillin and trimethoprim are frequently ineffective against isolates.

Cat influenza (flu)

A variety of pathogens may attack the respiratory tract in the cat to produce cat flu:

1. Feline reovirus which produces a mild condition.
2. Feline calicivirus which grows in the mucosa of the lung and mouth while leaving the upper respiratory tract and conjunctiva relatively unaffected. The signs usually include dyspnoea and severe ulceration of the tongue, hard palate, gums, nostrils and the nasal mucosa. The animal is depressed so that it does not eat, and there is a raised temperature.
3. Feline herpesvirus which invades the upper respiratory tract and conjunctiva and so produces a rhinotracheitis. The cat usually has a moderate fever, is depressed, shows anorexia and salivates. There is coughing and sometimes sneezing with a mucopurulent nasal and ocular discharge. Ulceration of the tongue and pharynx are not usually features of feline herpesvirus, unlike the ulceration which is seen with the feline calicivirus.
4. *Chlamydia psittaci*, a bacteria which grows inside cells and is the same organism which causes psittacosis. The symptoms usually include a bilateral conjunctivitis but the severity of the inflammatory response may vary between the eyes. There may be some blepharospasm and a serous or mucopurulent ocular discharge. A fever and anorexia can occur but are not always seen.

Treatment

Broad spectrum antibiotics are frequently used to control secondary bacterial pathogens. Useful antibiotics are ampicillin, amoxycillin and tetracycline. Tetracycline is specifically indicated for *Chlamydia psittaci*.

The conjunctivitis may be treated by applying antibiotic ophthalmic ointment up to six times daily. Useful antibiotics are neomycin or tetracycline. Again, if chlamydia is present, tetracycline is the preferred antibiotic. Keratitis is more difficult to treat because of the presence of the virus deep in the tissues: 0.5% idoxuridine (Kerecid or Dandrid) applied five times daily for 30 days is useful for this. Corticosteroids are contraindicated for the topical treatment of keratitis since they are immunosuppressant.

Sometimes cat flu produces a copious serous nasal discharge which can be treated with a topical paediatric preparation of 0.25% phenylephrine. When there is a thick mucopurulent nasal discharge these agents are probably contraindicated since the nasal mucus may become more viscous, making it more difficult for that cat to breathe.

Nursing is a very important aspect of treating cat flu. It is important to encourage the animal to eat with tempting food and to clean the eyes and nose several times daily. It is also important to keep the animal warm and in a comfortable environment. Intravenous fluids and feeding may be necessary.

Outbreaks of cat flu frequently occur in catteries. Disinfection is one part of controlling the spread of the disease. Two particularly suitable disinfectants which control the spread of the viruses are formaldehyde and sodium hypochlorite. A 1 in 30 solution of sodium hypochlorite is useful; a 4% solution of formaldehyde is adequate. Phenol and lysol solutions may not be adequate for killing the viruses associated with cat flu.

Pulmonary oedema

Pulmonary oedema occurs as a result of an undue accumulation of fluid in the extravascular spaces of the tissues of the lung. It may also arise as a result of an increase in the permeability of the pulmonary vasculature (noncardiogenic). Noncardiogenic pulmonary oedema can arise as a result of septicaemia and endotoxaemia, electric shock and smoke inhalation, microembolism, haemorrhagic shock and heat stroke. The clinical signs consist of tachypnoea with dyspnoea. There is often coughing associated with a blood-tinged foamy or frothy phlegm. Because of the poor oxygenation there is often a cyanosis. The pulmonary oedema gives rise to diffuse rales on auscultation.

Treatment (Table 13.2)

The treatment of cardiogenic pulmonary oedema will depend on the severity of the symptoms. Diuretics like frusemide are used

Table 13.2 Treatment of pulmonary oedema

Type	*Rest*	O_2	*Frusemide*	*Morphine*	*Xanthines*
Mild, cardiogenic	√	–	√	–	–
Severe, cardiogenic	√	√	√	√ (dog)	√
Mild, not cardiogenic	√	–	√	–	–
Severe, not cardiogenic	√	√	√	–	–

to help remove the excess fluid. Oxygen can be used to counteract the cyanosis and hypoxia. A xanthine derivative at doses of 0.01 mg/kg every two to three hours intravenously may be used until the dyspnoea and anxiety are reduced.

Noncardiogenic pulmonary oedema is often treated with the glucocorticoids. The rapidly-acting intravenous preparations like methylprednisolone sodium succinate at a dose rate of 30 mg/kg i.v. or prednisolone sodium succinate at a dose of 35 mg/kg i.v. are used. Although the glucocorticoids may prevent further endothelial damage, there is no conclusive evidence that they will restore the damaged endothelial tissue to normal. Oxygen is also useful. As with cardiogenic pulmonary oedema, it is important to avoid exciting the animal: enforced rest or sedation may actually be beneficial and reduce the oxygen demand.

Pneumonia (bacterial)

Pneumonia is defined as inflammation of the lungs. Bacterial pneumonia occurs as a result of the inflammatory response in the lung to a virulent bacterial attack. Clinical signs associated with this condition are a temperature, depression and restlessness. There is also a pain in the chest, giving rise to discomfort, coughing and difficulty in breathing. There may also be a mucopurulent nasal discharge. There are increased lung sounds on auscultation which are characteristic. Antibacterial agents are obviously indicated. If a Gram stain is made of the sputum or nasal discharge it may be possible to identify the pathogen. As a result of this, proper selection of the antibiotic may be achieved. If this is not possible then pneumonia should be treated empirically. A broad spectrum antibiotic like ampicillin or a combination of sodium penicillin G with kanamycin or gentamicin is indicated.

Oxygen therapy is particularly useful if there is a hypoxia. This may be administered using 100% oxygen delivered with a face mask for short-term therapy or 40–50% oxygen delivered in an oxygen cage for long-term therapy of more than several hours: 100% oxygen is not used for long-term therapy because it itself has a slight irritant effect on the respiratory tract.

Bronchodilators such as the xanthine derivatives (Millophyline or Theocardin) can be useful. Mucolytics and expectorants also have an indication.

Asthma

This condition is usually seen in young dogs but may also occur in cats. It is caused by hypersensitivity to a variety of allergens and is characterized by the sudden onset of wheezing and dyspnoea and occasionally cyanosis. There are characteristic fluid chest sounds. Treatment should involve the use of bronchodilators to counteract the effect of the bronchoconstriction produced by the immune response to the allergen. Corticosteroids are indicated. The most selective therapeutic agents to use are β_2-agonists, such as salbutamol (Ventolin). This is not licensed for use in small animals. Adrenaline may be used to produce brief bronchodilatation but suffers from the disadvantage that it has other effects when absorbed in the body, including stimulation of the heart. Long-term preventative measures, using the mast cell membrane stabilizer sodium cromoglycate (Intal), should be considered. Administration of this product by inhalation is difficult.

Further reading

Roudebush, P. (1982) Anti-tissue therapy in small companion animals. *Journal of the American Veterinary Medical Association*, **180**, 1105

Thayer, G. W. and Robinson, S. K. (1984) Bacterial bronchopneumonia in the dog. A review of 42 cases. *Journal of the American Animal Hospital Association*, **20**, 731

Ziment, I. (1978) *Respiratory Pharmacology and Therapeutics*, Saunders, Philadelphia

Chapter 14

The Reproductive System

This chapter describes the regulation and control of the oestrous cycle in the dog and cat and the therapeutics of the reproductive system.

Oestrous cycle in the dog

In the dog, oestrous cycles normally start at 6–7 months of age but the onset can range from 4 to 23 months. The oestrous cycle is divided into four stages:

1. The first stage, known as pro-oestrus, lasts 9 days (range 3–26 days). At this stage, vaginal smears are characterized by the presence of red blood cells, keratinized cells and, in early pro-oestrus, by the presence of leucocytes (Figure 14.1). In late pro-oestrus the leucocytes disappear.

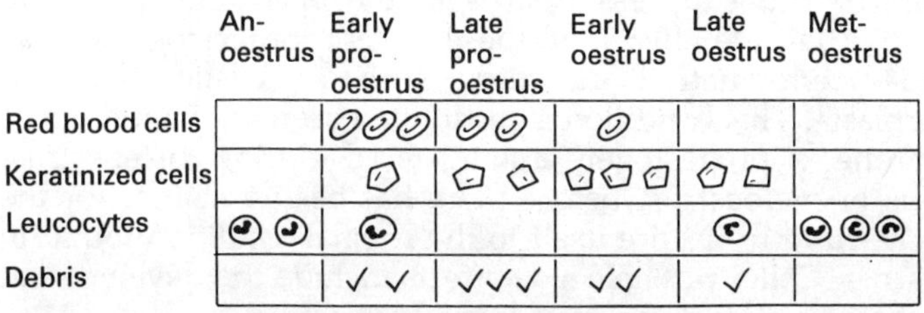

Figure 14.1 Vaginal smears during the oestrous cycle of a bitch

2. The next stage, oestrus proper, lasts 9 days (range 3–20 days). During this stage the bitch is sexually receptive and ovulation takes place. Vaginal smears are characterized by the presence of few, if any, red blood cells together with the presence of keratinized cells. There are no leucocytes during early oestrus; it is only during late oestrus that leucocytes are found sparsely.
3. Metoestrus follows oestrus; it lasts 75–95 days. The bitch is no longer sexually receptive and vaginal smears are

characterized by the absence of red blood cells and keratinized cells but the presence of many leucocytes.

4. Anoestrus lasts 3–4 months before the onset of the next pro-oestrus.

Pregnancy in the bitch lasts 63 days (range 53–73 days).

Oestrous cycle in the cat

The oestrous cycle of the queen cat takes place between January and September, with peaks of activity in February, May and June. There is usually an anoestrus which lasts from the end of September until January. The cycles last 14 days (range 9–23 days). Normally oestrus lasts 4 days but this period may be longer, up to 10 days if the queen is not mated. Ovulation is initiated as a result of coitus and occurs after 27–30 hours. Like the dog, the pregnancy lasts typically 63 days but the range is 60–70 days. Cats mature slightly later than dogs, with the cycles in the queen starting at about 9 months of age (range 5–18 months).

Therapeutic control of the oestrous cycle

Progestogens (many products are listed in Table 14.1) are used to control and suppress oestrus in the bitch and queen. In general, the side-effects of these potent progestogens have included endometrial disorders such as cystic glandular hyperplasia. This condition is most often seen after a high dose of synthetic progestogen administered during pro-oestrus, oestrus or metoestrus, before there has been a chance for the endometrium to restore itself to the normal condition found in anoestrus. Other possible side-effects include the development of diabetes mellitus and mammary neoplasia.

The preparations available for oestrous control are considered below.

Medroxyprogesterone acetate (Anoestrulin; Perlutex; Promone-E)

In the bitch, medroxyprogesterone acetete (Table 14.1) is administered during the second half of anoestrus. To obtain complete cessation of oestrous cycles, injections are given at six-month intervals. It is generally thought undesirable to extend the cessation of the oestrous cycle beyond two years.

Table 14.1 Oestrus control in bitches and queens

Generic name	*Products*	*Presentation/dose*	*Comment/uses*
Medroxyprogesterone acetate	Anoestrulin Perlutex Promone-E	Injectable Injectable or tablets Injectable Typically 50–75 mg/dog, 25 mg/cat. Single injection	For temporary and permanent oestrus suppression
Megestrol acetate	Ovarid Syntex Suppress	Tablets Tablets Normally 2 mg/kg daily for 8 days	For suppression of oestrus and temporary postponement
Progesterone	Progesterone Injection	Injectable 2.5–5.0 mg every 3 days starting well before oestrus	Used for temporary suppression of oestrus in queens only
Proligestone	Covinan Delvosteron	Injectable Injectable Bitches 33 mg/kg single injection. Queens 100 mg	Oestrus suppression, temporary and permanent
Testosterone	Androject	Injectable Bitch and queens 5–10 mg every 10–14 days	For suppression of oestrus at onset of pro-oestrus
HCG	Chorulon	Injectable 100–500 IU	Termination of oestrus in queens

Because of the possibility of development of cystic endometrial hyperplasia, it is recommended that medroxyprogesterone acetate should not be used:

1. In bitches before their first oestrus.
2. During pro-oestrus, oestrus or metoestrus.
3. If there is a history of previous genitourinary problems, persistent vaginal discharge, heat periods which are irregular or otherwise abnormal, or mammary tumours which are stimulated by progestogens.
4. In pregnant bitches.

Proligestone (Covinan; Delvosteron)

This is used for suppression and postponement of oestrus in the dog but is also used for oestrus control in the cat. The dose in bitches is up to 33 mg/kg body weight but the dose varies with body weight, with heavier animals receiving proportionately less. The dose for cats is normally 100 mg subcutaneously. The dose schedule consists of a first dose administered three months after the first oestrous cycle; a second dose after a further four months; a third and subsequent doses at five-monthly intervals. A similar dose schedule is also advised for queens. There is an exception though for queens, since it is possible to get a temporary postponement of calling by an injection of proligestone given in either dioestrus or anoestrus. Although it is possible that proligestone may give rise to endometrial changes, the overall incidence of uterine disorders following the use of proligesterone is very low (0.3% overall).

Progesterone

A dose of 2.5–5 mg administered every three days can be used to obtain temporary postponement of oestrus in the bitch.

Testosterone

It is possible to delay the onset of oestrus in the bitch by administering 10 mg every ten to fourteen days. In the queen cat, oestrus suppression may be obtained by administering a similar quantity every ten to fourteen days. Side-effects may include clitoral hypertrophy and vaginitis, together with an increase in the severity of pre-existing seborrhoeic dermatitis. It is also known that the fetuses of pregnant bitches will suffer severe masculinization.

Megestrol acetate (Ovarid)

Megestrol acetate is a progestogen with potent antioestrogenic properties. It may be given for the postponement of oestrus in the bitch. A course of tablets (available in 5 mg and 20 mg) is given at the onset of pro-oestrus, when a dose of 2 mg/kg daily for eight days is given. An extended period of oestrus suppression may be obtained by administering 2 mg/kg daily for four days followed by 0.5 mg/kg for sixteen days.

In cats, oestrus control is obtained by administering 2.5 mg per cat daily for up to two months, starting in dioestrus, or, starting in anoestrus, a dose of 2.5 mg per cat once weekly for up to eighteen months. It is also possible to prevent oestrus in the cat by administering 5 mg per cat daily for three days, beginning as soon as the signs of oestrus are observed.

Ovarid, like the other potent progestogens, may produce endometrial changes, particularly in bitches which have abnormal oestrous cycles. However, experience suggests that, if properly used, megestrol acetate is less likely to produce side-effects; oral administration allows the duration of the effect to be more easily controlled than with depot injections. Experience has also shown that it is possible to breed from queens and bitches that have received megestrol acetate treatment. In this, tablets appear superior to the use of depot therapy and the use of medroxyprogesterone acetate.

Human chorionic gonadotrophin (HCG; Chorulon)

A dose of 100–500 IU administered intramuscularly as a single dose is useful for the termination of oestrus in the queen cat. This product is a complex glycoprotein obtained from human urine during pregnancy. If administered on repeated occasions, it may give rise to an antibody–antigen reaction. The reaction may be seen shortly after injection of HCG and can be treated by the administration of 1 in 1000 adrenaline given intravenously or intramuscularly when the symptoms appear. Corticosteroids may also be given.

Misalliance

Misalliance or mismating should be treated as soon as is practical, at least within 72 hours of the mating. It can be treated with oestradiol.

Oestradiol benzoate

A dose of 5–10 mg given intramuscularly within four days of mating produces congestion and oedema of the uterotubal junction and so traps the egg, preventing it moving to the body of the fertilized uterus for implantation. Oestradiol, like all oestrogens, will produce suppression of bone marrow. Older dogs are more susceptible to this effect. Following the use of oestradiol for misalliance, there is an increased chance of the formation of cystic endometrial hyperplasia and subsequent pyometritis (incidence may be as high as 25%).

Induction of oestrus

In normal healthy bitches and queens that have had no history of reproductive disorders it is possible to induce oestrus by administering follicle-stimulating hormone (FSH) followed by HCG. There is considerable variation in the number of oocytes released from each ovary, so that it is likely that there will be considerable variability from animal to animal and from occasion to occasion. It is also likely that the potency of the various preparations varies from batch to batch.

Oestrus induction in the bitch

Doses of 50–200 IU of serum gonadotrophin (Folligon) are administered daily (subcutaneously) for ten days. This is then followed by HCG (Chorulon) using a dose of 100–200 IU/kg/day administered intramuscularly for three days, beginning on the tenth day. The bitch is mated whenever she will stand. Using this approach it has been possible to obtain good conception rates (75%).

Oestrus induction in the queen cat

FSH (at a dose rate of 2 mg/cat daily) for as long as five days will often induce oestrus in the cat. Mating should be permitted at the onset of oestrus.

Infertility in the dog

A variety of causes give rise to infertility in the dog. Those due to impotence and lack of libido are treatable with a variety of

Table 14.2 Agents used to treat infertility in the dog

Generic name	*Product*	*Dose*
Testosterone phenylpropionate	Androject	5–10 mg every 14 days
Testosterone	Testerone Implants	25–50 mg
Testosterone esters	Durateston	25–150 mg monthly
Methyltestosterone	Orandrone	5–30 mg daily reducing to 2–3 times weekly
Chorionic gonadotrophin	Chorulon, LH 1500	100–500 IU i.m. twice weekly for 4–6 weeks
Serum gonadotrophin	Folligon, Fostim	50–200 IU s.c. daily for 3 weeks (usually 8–10 days)

testosterone and gonadotrophic agents (Table 14.2). Defects of spermatogenesis, such as aspermia, low sperm counts and poor sperm motility, may be diagnosed on a basis of semen examination. Other causes include orcthitis due to bacterial infections or trauma and testicular atrophy due to hypoadrenocorticism and hypothyroidism. Hypothyroidism shows itself as myxoedema, obesity with unthriftiness, polydipsia and bilateral hair loss together with a poor coat colour, and reproductive dysfunction associated with loss of libido and polyuria. This condition may be treated with liothyronine (Tertroxin) at a dose rate of 20 μg three times daily (to the average 15 kg dog). This dose should be subsequently increased or decreased, according to the effect observed, until the lowest effective dose is established.

Infertility in the bitch

There are many causes of infertility in bitches; these include inflammation of all parts of the reproductive tract, i.e. metritis and vaginitis due to bacterial and viral infections. Any obstruction in the female reproductive tract, particularly at the uterotubal junctions, will also prevent fertilization. Other causes include poor timing of mating, abortion, fetal resorption and regression of the corpus luteum. Infections of the reproductive tract include herpesvirus, *Brucella canis*, streptococcal and staphylococcal infection and toxoplasmosis. Possible signs include pyrexia, anorexia and a vaginal discharge, together with the expulsion of any fetal material. Treatment is geared to correcting the underlying disorder.

Reproductive disorders of the female

Premature regression of the corpus luteum

Because the corpus luteum regresses prematurely there is a lack of progesterone. Diagnosis is based on a history of the bitch being susceptible to habitual abortion and the presence of a low serum progesterone concentration (necessarily measured by radioimmune assay) at the time of the abortion. Treatment consists of the intramuscular administration of progesterone, beginning about 14 days before the anticipated abortion (based on the patient's history). A dose of 1 mg/kg administered weekly until the 55th day of gestation appears to be appropriate. Caesarean section may be necessary.

Endometritis

A low-grade infection in the uterus or uterotubal junction will cause infertility. If the infection is low grade and chronic, symptoms may not be seen. It is sometimes possible to detect an excessively large number of neutrophils in the pro-oestral discharge and to recover significant growth of bacteria from the cervix during pro-oestrus. The therapy should be geared towards removing the bacteria by selecting an antibiotic on the basis of sensitivity tests. Treatment should normally be for a minimum of three weeks.

Persistent ovarian cysts (nymphomania)

If ovarian cysts persist longer than two weeks this will give rise to an enduring oestrus. Treatment consists of HCG (Chorulon) 50–200 IU/kg given intramuscularly daily for as long as nine days. Doses of 250 IU intramuscularly for two days may be administered in queens. This treatment to the bitch and the queen cat may be repeated after one week if necessary. An alternative approach is to use 50–200 μg buserelin (Receptal) administered intramuscularly daily for a period of up to five days in the bitch. In the queen cat a dose of 25 μg administered intramuscularly daily for two days may be useful. The use of buserelin in dogs and queen cats is not licensed at the moment.

Eclampsia

This is caused by hypocalcaemia, sometimes with a hypoglycaemia, and occurs in bitches just about to whelp, or in bitches feeding the pups. It is sometimes seen in queen cats. The symptoms include restlessness, panting, muscular spasms and, in extreme conditions, collapse and death. A variety of other conditions, including poisoning due to antifreeze, strychnine and metaldehyde, may mimic this condition. Response to treatment with calcium borogluconate is often diagnostic. Calcium borogluconate (10%) can be administered intravenously (must be slowly) to effect. A dose of 2–7 ml is usually adequate. A variety of calcium borogluconate preparations are suitable: one such compound which has been specifically licensed is Calcitad 50. The condition may be prevented by the administration of vitamin D together with a calcium supplement (Collo-Cal D Oral).

Agalactia

Agalactia results from a failure of the bitch to produce sufficient milk. There are a variety of causes including mastitis and possible systemic disease. This condition may be treated by using chorionic gonadotrophin (Chorulon) at a dose of 10 IU/lb for dogs or synthetic oxytocin (Oxytocin-S) at a dose rate of 2 IU/10 lb. The purpose of this treatment is to replace the natural posterior pituitary hormone, which may be deficient. It is also important that the pups or kittens should receive supplementary feeding if necessary.

Metritis

This condition is sometimes seen after parturition. It is characterized by a blood-stained vaginal discharge together with an anorexia, pyrexia, depression and agalactia. Therapy includes the use of antibiotics after bacterial culture together with electrolytes to compensate for the dehydration if necessary. Oxytocin (at a dose rate of 2.5 IU/10 lb) is useful as a uterine ecbolic to stimulate uterine contraction and the removal of the pathogenic material.

Pyometra

This condition is seen in the luteal phase of the oestrous cycle and is characterized by thirst, anorexia, abdominal swelling, and vulval discharge (in open pyometra). The treatment of choice is ovariohysterectomy in those animals that have no breeding value. Chemotherapy may be indicated in cases where there is a poor risk or where there is also intercurrent disease. Antibiotics may be used and should primarily be selected on a basis of culture results. However, gentamicin, and the cephalosporins are the initial drugs of choice. Prostaglandins ($F_{2\alpha}$) have luteolytic effects. A dose of 250 μg/kg once daily may be used until there is no discharge in the first hour after the injection. Prostaglandin $F_{2\alpha}$ acts by its luteolytic effect and its uterine ecbolic action to promote the removal of the uterine pathogenic material. Prostaglandin $F_{2\alpha}$ (dinoprost; Lutalyse) has been used in cases where surgery has to be avoided. It is suggested that success is likely to occur in over 90% of patients. Subsequently, it has been suggested that over 75% of these animals have had normal litters when treated in this manner.

Mammary tumours

The cause of mammary tumours is, in general, not known. The growth rate of some tumours is oestrogen dependent since their rate of growth can be reduced with progestogen therapy or the administration of testosterone. Temporary regression of some canine mammary tumours may be produced with the administration of the agents given in Table 14.3.

Table 14.3 Agents used to produce temporary regression of mammary tumours

Generic name	*Product*	*Dose*
Testosterone	Testosterone Implants	25 mg/10 lb dogs
Testosterone esters	Durateston	25–150 mg monthly, dogs 12.5–25 mg monthly, cats
Drostanolone propionate	Masteril	100 mg weekly, then gradually decrease dose in dogs
Megestrol acetate	Ovarid	1 mg/lb in dogs for 10 days

False pregnancy

This condition is fairly common. It is characterized by a distended abdomen, bed making and mammary development, together with the production of milk. It occurs about six to ten weeks after oestrus in the dog. Table 14.4 summarizes the therapeutic agents available and appropriate doses to be used.

Table 14.4 Agents used for the treatment of false pregnancy

Generic name	*Product*	*Dose*
Testosterone	Testosterone Implants	100–300 mg (s.c.)
Methyltestosterone	Methyltestosterone tabs Orandrone	5–30 mg daily for 5–7 days
Ethinyl-oestradiol (0.005 mg) + methyltestosterone (4.00 mg)	Sesoral tabs	Initial dose up to 8 tabs then 6 to 8 daily in divided doses, normally for 5 days
Proligestone	Covinan, Delvosteron	A single dose of 33 mg/kg
Megestrol acetate	Ovarid Syntex Suppress 20	2 mg/kg for 5–8 days

Reproductive disorders of the male

Aggression/excessive libido

A variety of causes may give rise to an unnecessarily aggressive dog or a dog which is hypersexual. A variety of treatments are available. Initially, behavioural methods may be tried or, alternatively, therapeutic agents consisting of a variety of progestogens are available and listed below.

Megestrol acetate (Ovarid)

This may be used at a dose rate of 2 mg/kg daily for seven days. If the condition improves this dose may be reduced to 1 mg/kg daily for a further fourteen days. If, however, it fails to respond to the initial dose, the dose may be increased to 4 mg/kg daily for seven days. Should this subsequent increase in megestrol administration fail to be successful, treatment should be stopped. If the second, higher dose of 4 mg/kg daily for seven days proves successful, a further dose of 1 mg/kg daily for fourteen days may be given. This dose schedule, however, is only given as a guide since it may be adjusted according to response. In a minority of animals it may be necessary to prescribe a low maintenance dose once weekly.

Medroxyprogesterone acetate (Perlutex)

This may be given by injection at a dose rate of 10 mg/kg every four to six months as necessary. It is suggested that this preparation is useful for the control of excessive barking in dogs and hypersexuality in postpubescent dogs. In neutered female cats and neutered or entire male cats medroxyprogesterone acetate at a dose rate of 10 mg/kg may be given and repeated every three to six months to control certain behavioural problems.

Delmadinone acetate (Tardak)

This compound is a synthetic progestogen but it has antioestrogen and antiandrogen properties. It is not an anabolic but has, interestingly enough, anticonvulsant properties. It is used at a dose rate of 1–2 mg/kg body weight and administered intramuscularly or subcutaneously for the treadtment of hypersexuality and excessive aggression. It is also useful for certain forms of nervousness and epileptiform seizures.

Castration may also prove to be beneficial and is a permanent answer should the chemotherapeutic measures indicate that this approach would be helpful.

Balanoposthitis/balanitis

These conditions are caused by bacterial infection, herpesvirus (dog pox) or overexcitement. They are characterized by reddening and swelling of the prepuce together with discharge and possible vesiculation. A variety of topical antiseptic agents have proved successful. Metronidazole (Torgyl) applied topically may be useful. Metronidazole is also available in injection and tablet form. A dose rate of 20 mg/kg administered daily for five to seven days is usually regarded as sufficient.

Prostate enlargement

This condition is seen in older male dogs and is characterized by constipation and ribbon-like faeces and tenesmus; very occasionally it gives rise to a perineal hernia. Diagnosis is usually made on a basis of rectal palpation and occasionally radiography. Delmadinone acetate (Tardak) can be used at a dose rate of 1–2 mg/kg body weight as a single dose. It is usually necessary to allow up to four days to pass before the effects of treatment can be observed. In those dogs that do not show an improvement after eight days, a second treatment may be tried. In those animals which do show a response, a second treatment following three to four weeks after the initial injection will be required. Subsequent redosing when symptoms show their first sign of reappearance will control the condition effectively. Oestradiol benzoate (Oestradiol Benzoate) at a dose rate of 1 mg per animal daily or 5 mg weekly is also useful.

Anal adenomas

The cause of this condition is not known. It is recognized around the anus in older dogs and is seen as a multilobular swelling often predisposed towards bleeding. The condition may be treated with delmadinone acetate or oestradiol benzoate at the same dose rate as that required for the treatment of prostatic enlargement.

Further reading

Jones, D. E. and Joshua, J. O. (1982) *Reproductive Clinical Problems in the Dog*, Wright, Bristol

Lamming, G. E., Foster, J. P. and Bulman, D. C. (1979) Pharmacological control of reproductive cycles. *Veterinary Record*, **104**, 156–160

Chapter 15

The Urinary Tract

This chapter discusses the therapeutic aspects of the urinary tract. It considers urinary incontinence, cystitis, feline urolithiasis syndrome, urolithiasis and renal failure (acute and chronic).

Urinary incontinence

This condition has a variety of causes and is characterized by the unconscious passing of urine at inappropriate times or places. The causes include low hormone levels, irritability of the detrusor muscle of the bladder, weakness of the urethral sphincter, and inflammation of the urinary tract.

Figure 15.1 summarizes the pharmacological and physiological control of the bladder. The cholinergic parasympathetic nervous supply to the bladder acts by releasing acetylcholine which stimulates muscarinic receptors on the detrusor muscle, causing contraction and release of urine. At the same time there

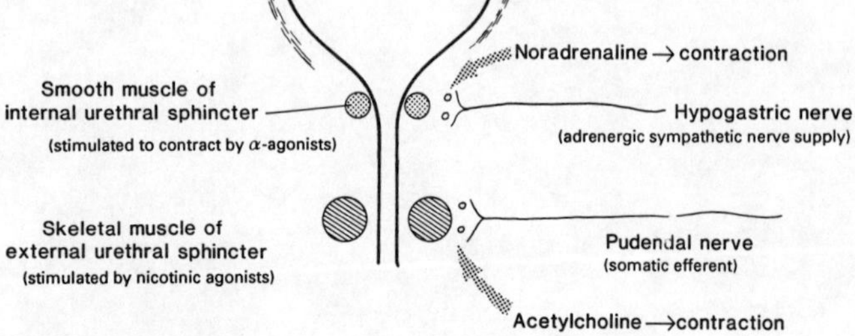

Figure 15.1 The efferent control of the bladder and the pharmacological receptors involved

is a relaxation of the urethral sphincters. To prevent urination, the internal urethral sphincter is normally closed and is so maintained under the influence of the sympathetic nervous input which releases noradrenaline to stimulate α-receptors causing contraction of the smooth muscle of the internal urethral sphincter and inhibition of urination. The pudendal nerve, which releases acetylcholine to cause contraction of the skeletal muscle of the external urethral sphincter, is also involved in maintaining continence.

Oestrogen-treatable incontinence

This condition is seen in bitches months or several years after speying. Typically it is precipitated by a polyuria due to any cause. Weakness of the urethral sphincter makes it difficult for the urine to be retained and as a result there is an incontinence. The signs then consist of involuntary urination with constant and intermittent dribbling of urine.

Oestradiol benzoate may be used for the treatment of this condition. It is suggested that a dose of 1 mg daily for 3 days should be followed by a dose of 1 mg every third day. Alternatively, diethylstilboestrol may be used at a dose rate of 0.1–1 mg/day for 3–5 days followed by a maintenance dose of approximately 1 mg/week. Some bitches may require higher therapeutic doses. Toxic doses of oestrogens can cause the induction of oestrus and damage to bone marrow. This second effect may give rise to leucocytosis and thrombocytopenia. If the use of oestrogens alone is not successful, α-agonists like ephedrine or phenyl propanolamine may be used as alternatives in some animals. The suggested dose for ephedrine is 2–4 mg/kg t.i.d. orally, and, for phenylpropanolamine, 12.5–50 mg t.i.d. orally in dogs and cats. Side-effects of α-stimulation are likely. They include increased heart rate, raised blood pressure, restlessness, irritability and apparent anxiety.

Testosterone-treatable incontinence

This condition is seen less frequently but occurs occasionally in the castrated male dog. Diagnosis is made on the basis of the exclusion of other causes of incontinence and response to testosterone therapy. Testosterone propionate can be administered three times a week either intramuscularly or subcutaneously at a dose of 2 mg/kg body weight. A 25 mg implant will remain active for 60 days; a dose of 25–100 mg can be used in the dog.

Detrusor irritability

Contraction of the detrusor muscle will produce urination. Irritability of this muscle (a tendency for this muscle to contract spontaneously) will bring about an incontinence. Since the detrusor muscle is stimulated by acetylcholine, which acts on muscarinic receptors to produce contraction, an appropriate treatment for detrusor irritability is to use a muscarinic antagonist (atropine-like drugs).

A proprietary preparation (Renachek) which contains hyoscyamine, atropine, scopolamine, sulphafurazole and ammonium chloride may be used for the treatment of this condition. It is suggested that a dose (in the dog) of 1 tablet/20 lb three times daily is used. In the cat, a dose of half a tablet three times a day may be used. Alternatively propantheline (Pro-Banthine) can be used. This compound is also an anticholinergic drug. It has atropine-like actions and weak ganglion-blocking properties. It is useful for the treatment of many conditions which require a spasmolytic. In the dog it can be given at a dose rate of 0.2 mg/kg orally three times a day. In the cat a dose of 7.5 mg can be given every third day. It is possible to increase the dose to control the detrusor irritability. An overdose of the anticholinergic agents is characterized by urinary retention, due to paralysis of the bladder, and other effects like restlessness, excitement, paralysis and coma. Other possible side-effects include a dry mouth, constipation and a disturbance of vision.

Urinary retention

Detrusor paralysis

This condition may arise as a result of overdistention of the bladder which uncouples the smooth muscles of the bladder as a result of the prolonged stretching; they are normally electrically coupled so that they contract together. Coordinated contractions of the bladder muscle are no longer possible. To treat this condition it is necessary to remove the cause of the urinary retention (say a bladder stone) and to empty the bladder at least three times a day. Normally manual expression is the preferred method, particularly when there is a low tone on the urethral sphincter. However, if there is an excessive tone on the urethral sphincter it may be necessary to use a catheter intermittently to empty the bladder. An indwelling catheter should be avoided since it predisposes towards infection in the urinary tract. Generally, it is advisable to use antibiotic cover for the control and prevention of urinary tract infection, which is particularly likely to occur when there is urinary retention.

Once evidence of partial recovery of the detrusor muscle is seen, it is possible to stimulate contraction using a cholinergic agent (bethanechol; Myotonine). This can be used to enhance but not initiate the detrusor reflex. It can be used at a dose of 2.5–10 mg per animal every eight hours subcutaneously or at a dose of 5–25 mg per animal every hours orally. In cats, a dose of 2.5–5 mg per animal can be given orally twice a day. It is pointed out that bethanechol should not be used when there is evidence of urethral resistance. Bethanechol has a relatively selective action on the bladder but will also act on the other muscarinic receptors of the body. Thus, there may be an increase in gut activity, producing vomiting and diarrhoea, especially if excessive doses are given. Salivation may also be seen. A slowing of the heart rate can also occur.

Excessive tone of the urethral sphincter

This condition is characterized by excessive resistance to manual emptying of the bladder and urinary retention. It is logical to use α-blockers to treat this condition. One such drug is phenoxybenzamine (Dibenyline). This drug is closely related to nitrogen mustard and is a powerful α-blocker but has a slow onset of action even after intravenous injection. Its effects can last for several days. It acts, following metabolism, as an alkylating agent. Once blockade has been established it is resistant to displacement from the receptor. Phenoxybenzamine causes a moderate fall in the diastolic blood pressure as well as relaxing the urethral sphincter muscles. It is suggested that an initial dose in dogs is 10 mg given orally once daily. If no response is observed after four days then the dose may be increased to 10 mg every 12 hours. If no response is seen after another four days, the dose may be increased again by 10 mg every 8 hours for 1 day. In the cat the initial suggested dose is 0.25 mg/kg given orally every 8 hours if necessary. Alternatively, the tone on the urethral sphincter may be controlled using diazepam (Valium) at a dose rate of 2–10 mg every 8 hours in the dog; excessively high doses will produce sedation.

Prostatitis (bacterial)

Bacterial prostatitis is produced by bacterial invasion of the prostate gland; it does not include prostatic hyperplasia and cystic hyperplasia. This condition frequently gives rise to a recurring cystitis in the male dog. The condition is characterized by a urethral discharge without urination and an enlarged, painful prostate gland. Sometimes there is straining and constipation with an abnormal walking pattern. The diagnosis of bacterial prostatitis in the dog can be confirmed by the presence of large numbers of pathogenic bacteria in prostatic fluid or semen.

Antibiotics which may be useful for the treatment of this condition include trimethoprim/sulphadiazine, erythromycin and tetracycline. The duration of antibiotic therapy should be at least 14 days; it may be beneficial to continue for 21 days. The problem with prostatitis is that in the chronic condition penetration of the antibiotic into the infected gland is difficult. Castration is effective in decreasing the recurrence of this condition. Since the beneficial effects of oestrogens have not been established, and there is a toxic effect of oestrogens on the bone marrow of dogs, it may be advisable to avoid the use of these substances.

Cystitis/urinary tract infections

Infection of the urinary tract or bladder can give rise to acute or recurrent conditions. Acute and uncomplicated cystitis usually occurs without the development of chronic inflammatory lesions in the urinary tract. The recurrent urinary tract infections will usually return following withdrawal of therapy. The condition is characterized by frequent urination, dysuria, haematuria and incontinence. The urine can be cloudy and foul smelling. If the kidneys are involved, so that there is a pyelonephritis, there is usually a raised temperature, depression, vomiting and pain in the upper abdomen. These conditions are usually treated with antimicrobial agents which are secreted in high concentrations in the urine. This means that a low therapeutic level, producing a low plasma concentration, may produce adequate therapeutic levels in the urine. However, when a kidney infection is being treated, the level of antibiotic in the urine is unimportant: an adequate tissue concentration in the kidney is required.

Antibacterials for cystitis

Penicillin is actively secreted in the urine in high concentrations and even though it is a narrow spectrum antibiotic it may reach the concentration to kill normally insensitive bacterial species like *E. coli*. In order to gain the highest concentration of the antibiotic in the bladder, it is suggested that the penicillin should be administered three or four times daily and opportunities for urination should be restricted to about 15 minutes before the administration of the next dose of antibiotics. Penicillin G or ampicillin are suitable agents for this purpose (Table 15.1). Usually this treatment is very effective, except where the organism which causes the infection is *E. coli* which has undergone previous exposure to antibiotics. Proteus and strains of klebsiella and pseudomonas are also organisms which are likely to give rise to resistance.

Table 15.1 Therapeutic agents for bacterial cystitis

Generic name	*Product*	*Dose*
Penicillin G	–	110 000–165 000 units/kg dog and cat. 3 or 4 times daily
Ampicillin	Penbritin	77–110 mg/kg orally, dog and cat. 3 or 4 times daily
Amoxycillin	Clamoxyl	4–10 mg/kg 3–4 times daily
Amoxycillin + clavulanic acid	Synulox	15 mg/kg 2–3 times daily
Trimethoprim/ sulphadiazine	Tribrissin	Dogs, 30 mg/kg twice daily Cats, 20 mg daily
Nitroxoline	Nibiol-V 50 mg tablets	10 mg/kg daily dog and cat
Nitrofurantoin	Berkfurin 50 mg and 100 mg tablets	4 mg/kg dog and cat 3 times daily
Ethylenediamine (urinary acidifier)	Chlorethamine 90 mg tablets	Up to 90 mg three times daily
Hexamine BP/sodium acid phosphate	Hexamine/Sodium Acid Phosphate tablets	300–600 mg daily

Amoxycillin (Table 15.1) gives a much higher concentration in the urine in the dog than ampicillin, for the same dose administered, but is excreted at the same rate; this means that higher urine levels are achieved with amoxycillin. Amoxycillin can now be regarded as the drug of choice because of its more rapid bactericidal action and the higher urine concentration achieved.

Often, recurrent urinary tract infection can be associated with chronic bacterial infection of the prostate gland. Since trimethoprim is concentrated in the canine prostate, unlike most other antibacterial agents, it is very useful with sulphadiazine for the treatment of chronic or recurrent urinary tract infections especially in the male (Table 15.1). Trimethoprim is a weakly basic drug, while sulphadiazine is a weakly acidic drug, so that variations of the pH in the urine will alter the ratio of one or other of these drugs within it. In addition, trimethoprim appears to be extensively metabolized in the dog, so that urine levels tend to be low. This means that optimum ratios of trimethoprim and sulphadiazine may not be achieved in the urine. Despite these drawbacks, the combination does appear to be quite effective in clinical conditions, possibly because of the penetration of the two components from the plasma into the urinary tract mucosa. Amoxycillin combined with clavulanic acid (Synulox) is also very useful for the treatment of recurrent cystitis. The clavulanic acid acts to antagonize the β-lactamase enzymes which may destroy the amoxycillin; the β-lactamase enzymes are produced by some resistant organisms. Synulox is particularly useful for the treatment of recurrent urinary tract infections since the two compounds in this preparation are delivered at the same rate in the urine because they have very similar pharmacokinetic properties and have similar distributions and half-lives. If culture tests suggest that neither amoxycillin nor trimethoprim are likely to be effective, other antibiotics will have to be given. Erythromycin, gentamicin and streptomycin are most effective in urine which is alkaline (pH 7.5–8.0). On the other hand, hexamine and nitrofurantoin are most effective in acid urine. If hexamine is to be used (Table 15.1) the pH should be maintained below 5.5 and at this pH the compound dissociates, releasing mandelic acid and formaldehyde. Hexamine is usually given in combination with sodium acid phosphate to acidify the urine but it is necessary to confirm that the urine is sufficiently acid by measuring the pH. This preparation may give rise to a chemical cystitis, despite being effective against bacterial cystitis.

If there is renal failure there may be a marked alteration of the excretion of antibacterial agents. Under these conditions it is wise to use a nontoxic agent such as amoxycillin.

Cystitis due to candidiasis

This condition can only be diagnosed following culture of the urine from cases of cystitis. Sometimes the yeast (candida) may be recovered transiently in the urine. If the candida is not producing a clinical condition it may be sufficient to remove the predisposing causes, such as the administration of corticosteroids and immunosuppressive drugs. Perhaps the inappropriate administration of an antibiotic may be stopped. Diabetes mellitus may also be present and needs to be considered. Alkalinization of the urine is also helpful, using administration of sodium bicarbonate at a dose rate in the region of 325 mg three times daily (orally) to increase the pH above 7.5.

If there is evidence of candiduria and the animal is in a poor condition, then the therapy has to be more aggressive. Initially the urine can be made alkaline as before and the predisposing factors removed. 5-Fluorocytosine may be used at a dose rate of 60 mg/kg (orally) every eight hours. It is excreted in the urine in an active form and may be useful for the treatment of this condition. However, side-effects which may occur occasionally include depression of the bone marrow, dermatitis and liver toxicity. In animals which show evidence of kidney failure, reduced doses should be used. Ketoconazole may also be used instead of 5-fluorocytosine at a dose of 10 mg/kg (orally) given every eight hours. Treatment for systemic candidiasis should last (in general) for 4–6 weeks.

Canine urolithiasis

A variety of causes can give rise to the formation of stones in the bladder and urine. Eventually this condition shows itself as a dysuria, haematuria, pain, anuria, depression and inappetence. Sometimes the stones are sufficiently large to be palpated in the bladder or they may be passed unnoticed in the urine. X-ray can usually identify these uroliths. The male animal may show anuria due to a blockage as a stone enters the urethra. The bitch may show signs of chronic and persistent cystitis. There are six types of bladder stone (uroliths). The nature of the uroliths is determined from the chemical analysis of stones which have been passed or collected during surgery. The treatment and prevention of these stones to some extent depends on their chemical nature and how they have been formed.

Magnesium ammonium phosphate (struvite) uroliths

Struvite uroliths are the most commonly occurring stone in the dog and cat (about 80% of cases). In dogs it is believed that the most common predisposing cause is the presence of urease-positive staphylococcus or proteus organisms in the bladder.

These organisms act on the urea to release ammonia and raise the pH. If, in addition, there is a low urine output so that the concentration of the salts (magnesium, ammonia and phosphate) in the urine is relatively high, it is then possible that struvite uroliths will be formed. Treatment often consists of surgical removal of the uroliths. Following a successful surgical operation for removal, it is necessary to prevent recurrence. This is usually carried out by:

1. Increasing the volume of urine. This aims to prevent stagnation of the urine and dilutes the concentration of the crystalloids which cause the uroliths. Obviously an adequate water supply must be ensured. An increase in the consumption of water may be encouraged by the administration of 0.5–10 g sodium chloride daily in dogs which have a healthy cardiovascular and renal status. The aim should be to decrease the specific gravity of the urine to less than 1.02.
2. Eradicating the urease-producing bacteria. This may be achieved by an appropriate aggressive antibacterial regime (Table 15.1).
3. The use of acetohydroxamic acid (Lithostat). At a dose rate of 25 mg/kg/day this can be given as a urease inhibitor. It is best given in divided doses twice daily. Acetohydroxamic acid retards the alkalinization of the urine caused by the growth of the urease-producing bacteria. It is fairly rapidly absorbed from the gastrointestinal tract and is excreted unchanged in the urine. It has a dose-dependent bacteriostatic effect on the bacteria in the urine and can potentiate the antibacterial effects of other antibiotics. At very high doses it may produce a haemolytic anaemia.
4. The use of urinary acidifiers if the pH of the urine remains alkaline despite the administration of antibacterial compounds. Ethylenediamine (Chlorethamine) is useful for this purpose. Up to 90 mg can be given three times daily. The aim of the treatment should be to reduce the pH below 6.5.

It may also be an advantage to modify the diet in an attempt to reduce the amount of phosphorus and magnesium which appears in the urine. Thus, dietary protein should be reduced and a small amount of salt may be added to the diet to stimulate urine production.

Urate uroliths

These are of two types, ammonium acid urate uroliths and uric acid uroliths.

The ammonium acid urate uroliths are more common than the simple uric acid uroliths in all dogs except the Dalmatian where the reverse is true. Ammonium acid urate uroliths are more likely to occur in dogs which have abnormalities of the portal vasculature. In these animals there is an abnormal ammonia concentration in the blood as well as an abnormally high uric acid concentration. This presumably predisposes towards the development of the ammonium acid urate uroliths in the bladder.

Uric acid uroliths are more soluble in more alkaline (pH 6.5–7.0) urine. Ammonium acid urates are little affected by changes in pH. Prevention of recurrence of urate uroliths may be achieved using the following approaches:

1. Making the urine more alkaline by administering sodium bicarbonate, either as tablets or baking soda, mixed with the food so that the urine achieves a pH of 6.5–7.
2. The administration of allopurinol (Zyloric). This can be administered at a dose rate of 10 mg/kg every eight hours for a month. The dose may then be reduced to 10 mg/kg twice daily thereafter. Allopurinol acts to reduce the plasma uric acid concentration and the urinary output of the urates by inhibiting an enzyme (xanthine oxidase). Allopurinol is a competitive antagonist of xanthine oxidase and leads to a much lower concentration of uric acid in the urine. It is interesting that allopurinol is also acted on by the xanthine oxidase and that the metabolic product alloxanthine itself further inhibits the action of xanthine oxidase. The net effect is that the secretion of uric acid falls and there is a compensatory increase in the amount of hypoxanthine, xanthine, allopurinol and alloxanthine in the urine. Adverse effects may include skin rashes and possible hypersensitivities. The dose of allopurinol should be reduced in animals with renal failure.
3. A diet with a low purine concentration should be used. This means that the diet should consist of an all-vegetable source.
4. Urinary tract infections are usually secondary to the development of urate uroliths. Treatment of the urinary tract infection is usually fairly simple.

Cystine uroliths

Cystine uroliths may result from a cystinuria which arises as a result of an inherited renal tubular defect. It may occur in a variety of breeds, especially the dachschunds. It can occur in both sexes but is seen predominantly in the male dog, presumably because of the narrow urethra. The following treatment may be useful in preventing recurrence:

1. Maintaining the pH at an alkaline state (above 7.5) by the addition of sodium bicarbonate tablets or baking soda mixed in the food.
2. The administration of penicillamine (Distamine or Cuprimine) orally at a dose rate of 15 mg/kg twice daily mixed in the food. The D-isomer is the least toxic (L-isomers also occur). It is a readily absorbable compound and passes from the gut into the plasma and forms a dimer with cystine which consists of cystine-D-penicillamine disulphide. This disulphide is much more soluble than the dimer cystine-cystine which would normally occur. There is an advantage in maintaining the urine at an alkaline pH even when this substance is administered, since the new dimer formed with D-penicillamine is also more soluble in high pHs. Side-effects may occur with this compound and these consists of vomiting and anorexia. If these signs do occur, the dose can be reduced to about 10 mg/kg/day. Side-effects reported with D-penicillamine include vomiting, rashes, fever and, very rarely, a nephrotic syndrome. D-penicillamine is useful in controlling cystine uroliths in man.

Calcium oxalate uroliths

Oxalic acid is normally excreted in the urine and arises as a result of metabolism in the liver. For unknown reasons in some animals there may be a high oxalic acid concentration and a high calcium concentration in the urine which predispose towards these uroliths. Prevention of recurrence of these uroliths is difficult. The following approaches may be tried:

1. The chronic long-term administration of hydrochlorothiazide (Vetidrex) at a dose rate of 2 mg/kg twice daily (orally) may be useful for animals which have a high calcium secretion in the urine due to some unknown defect of tubular resorption. The thiazide diuretic decreases the calcium excretion by increasing renal tubular resorption.
2. Increase the urine output by the administration of salt in the diet as before; in addition, the amount of calcium added to the diet should be restricted.

Silica uroliths

Silica uroliths are found predominantly in the male Alsatian. They can occur in other species. The cause of silica uroliths is not known so that it is difficult to control and prevent their recurrence. It is suggested that the following treatments may be useful in preventing recurrence:

1. Polyuria should be induced by the administration of salt to the diet as before.
2. The diet of the animal should be changed, since it is reasonably likely that this may be a predisposing factor. The pH does not appear to influence the precipitation of uroliths.

Calcium phosphate (apatite) uroliths

These stones are more likely to occur when there is a high urinary concentration of calcium phosphate and a high urinary pH. Since they are more soluble in acid pH, it is useful to ensure that the urine has a pH below 6.5. This may be achieved by the addition of hexamine (Table 15.1) or ammonium chloride to the diet. It is also an advantage to ensure a polyuria in preventing this type of stone. Apatite uroliths are often seen when there are metabolic disorders such as primary hyperparathyroidism or excessive calcium or phosphorus in the diet.

Kidney failure

Kidney failure can be classified on clinical grounds into acute renal failure or chronic renal failure.

Acute renal failure

Acute renal failure, due to leptospirosis, bacterial infection (often *E. coli*, staphylococci or proteus), ischaemia, acute tubular necrosis or glomerulonephritis, shows the following signs: inappetence, loss of weight, malaise, increased thirst, abdominal pain, oliguria, intermittent vomiting, constipation, sometimes diarrhoea, uraemia, convulsions and occasionally sudden death.

Chronic renal failure

Chronic renal failure may be due to a variety of causes such as chronic interstitial nephritis, glomerulonephritis, canine adenovirus, pyelonephritis, nephrolithiasis, poisoning, amyloidosis, urinary tract obstruction, neoplasia, ischaemia or as a sequel to acute renal failure. The signs of chronic renal failure include: polydipsia, vomiting, uraemia, polyuria, dehydration, depression, oral ulceration, anaemia, diarrhoea and a rough coat.

Treatment of acute renal failure

The treatment of acute renal failure consists of aggressive symptomatic treatment. It is important to assess the body weight, fluid intake and urine output, degree of hydration, the colour of the mucous membranes, pulse rate, capillary refill time, temperature, respiratory rate, blood urea nitrogen, total plasma proteins, packed cell volume and serum sodium, potassium chloride, bicarbonate, calcium and phosphorus concentrations. Any abnormality of these should be corrected.

Correction of dehydration

An appropriate volume of fluid (often lactated Ringer's solution) can be administered by an intravenous catheter (see Chapter 10). Due care should be taken if there is any cardiac problem. The time taken for the correction of the dehydration can be three hours, providing there is no cardiac condition. A mild overhydration may have little effect and even be desirable.

Measurement of the rate of urine production

The measurement of urine production is useful for a guide to supplementary fluid administration. It is recommended that an indwelling catheter be avoided. A metabolism cage is useful for the collection of urine. It does not predispose towards production of urinary tract infection.

Correction of hyperkalaemia

It is possible to drive the potassium intracellularly by the administration of an intravenous solution of sodium bicarbonate. A dose of 1 mEq/kg body weight intravenously is suggested. It is recommended that half the calculated dose is given by a slow intravenous injection and the remaining half given slowly over the next four hours.

Correction of metabolic acidosis

Sodium bicarbonate may be given to correct metabolic acidosis. This is only possible if plasma bicarbonate levels can be measured which is not usually possible in routine small animal practices.

Increasing the urine output

It is useful to encourage urine production so that the kidney, even though it is not functioning properly, may make some corrections to the body pH and mineral levels. Initially it is important to establish and correct any fluid deficit. If this does not correct the oliguria, frusemide (Lasix) at a dose rate of 2 mg/kg given intravenously is useful. This may be supplemented by the intravenous administration of dopamine (50 mg of dopamine in 500 ml of lactated Ringer) to increase the renal blood flow and glomerular filtration rate. Dopamine acts on renal dopamine receptors and produces renal vascular dilatation. If there is no diuresis as a result of this therapy, the dose of frusemide may be increased. However, if this dose of frusemide and dopamine is adequate, the treatment may be continued every eight hours.

The control of uraemic symptoms

Uraemia may be controlled and limited by reducing the amount of protein in the diet. One way of achieving this is to use a nephritis diet which has only 5% of the diet as protein. Adequate energy is available as carbohydrate and fat to minimize protein as an energy source.

In addition to controlling protein in the diet, cimetidine (Tagamet) can be used for the control of haemorrhagic gastritis induced by the uraemia. Cimetidine acts by blocking H_2-histamine receptors on the parietal cells of the stomach. It acts to decrease acid secretion following stimulation by gastrin and histamine. It is suggested that a dose of 10 mg/kg is given intravenously to uraemic dogs and that this is followed by a dose of 5 mg/kg body weight intravenously every twelve hours. After the uraemic crisis producing the gastritis has been controlled, it is possible to administer the cimetidine orally at a dose of 5 mg/kg twice daily for 2–3 weeks for further control of the uraemic gastritis. A dose of 5 mg/kg body weight given intravenously and followed by 2.5 mg/kg every twelve hours can be used in the cat. This is then followed by a dose of 2.5 mg/kg body weight given twice daily for two weeks.

Treatment of chronic renal failure

Usually chronic renal failure is treated symptomatically but the underlying cause should not be ignored. The treatment can consist of the following approaches:

1. *Free access to water* Animals must have free access to clean water at all times in order to minimize the risk of dehydration.
2. *The administration of nephritis diets* It is an advantage to reduce the amount of protein in the diets of animals suffering from chronic nephritis so that there is not a high output of nitrogenous metabolic waste. One such diet is Pedigree Petfoods Nephritis Diet which contains approximately 5% protein essential for replacing body tissue. In addition, there is an adequate energy supply in the form of fat and carbohydrate to minimize the use of protein as an energy source.
3. *Salt intake* The administration of excessive amounts of sodium chloride in the diet may lead to a volume overload and hypertension. Usually dogs with chronic renal failure can adjust to a wide variety of salt levels in the diet providing changes are made slowly over a period of about 14 days. However, animals which have congestive heart failure, nephrotic syndrome or hypertension may benefit from the administration of a diet with a reduced salt concentration.
4. *The administration of sodium bicarbonate to control acidosis* Sodium bicarbonate may be administered to control metabolic acidosis associated with renal failure. It is suggested that a dose of about 8–12 mg/kg body weight be given initially every eight hours. Subsequently the dose can be adjusted according to needs. As a general guide it is useful to adjust the urinary pH between 6.5 and 7.0. Values greater than 7.5 suggest an overdose of sodium bicarbonate; values less than a pH of 6.0 suggest an inadequate dose. Care must be taken to avoid an excessive dose of sodium bicarbonate and the induction of metabolic alkalosis.
5. *The administration of anabolic steroids* (Finajet or Norandrolin) Anabolic steroids are useful for treating anaemia in animals with chronic renal failure. They stimulate a positive nitrogen balance and the deposition of calcium in bones.
6. *The administration of vitamin supplements* A variety of water-soluble vitamins (B and C) are useful for treating dogs and cats with renal failure because of their excessive excretion in urine. It is also useful to avoid multivitamin preparations

which contain vitamins A and D because these may have an adverse action on the calcium–phosphorus balance.

7. *The control of hyperphosphataemia* To control and minimize the levels of phosphate in the blood, diets with a low protein/phosphorus content can be used. They may be given in combination with substances which bind phosphate. Thus, aluminium hydroxide (Asilone) can be used. They are particularly useful if a reduction in the protein of the diet fails to reduce serum phosphorus levels to a desired level of 3–5 mg/100 ml. An initial dose of aluminium hydroxide of 30–90 mg/kg body weight per day is suggested. This must be varied according to the response. It is important to retest the serum phorphorus levels every 14 days until a proper dose of aluminium hydroxide binding agent is determined.
8. *The control of hypercalcaemia* Sometimes low levels of calcium occur in the plasma of animals suffering from chronic renal failure. To control this, calcium supplements and vitamin D therapy may be useful.
9. *Minimizing stress* It is obvious that an animal suffering from chronic renal failure is not able to adapt to changing metabolic requirements. Thus, changes like pregnancy, anaesthesia and surgery may precipitate another uraemic crisis.

Feline urolithiasis syndrome

This condition is seen in the cat, predominantly in the castrated male. It is also seen in those animals which have been fed on dry cat food and which lead a sedentary life. It is the result of a blocked urethra due to the presence of uroliths or sloughed tissue. The signs consist of crouching, increased frequency of urination, haematuria with small amounts of urine, and abdominal discomfort. There is a palpably enlarged bladder due to urethral obstruction. This condition may progress giving rise to depression, dehydration and eventually death. Treatment consists initially of removing the obstruction by flushing or urethral massage. Once the blockage has been removed, antibiotic therapy may be instituted to control the infection in the urinary tract. Alternatively, urinary antiseptics may be used. If dehydration is present because the condition has been there for a long time, fluid replacement may be necessary. The administration of proquamezine (Myspamol) (Table 15.2) may

Table 15.2 Agents suitable for the treatment of feline urolithiasis syndrome

Generic name	*Product*	*Dose*
Proquamezine	Myspasmol injection	3 mg/kg
Methyltestosterone	Orandrone 5 mg tablets	5 mg daily
Testosterone	Testosterone 25 mg implant	Lasts about 60 days

be considered during acute episodes for the symptomatic treatment of dysuria in those cats where the obstruction is incomplete. A dose of 3 mg/kg injected intramuscularly may be useful. Care must be taken to avoid excessive urinary retention.

Prevention consists of changing the diet from dried cat food and increasing the urine flow by ensuring ready access to plenty of water. Small amounts of salt may be added to the diet to encourage drinking.

Further reading

Cowgill, L. D. (1983) Diseases of the kidney. In *Textbook of Veterinary Internal Medicine*, 3rd edn, vol. 2 (ed. S. J. Ettuger), Saunders, Philadelphia

Hardy, R. M. (1982) Disorders of water metabolism. *Veterinary Clinics of North America*, **12**, 353

Lindner, A., Cutler, R. E. and Goodman, W. G. (1979) Synergism of dopamine plus frusemide in preventing acute renal failure in the dog. *Kidney International*, **16**, 158

Ling, G. V. (1983) Treatment of urinary tract infections with antimicrobial agents. In *Current Veterinary Therapy VIII* (ed. R. W. Kirk), Saunders, Philadelphia, p. 1051

Oliver, J. E. (1983) Dysuria caused by reflex dyssynergia. In *Current Veterinary Therapy VIII* (ed. R. W. Kirk), Saunders, Philadelphia, p. 1088

Osborne, C. A. and Klausner, J. S. (1980) Calcium oxalate urolithiasis. In *Current Veterinary Therapy VIII* (ed. R. W. Kirk), Saunders, Philadelphia, p. 1055

Thornhill, J. A. (1983) Control of vomiting in the uremic patient. In *Current Veterinary Therapy VIII* (ed. R. W. Kirk), Saunders, Philadelphia, p. 1022

Chapter 16

The Endocrine System

This chapter considers therapeutic aspects of disorders of the pituitary, the insulin-producing cells in the pancreas, the thyroid and the parathyroid gland.

The pituitary gland

Disorders of growth hormone (somatotrophin) production

Growth hormone is produced in the anterior pituitary; it is a protein of 188 amino acids and exists in three or four forms which can be separated by electrophoresis. The control and release of growth hormone from the anterior pituitary is believed to be by an as yet uncharacterized growth hormone releasing factor which is secreted by the hypothalamus.

Growth hormone is responsible for growth in young animals and for protein formation (anabolism). It increases the transport of neutral and basic amino acids and stimulates their cellular uptake and incorporation into proteins. It also acts on blood sugar to increase liver glycogen production; it therefore has an anti-insulin effect. It increases blood lipids and produces a reduction in body fat.

The normal plasma level of growth hormone is less than 10 ng/ml. This level fluctuates and peaks occur during exercise, stress, sleep and hypoglycaemia; glucocorticoids will increase the level of growth hormone. Growth hormone cannot be administered orally since it is a protein and is broken down in the gut; it is administered parenterally and has a plasma half-life of 30 minutes.

Pituitary dwarfism

This condition is due to a lowered secretion of growth hormone from the anterior pituitary in a young animal. The signs and symptoms are caused by the deficiency. The condition occurs rarely but predominantly in the Alsatian; it may be caused by a hypoplasia of the pituitary or a cystic deformation of the craniopharyngeal duct. Other unknown causes may contribute to the condition.

The clinical symptoms consist of lethargy and listlessness. Usually there are bilateral symmetrical areas of alopecia which are found on the head, top of the shoulders and on the medial aspects of the legs. These skin areas are often hyperpigmented, with hyperkeratosis being present on the abdomen and inguinal area. Often the puppy coat is retained for longer than usual.

The diagnosis can be confirmed with a radioimmune assay to measure plasma growth hormone levels. Treatment is not usually carried out but may be attempted with bovine or pig growth hormone. Dosages of 5–10 units subcutaneously given every other day for ten injections may be useful. Normally a response should be seen in two months, a remission may last for over three years.

Acromegaly (canine)

This condition arises as a result of overproduction of growth hormone in a mature dog. This can result from a growth in the pituitary gland or from the administration of potent progestogens. The condition is recognized by a thickened skin and an increase in hair growth, together with an abdominal enlargement. There is also an increase in drinking and passing of urine; the animal is generally easily fatigued. Diagnosis is usually confirmed on the basis of a radioimmune assay to measure growth hormone levels in the plasma. Raised levels cannot be suppressed by the intravenous administration of glucose (1 g/kg). Treatment will vary according to the predisposing factors; if they have been initiated by an overadministration of progestogens for oestrus control, these must be withdrawn.

Antidiuretic hormone (vasopressin) disorders

Antidiuretic hormone (ADH) is a peptide made up of eight amino acids. It is released from the posterior pituitary as a result of a rise in plasma osmolarity (detected by osmoreceptors in the anterior hypothalamus). Another factor which can stimulate its release is a fall in plasma volume, which is detected by receptors in thoracic veins. It may also be stimulated by the administration of morphine and other opiates.

ADH will concentrate urine by increasing the water permeability of the distal tubules and collecting ducts of the kidney, bringing about an increase in water reabsorption. In massive doses, ADH will cause smooth muscle contraction by direct action on the blood vessels, gut and bladder.

ADH cannot be administered by mouth since it is broken down by proteolytic action in the gut. It has to be administered parenterally and has a half-life of 15 minutes, since it is rapidly inactivated by the liver and kidneys.

Central diabetes insipidus

This condition arises because of failure of the posterior pituitary to release adequate amounts of ADH. It is occasionally seen in the dog but very rarely in the cat. The cause of the condition is usually not known but is obviously related to some disturbance in pituitary function. Clinical signs consist of a sudden onset of a marked polyuria and secondary polydipsia. Some animals become severely dehydrated as a result of the polyuria; some dogs will vomit because they drink too much water. Other signs include weight loss, poor appetite and depression. The differential diagnosis includes diabetes mellitus, pyometra, hyperadrenocorticism, renal tubular failure, chronic renal disease and hyperthyroidism.

To confirm the diagnosis it is usually best to demonstrate that water restriction does not cause a significant antidiuresis or a hypertonic urine. Administration of ADH also produces dramatic improvement in the condition.

ADH may be given in the form of vasopressin injection BP (Pitressin) as an aqueous solution which has a very brief duration of action (about two hours, following intramuscular administration). Vasopressin tannate injection (Pitressin Tannate) is an oily suspension which must be shaken thoroughly and warmed before use. Its effects last two or three days following intramuscular administration; it must not be given intravenously. Doses vary with the individual patient. It is usual to start at 1–2 IU intramuscularly every three days. This dosage and frequency is then adjusted according to response. An overdose of ADH can lead to water intoxication.

The condition may also be treated by non-ADH compounds like chlorothiazide or chlorpropamide. These drugs have the advantage, if effective, of being administerable by mouth. Doses will depend on the response of the animal. Initially, 50–150 mg every 12 hours can be given. In human patients the thiazide diurectics, if given chronically, can produce a 50% reduction in urine volume. To control the diabetes insipidus it is also necessary to control rigidly the salt intake in the diet.

Nephrogenic diabetes insipidus
This condition is similar, with symptoms of polyuria, etc., but arises as a result of the kidney failing to respond to normal levels of plasma ADH. Treatment is aimed at correcting the renal pathology, since increasing ADH is unlikely to be effective.

The thyroid gland

The thyroid gland is found at the junction of the larynx and the trachea. It secretes thyroxine (T_4) and tri-iodothyronine (T_3) and is controlled by stimulation by thyroid-stimulating hormone (TSH) which is released from the pituitary. In addition, it secretes calcitonin.

Thyroxine and tri-iodothyronine are tyrosine derivatives and contain iodine. Thus, a regular intake of iodine (normally 10–20 μg/day) is required. Iodine is absorbed from the upper gastrointestinal tract and actively transported into the thyroid gland. Once it reaches the thyroid gland, it is oxidized and coupled to tyrosine to form monoiodotyrosine and di-iodotyrosine. These two compounds then combine to form thyroxine and L-tri-iodothyronine (Figure 16.1). Thyroxine and L-tri-iodothyronine are the active hormones and are stored in combination with a protein, thyroglobulin. This protein can be hydrolysed to release the active hormones into the bloodstream. All these processes are under the control of TSH, which stimulates production and release.

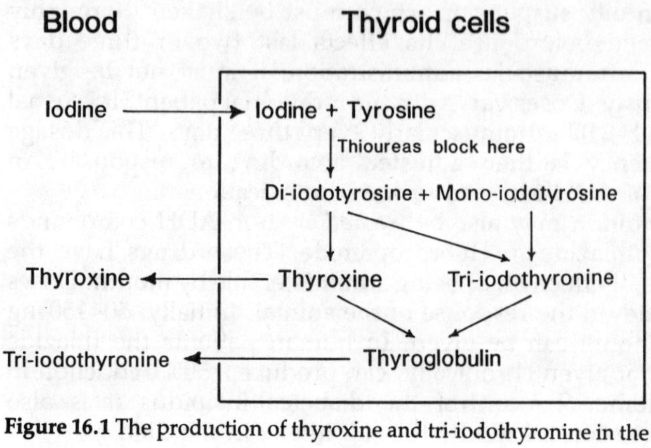

Figure 16.1 The production of thyroxine and tri-iodothyronine in the thyroid

Thyroid hormone transport

Thyroid hormones are carried in the blood, mostly protein bound; 80% of the hormones consist of thyroxine and 20% tri-iodothyronine. The specific protein which carries the thyroid hormones is known as thyroxin-binding globulin (TBG). The concentration of TBG is increased by pregnancy, oestrogens or phenothiazines; the total level of thyroid hormones in the blood also increases, although the free concentration remains constant. If the concentration of TBG falls as a result of stimulation from androgens, corticosteroids or in hypoproteinaemia, there will be a fall in the total level of the hormones. Compounds like aspirin, phenytoin and warfarin (acidic drugs) can compete for the thyrosine-binding sites and so reduce the blood thyroxine levels.

Thyroid hormone measurement

Protein-bound iodine measures the concentration of the organically bound iodine in blood. It can be raised by material from radiographic contrast media, giving false results. The resin uptake tests measure the saturation of the binding sites on the transport proteins and can be affected by changes in plasma TBG concentrations. Serum free thyroxine, which measures the free level of thyroxine, can also be affected by changes in TBG concentrations but not by the presence of free iodine. The free thyroxine index and effective thyroxine ratio tests consider both the TBG level and the organically bound iodine and give more consistency in their results.

Thyroid hormone actions

Generally the actions of thyroid hormones can be described as an ability to increase oxygen consumption and to stimulate the metabolic rate in all tissues. The hormones are important for the development of normal growth, are associated with an increase in peripheral utilization of glucose and will stimulate the breakdown of protein, especially in hyperthyroid states. They are concerned in tissue differentiation and maturation: in fetal and newborn animals thyroid deficiency leads to an underdevelopment of the central nervous system. Thyroid deficiency also produces a failure of growth in the skin and hair and an increase in protein leakage from blood capillaries. A number of the metabolic effects produced by the thyroid hormones may be related to their action on β-adrenoreceptors; they are able to stimulate these receptors and may give rise to an increase in the heart rate (tachycardia) and arrhythmia. This latter effect occurs in severe thyrotoxicosis and can lead to heart failure (seen in cats). Other effects which may be mediated by the adrenoreceptors include a breakdown of fat and glycogen.

Production disorders

An overproduction of thyroid hormones leads to hyperthyroidism or thyrotoxicosis. There is a direct increase in the circulating thyroxine and tri-iodothyronine; this condition may be caused by excessive production by the gland itself or due to excessive stimulation by TSH from the pituitary. Underproduction can lead to myxoedema, brain disorder in young animals or hypothyroidism in adults.

Hypothyroidism

This condition may arise as a result of a deficiency of TSH from the pituitary or a deficiency of the thyroid gland itself. The clinical signs usually develop slowly over a period of several months. There is often a history of slow physical movements, cold intolerance, weight gain and general indolence. The rectal temperature may be 1–2°C lower than normal; there is often a reduced exercise tolerance. The skin and hair may show characteristic changes: sometimes there is an alopecia, often on the chest, flanks and thighs; sometimes there is a pigmentation in those areas of alopecia. There is often thickening of the skin and puffiness of the skin of the face and forehead. The heart is affected with the pulse rate being lower than normal. The gut may be affected, with an increase in appetite of some animals; occasionally there may be diarrhoea. In the female there may be irregular or abnormal oestrous cycles or complete anoestrus. In the male there is a lack of libido and hypogonadism.

The diagnosis is usually made on the basis of clinical signs and a laboratory evaluation. In general, the levels of tri-iodothyronine and thyroxine are estimated by radioimmune assay. It has already been pointed out that these may be affected by a variety of factors.

Treatment

Treatment consists of using a thyroid hormone replacement, liothyronine (L-tri-iodothyronine; Tertroxin), for the rest of the patient's life. The dose is usually determined on the basis of clinical response. Thus, an appropriate dose would be expected to alleviate the signs of obesity and skin disease and also to control the heart rate of the animal. An initial dose of 20 μg may be given 1–3 times daily to the average 15 kg dog. This may be increased or decreased according to the effects observed until the lowest effective dose is established. Liothyronine 20–30 μg is equivalent to 1–1.5 tablets of Thyroid BP (dry preparation).

Hyperthyroidism

Hyperthyroidism is also known as thyrotoxicosis. This condition is often associated with an enlarged thyroid gland (goitre), polydipsia, polyphagia, weight loss, weakness and fatigue. Sometimes there is a certain nervousness and tremor together with an intolerance of a hot environment. Occasionally there may be an absence of the oestrous cycle in unneutered bitches. In dogs (most commonly seen in the boxer) it is often associated with neoplasia of the thyroid but, in the cat, with hyperplasia. In the dog the thyroid neoplasm is usually malignant and spreads rapidly to the lungs. Thyroidectomy is the treatment of choice and is often curative in the cat. Propranolol (a β-blocker) is useful in controlling the tachycardia, especially prior to surgery. It is important to preserve the parathyroids at thyroidectomy.

Synthetic goitrogens such as propylthiouracil and the longer acting methimazole inhibit thyroid synthesis by blocking the iodine uptake by the gland (Figure 16.1). They have the effect of reducing the release of thyroxine from the thyroid gland. Thus, in the case of thyroid neoplasia these substances may be of some short-term beneficial effect since they will reduce the amount of thyroxine secreted by the thyroid neoplasm. They can also be used as a preoperative prophylactic against a thyroid crisis provoked by surgical trauma; adding potassium iodine to the diet for a week before surgery to normalize thyroid activity is preferable.

The parathyroid gland

The parathyroid gland secretes parathormone which is a protein with a molecular weight of about 8500 and affects calcium and phosphate metabolism in the body. It increases the rate of resorption of calcium and phosphate from bone and increases active absorption of calcium from the upper gastrointestinal tract. Further, it increases renal tubular absorption of calcium and excretion of phosphate. All these actions lead to an increase in the plasma calcium concentration. As the plasma calcium concentration rises, this leads to an inhibition of parathormone secretion. Parathormone is destroyed by the gut bacteria if it is administered orally. Following injection it has a plasma half-life of about 20 minutes.

Hyperparathyroidism

This condition is rare and is usually due to hyperplasia or tumour of the parathyroid gland. It causes a hypercalcaemia, bone cysts and renal calculi. Treatment is usually surgical (removal of the affected gland). It is also possible to treat the condition symptomatically by trying to control the hypercalcaemia. This may be achieved by promoting urinary excretion of calcium by the administration of frusemide 5 mg/kg initially and then 5 mg/kg/hr thereafter. Glucocorticoids may also be used since they will limit bone resorption and decrease the intestinal absorption of calcium. Further, they increase the kidney excretion of calcium. Sometimes there is a direct cytolytic effect on the tumour cells.

Hypoparathyroidism

This condition occurs infrequently but can arise as a result of accidental removal of the gland during thyroid surgery. Symptoms can be life threatening due to hypocalcaemia leading to tetany and convulsions. Treatment of this condition may be by parathormone but more rapid control is achieved by the intravenous administration of calcium and dihydrotachysterol vitamin D (intravenous 10% calcium borogluconate 0.5–1.0 ml/kg up to 10 ml total; in addition dihydrotachysterol 0.07–0.01 mg/kg administered orally, and daily). These can be continued for a period of two weeks to restore normal levels of calcium in the plasma.

The pancreas

Diabetes mellitus

This condition arises as a result of a deficiency in insulin production by the β cells of the pancreatic islets of Langerhans.

Insulin is a protein which has molecular weight of 6000 and is made up of two amino acid chains linked by disulphide bridges. It is produced in the β cells from a precursor protein known as proinsulin. The concentration of glucose in the blood which perfuses the pancreas directly controls the release of insulin. Other controlling factors include amino acid and fatty acid concentrations and the activity of the vagus nerve. Secretion can be inhibited by α-adrenergic actions of adrenaline and noradrenaline.

Insulin actions

Insulin causes a number of effects, mainly by acting on cell membranes. It dramatically influences the metabolism of carbohydrate and fat:

1. The blood sugar concentration is reduced by insulin since it increases the uptake of glucose and decreases hepatic release.
2. Insulin inhibits the uptake of amino acids into cells and stimulates their incorporation into proteins.
3. Insulin decreases the rate of fatty acid production from triglycerides.
4. It increases the cellular uptake of potassium.

Insulin is broken down in the body and has a half-life of about 20 minutes. It is secreted from the pancreas, which releases about 25% of its total insulin content each day, and is distributed throughout the extracellular fluid. It is excreted in the bile and urine and is reabsorbed from the kidney. The liver is the main organ responsible for its breakdown: 40% of the amount in the hepatic artery is extracted in a single passage through the liver.

The relationship between insulin and other hormones acting on carbohydrate metabolism is complex. Glucagon is another pancreatic hormone and is released from the α cells of the islets of Langerhans. It, too, responds to a fall in plasma glucose or free fatty acid concentrations. Glucagon decreases cellular glucose and free fatty acid uptake and increases gluconeogenesis. It raises the plasma glucose and free fatty acid levels and so tends to remove its own stimulus for release. It has the opposite effect to insulin.

Overproduction of insulin is rare and is occasionally associated with a secretory neoplasm in the pancreas. The symptoms of this include epilepsy due to hyperglycaemia:

treatment requires surgical removal of the neoplasm. Diazoxide can be used as a chemical substance which will suppress insulin production. Streptozotocin can accomplish a similar effect by permanently destroying the β cells; this drug is an antimitotic drug derived from *Streptomyces achromogenes*.

Underproduction of insulin leads to the condition known as diabetes mellitus. Two types of diabetes mellitus are recognized:

1. Type I or juvenile onset diabetes, seen when there is a low insulin level in the plasma and hyperglycaemia is present; most common in animals.
2. Type II diabetes characterized by normal or high insulin levels and hyperglycaemia. It corresponds to the human, maturity onset classification. In both conditions the plasma insulin level is unresponsive to changes in plasma glucose levels. It has occasionally been suggested that damage to the islet β cells by autoimmunity or overstimulation can lead to defective insulin secretion.

Signs of uncomplicated, insulin-dependent (type I) diabetes mellitus

Animals with this condition have a normal appetite and do not vomit or dehydrate. They appear well but have the characteristic polyuria and polydipsia, and sometimes associated weight loss. They may have a moderate ketonaemia or ketonuria. There is a hyperglycaemia and a glycosuria. There may be cataracts as well.

It is preferable to use an insulin preparation for treatment rather than oral hyperglycaemic drugs, which are rarely successful in controlling diabetes mellitus in dogs and cats. It is also important to control carbohydrate intake. This alone may be effective in very mild cases. In bitches ovariohysterectomy is often helpful. Chemical control of oestros should be undertaken with great care since progestogens (e.g. Ovarid) may aggravate the condition.

Insulin preparations (Table 16.1)

Insulin preparations have been obtained from the pancreas of cattle (Nuso) and pigs (Actrapid). More recently, human insulin has been obtained by recombinant DNA technology; it is expensive and has no theoretical advantage in the dog and cat. Insulin obtained from the pig, e.g. Actrapid, may be advan-

Table 16.1 Insulin preparations

Preparation	*Peak effect* (h)	*Duration of action* (h)
Short acting		
Soluble (Regular)	6–8	6–12
Actrapid	6–8	6–12
NUSO	6–8	6–12
Long acting		
Lente	6–12	24–30
Semilente	8–10	12–16
Ultralente	7–10	24–36
PZI	6–10	24–36
Isophane (NPH)	8–12	12–24
Globin zinc	8–12	18–24
Biphasic (Rapitard)	6–12	20–24

tageous in the dog since the amino acid sequences in the pig and the dog are the same. This means that the development of antibodies to insulin may be less likely to occur. The amino acid sequence of feline insulin is not known. A number of insulin preparations are available which have different durations of action (Table 16.1).

Soluble insulin (regular SI)
This is rapidly acting and will reduce blood sugar within 30 minutes. The peak of action of the soluble insulin occurs at about six hours. The duration of action is about twelve hours. Soluble insulin is used for emergency treatment of diabetic ketoacidosis; treatment of this condition requires intravenous administration of doses of up to 30 units at half to one hour intervals until the blood sugar is reduced to acceptable levels. Because of its rapid and short action its use is limited in veterinary practice to hospital situations.

Protamine zinc insulin (PZI)
This preparation is made of a combination of insulin with zinc chloride and protamine; protamine delays the absorption of insulin from the injection site. It should not be given with soluble insulin in the same syringe since the excess protamine present converts the soluble insulin into PZI. Its duration of action in the dog and the cat is usually shorter than in the human and lasts about 24 hours. The peak action of PZI occurs 6–10 hours after administration. The properties of PZI make it

suitable for a single daily injection so that many veterinary surgeons and owners find it a particularly satisfactory preparation for routine use.

Neutral protamine Hagedorn (NPH) insulin (isophane insulin)
This preparation is similar to PZI but there is not an excess of protein so it can be safely mixed with a soluble insulin preparation. Its duration of action in dogs is thought to be about 12 hours, rather than 24 hours as in the human: in the cat the duration of action is slightly less than 12 hours. This means that most dogs and cats will require two rather than one daily injection of NPH insulin. The peak onset of action for NPH insulin is quite variable so that it is not possible to predict when the lowest levels of blood glucose are likely to occur.

Dose
Insulin preparations are available in concentrations which are indicated as U-100 and U-500. This notation refers to the number of units per ml. It is unlikely that preparations with U-500 will be used in dogs and cats because they are too concentrated. The U-100 preparations are particularly easy to use because of the simplicity of the metric system.

An initial dose of PZI in the dog is suggested as 1 unit/kg body weight administered in the morning, once daily. If NPH is used, adequate control of the blood glucose levels will be achieved by twice-daily NPH insulin injections. The cat is more sensitive to insulin so that an initial dose of PZI should not be more than 0.5 unit/kg body weight. Normally a single daily injection of PZI is adequate for control of glucose.

Feeding and insulin administration routine

One approach which appears to be most convenient is to monitor the glucose in the urine in the morning and to follow this by feeding and the administration of the daily dose of PZI. In the evening the second meal, which contains half the calorific values, can be given. The blood glucose should be measured every morning. If small amounts of urinary glucose are detected it means that it is unlikely that there will be a hypoglycaemia throughout the day. If no glucose is detected in the urine, it may mean that at some period during the day the animal will be hypoglycaemic. Appropriate glucose levels to aim for in the urine are between 100 mg/100 ml to 250 mg/100 ml. If the urine glucose varies outwith this limit, then the dose of insulin may be increased or decreased by 5 or 10%.

It is normal to feed the animal twice a day, giving half of the calorific requirements in the morning and the remainder in the evening. If the animal's appetite is good in the morning, then the full insulin dose may be administered. If the animal refuses food in the morning, approximately one-half of the usual insulin dose may be given.

If NPH insulin is used, with administration twice daily, then similar concentrations of urine glucose can be aimed for.

Insulin-induced hyperglycaemia

This paradoxical effect occurs when the animal responds to an overdose of insulin and produces a hypoglycaemia, which causes the release of adrenaline and noradrenaline and a certain amount of glucagon. These combine to produce a rebound hyperglycaemia. This rebound hyperglycaemia often occurs in the evening and causes a glycosuria in the morning. It may lead the owner to increase the dose of insulin, which further aggravates the situation. In the end, signs of hypoglycaemia occur during the day.

Diabetic ketoacidosis

This condition is more serious and is characterized by an animal which is obviously ill and anorexic, as well as possessing ketones in the blood and urine. Sometimes the animal may be dehydrated. Animals may be dehydrated down to levels equivalent to 10–15% of their body weight; fluids should be administered intravenously. An isotonic fluid, such as lactated Ringer or 0.9% NaCl, is the preferred solution. Regular insulin (soluble insulin) should be administered to correct the diabetic ketoacidosis. A dose of 2 units of regular SI insulin for dogs under 10 kg and 0.25 unit/kg for dogs over 10 kg should be used. Afterwards a dose of 1 unit for dogs under 10 kg and 0.1 unit/kg for dogs over 10 kg of body weight can be administered hourly. Blood glucose concentrations should be determined hourly and administration of insulin ceased when the blood glucose level drops to between 200 and 250 mg/100 ml. Typically this occurs after 4 hours of starting the insulin therapy.

Secondary diabetes mellitus

This condition can follow several diabetogenic factors, e.g. excess progestogens, oestrogens, glucocorticoids, thyroxine, growth hormone and glucagon; the most common is following chronic administration of a potent progestogen like medroxy-progesterone acetate (e.g. Promone-E). The condition arises because progestogens stimulate an excessive release of growth hormone from the pituitary, giving rise to a peripheral insulin resistance. This peripheral insulin resistance is then followed by an ineffective hyperinsulinaemia and hyperglycaemia. In the early stages treatment is simple: the administration of the progestogens can be stopped. In bitches producing excessive progesterone from the ovary, ovariohysterectomy is effective. Thus in an old bitch, approximately 200 units of insulin per day may be required to control ketoacidosis before speying but the requirement for insulin may drop to zero within five days of the operation. However, in cases which have been untreated for a considerable time, the requirement for insulin may not drop to zero following the removal of the progestogen.

Oral hypoglycaemic drugs

These compounds reduce the plasma glucose concentration and are used in human practice for the treatment of maturity onset (type II) diabetes. They are not very effective in veterinary practice. A diagnosis of type II diabetes mellitus is infrequently made because the hyperglycaemia is insufficient to cause diuresis. Examples of these oral hypoglycaemic drugs include tolbutamide (Rastinon), chlorpropamide (Daonil) and metformin (Glucophage).

Hyperinsulinism

This condition is not common in small animal practice but has been observed in boxers and standard poodles. The clinical signs which arise from the hypoglycaemia consist of weakness, loss of balance, generalized seizures with some fainting and muscle fasciculation. This is provoked by events which further depress the blood glucose such as fasting, exercise or excitement. A diagnosis is made on the basis of the blood glucose concentration and a radioimmune assay of the insulin concentration. Treatment consists of controlling the hypergly-caemia by the intravenous administration of 50% dextrose solution to effect. It is also interesting that the CNS depressant and α_2-agonist xylazine at a dose of 1.1 mg/kg given intramuscularly may help, in that it suppresses the insulin release from normal β cells. Substances which are diabetogenic (diazoxide and streptozotocin) may be used for medical treatment of this condition. Diazoxide (10 mg/kg b.i.d. orally, up to 20 mg/kg b.i.d.) induces the release of insulin but may decrease in effectiveness over a period of months. Streptozotocin (14 mg/kg) may be given i.v. (by infusion pump over 1 hour) on two successive days every month.

Further reading

Allen, T. A. (1983) Canine hypoglycaemia. In *Current Veterinary Therapy VIII* (ed. R. W. Kirk), Saunders, Philadelphia, p. 845

Belshaw, B. G. and Rynberk, I. (1979) Radioimmunoassay of plasma T_4 and T_3 in the diagnosis of primary hypothyroidism in dogs. *Journal of the American Animal Hospital Association*, **15**, 17

Chew, D. J. and Meuten, D. J. (1982) Disorders of calcium and phosphorous metabolism. *Veterinary Clinics of North America*, **12**, 411

Church, D. B. (1983) Diabetes mellitus In *Current Veterinary Therapy VIII* (ed. R. W. Kirk), Saunders, Philadelphia, p. 838

Eigenmann, J. E. (1981) Diabetes mellitus in elderly female dogs: recent findings on pathogenesis and clinical implications. *Journal of the American Animal Hospital Association*, **17**, 805

Feldmann, E. C. and Nelson, R. W. (1982) Insulin-induced hypoglycaemia in diabetic dogs. *Journal of the American Veterinary Medical Association*, **180**, 1432

Kaneko, J. J. *et al.* (1978) Glucose tolerance and insulin response in diabetes mellitus of dogs. *Journal of Small Animal Clinical Practice*, **19**, 85

Lees, G. E. (1983) Hypoparathyroidism. In *Current Veterinary Therapy VIII* (ed. R. W. Kirk), Saunders, Philadelphia, p. 876

Milne, E. M. (1987) Diabetes mellitus. An update. *Journal of Small Animal Clinical Practice*, **28**, 727

Mulnix, J. A. (1983) Diabetes insipidus. *Current Veterinary Therapy VIII* (ed. R. W. Kirk), Saunders, Philadelphia, p. 850

Nelson, R. W. (1984) Use of insulin in small animal practice. *Journal of the American Veterinary Medical Association*, **185**, 105

Parker, W. M. and Scott, D. W. Growth hormone responsive alopecia in the mature dog: a discussion of 13 cases. *Journal of the American Animal Hospital Association*, **16**, 824

Chapter 17

The Eye

This chapter considers therapeutics of the eye. A brief description of the physiology of the eye is followed by a description of the pharmacology of therapeutic agents used for treatment of eye conditions. The final section in this chapter covers the therapeutic aspects of some specific conditions.

Aqueous humour production and accommodation

Figure 17.1a illustrates the production of aqueous humour in the eye. Aqueous humour is secreted by the epithelium of the ciliary body and passes round the pupil to the vessels of the trabecula.

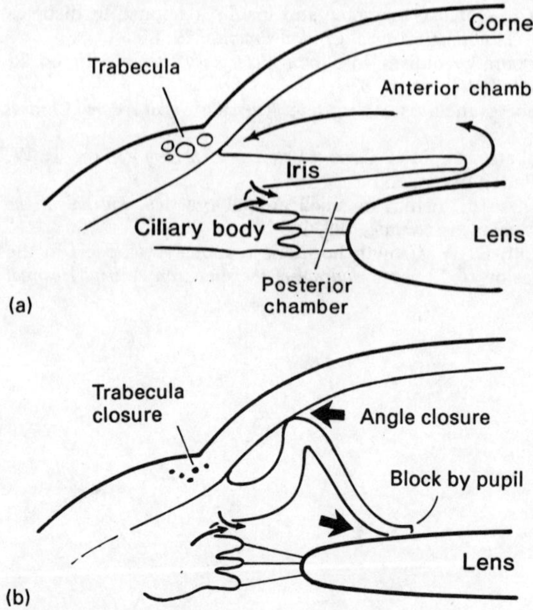

Figure 17.1 (a) The production and drainage of aqueous humour in the eye. (b) The effect of atropine can lead to reduced drainage and the production of narrow-angle glaucoma

Atropine relaxes the ciliary muscle and the lens focuses to a distance; in some animals it can lead to a rise in intraocular pressure. This is known as a narrow-angle glaucoma.

Normally acetylcholine, which is released from the oculomotor nerve, acts on muscarinic receptors in the ciliary body to produce relaxation of the muscle so that the lens becomes focused to a distance (cycloplegia). Constriction of the pupil is brought about in a reflex way if a bright light reaches the retina. Activity in the optic nerve gives rise to reflex activity in the oculomotor nerve. The pupillary light reflex is often used for diagnostic purposes.

The sympathetic nerve supply from the cranial cervical ganglion via the cervical sympathetic trunk reaches the pupil, where the release of adrenaline and/or noradrenaline brings about dilatation of the pupil (mydriasis). Stimulation of adrenoreceptors on the pupil with phenylephrine will produce dilatation of the pupil.

The sympathetic nerves which supply the ciliary body are believed to be limited to the vessels and epithelium of the ciliary processes. Stimulation of α-receptors will produce vasoconstriction in the ciliary body and reduce the production of aqueous humour. Stimulation of β-receptors will produce vasodilatation in the ciliary body and increase the rate of formation of aqueous humour, possibly giving rise to an increase in intraocular pressure. There are also adrenoreceptors localized in the tissue of the trabecula so that sympathomimetic amines and their antagonists can affect the drainage of the aqueous humour from the eye. The secretion of aqueous humour also involves the activity of the enzyme carbonic anhydrase which catalyses the formation of carbonic acid from CO_2 and water. If this enzyme is blocked with an inhibitor like acetazolamide, it reduces the rate of production of aqueous humour.

The actions of some drugs used for therapeutics of the eye

Pilocarpine (Isopto Carpine)

This compound is an alkaloid which has strong muscarinic and weak nicotinic actions. It will stimulate exocrine glands and increase tear production, as well as producing constriction of the pupil. A solution of pilocarpine (about 1%) is applied to the eye to reduce intraocular pressure during glaucoma; it is also used to reduce and antagonize the cycloplegia and mydriasis produced by drugs like atropine and tropicamide.

Physostigmine (eserine)

This drug inhibits cholinesterase, which is responsible for the breakdown of acetylcholine. It readily crosses the blood–brain barrier, and parenteral administration of large doses can give rise to depression of the respiratory centre. However, it is usually applied to the conjunctiva in a solution of 0.1–1% since it acts to produce pupillary constriction (miosis): this effect is beneficial in facilitating the drainage of aqueous humour in the treatment of certain types of glaucoma.

Ecothiopate (Phospholine)

This drug acts as a long-acting miotic. It is an organophosphorus compound which combines irreversibly with cholinesterases and potentiates the normal effects of acetylcholine. The drug acts on the ciliary muscles and causes contractions which pull on the trabecula and open up this structure, facilitating drainage of aqueous humour from the eye. It may produce a painful spasm of the ciliary muscle. A single application to the eye will lower intraocular pressure for about one week.

Demecarium (Tosmilen)

Chemically this drug is made from two molecules of neostigmine with a decamethylene chain interposed. It has an intermediate duration of action between those of physostigmine and ecothiophate. It is used as a long-acting miotic for glaucoma. It acts as an antagonist of cholinesterase.

Atropine sulphate

Atropine combines reversibly with muscarinic receptors which are found in a variety of tissues including the ciliary body and iris. Atropine antagonizes the efferent pathway in the parasympathetic nerve (oculomotor nerve) and inhibits the constriction of the pupil after exposure of the retina to bright light. It produces mydriasis and is accompanied by a marked rise in intraocular pressure in those animals which are predisposed towards narrow-angle glaucoma (Figure 17.1b). As a result of the action of atropine, the iris may block the filtration angle in the anterior chamber of the eye. The effects of atropine also relax the ciliary muscle so that the lens becomes focused for distant vision (cycloplegia) and accommodation stops.

Although atropine can be used to produce dilatation of the pupil and inhibition of accommodation, its effects may last for up to one week following topical application. Shorter-acting drugs are usually used, especially if there is a predisposition towards a narrow-angle glaucoma.

Tropicamide (Mydriacyl)

The pharmacological effects of tropicamide are very similar to those of atropine. The main difference is its shorter duration of action. If it is applied topically to the eye it produces a dilatation within about fifteen minutes and its effects last for only about eight hours. It is suitable for producing dilatation of the pupil for examination of the retina.

Carbonic anhydrase inhibitors

These act in a general way to inhibit the formation of carbonic acid (H_2CO_3) in the tissues. In the eye, this gives rise to a reduced rate of formation of aqueous humour and reduction in intraocular pressure. Other effects in the body include a reduction in the formation of gastric HCl, but only in excessive doses, and a metabolic acidosis from increased urinary excretion of sodium bicarbonate. The latter effect is usually associated with a transient diuresis lasting about seven hours.

Acetazolamide (Diamox)

This agent is active after oral or parenteral administration. Peak plasma levels are found within two hours of oral administration. Acetazolamide inhibits carbonic anhydrase-mediated movement of bicarbonate across membranes through the body and depresses aqueous humour secretion, as well as the formation of parotid saliva and pancreatic juices.

Dichlorphenamide (Daranide)

This agent is similar to acetazolamide except that it causes excretion of chloride as well as bicarbonate and is slightly more potent.

Drugs acting on adrenoreceptors

Adrenaline

Adrenaline can be instilled into the eye for the treatment of simple open-angle glaucoma; it is contraindicated in narrow-angle glaucoma since it is likely to produce a dilatation of the pupil and an increase in intraocular pressure. It is known from human studies that adrenaline may produce an increase (a β-effect) or a decrease (an α-effect) in the rate of production of aqueous humour, as well as a decrease in the resistance of the drainage pathway formed by the trabecula. Intraocular pressure will fall, providing the pupillary dilatation does not prevent the drainage of aqueous humour.

Timolol (Timoptol)

This drug is a β-antagonist and is about five times more potent than propranolol. It reduces the intraocular pressure without affecting the resistance of the drainage system at the trabecula. It is more potent in the cat in its action on intraocular pressure than it is in man. In man it is known that, if timolol is used for many months, there may develop a slowly increasing intraocular pressure as a result of the change in the nature of the adrenoreceptors controlling the formation of aqueous humour. Timolol has an advantage over propranolol in that it does not have a marked local anaesthetic effect. However timolol will inhibit tear production.

Guanethidine (Ismelin)

This drug acts in a distinctive way by inhibiting the release of noradrenaline from sympathetic nerve terminals. It acts to reduce the resistance to drainage at the trabecula. It can be used either alone or together with adrenaline for the treatment of open-angle glaucoma. An interesting action of guanethidine is that it increases the sensitivity of the effector cells in the eye which becomes supersensitive to adrenaline and noradrenaline.

Thymoxamine (Opilon)

This agent is an α-antagonist. It blocks the effect of sympathetic innervation to the pupil. It can be used to treat narrow-angle glaucoma and reverse the mydriasis produced by sympathomimetic amines. It has little action on ciliary muscles and does not produce any discomfort or restrict accommodation.

Phenylephrine

This agent acts as an α_1-agonist and has a biphasic effect (a rise followed by a fall) on intraocular pressure. It is not used for the treatment of glaucoma but it may be used to produce dilatation of the pupil.

Antibiotics for the eye

Topical application of antibiotics to the eye has to take into account the production of tears which wash the eye fairly frequently. Thus, drops may stay on the surface of the cornea for periods of less than twenty minutes; in fact, some may disappear within thirty seconds. Ointment formulations may remain longer, up to about an hour, in the conjunctival sac. When there is a purulent infection of the conjunctiva, eye drops have the advantage in that they will tend to wash the discharge and the mucus from the surface of the cornea. When there are penetrating lesions of the cornea and conjunctiva, ointment bases may enter the anterior chamber and perhaps produce an inflammatory lesion, further aggravating the condition. Drops are usually considered to be easier to administer by the owners and ideally should be instilled hourly. Table 17.1 summarizes some of the antibiotic preparations which are available for topical application to the eye.

Table 17.1 Topical preparations for the eye: antibacterials only

Generic name	*Product*
Chlortetracycline	Aureomycin Eye Ointment 1%
Chloramphenicol	Chloromycetin Ophthalmic Ointment 1%
Neomycin	Neobiotic Eye Ointment or Neomin Eye Drops
Miconazole, polymixin B and bacitracin	Oftentral Ointment
Cloxacillin	Orbenin Ophthalmic Ointment

The antibiotics which, if given systemically, are capable of crossing the blood–aqueous barrier and entering the eye in therapeutic concentrations are chloramphenicol, kanamycin, erythromycin and the sulphonamides. Sulphacetamide, which is not irritant, can be applied topically and will penetrate the globe.

Corticosteroids

Table 17.2 summarizes topical preparations which are available for the eye and which include antibiotics and glucocortico-

Table 17.2 Topical preparations for the eye: antibiotics plus steroids

Generic name	*Product*
Neomycin + betamethazone sodium phosphate	Betsolan Eye and Ear Drops
Chloramphenicol + hydrocortisone acetate	Chloromycetin Hydrocortisone Ophthalmic Ointment
Neomycin + hydrocortisone	Cortocaps or Neobiotic HC Drops 0.5%
Neomycin + thiostrepton + nystatin + triamcinolone	Panalog Ophthalmic Ointment
Neomycin + betamethazone 17-valerate	Vetsovate Eye and Ear Drops

steroids. The most potent corticosteroid preparation which is available is the one which contains betamethazone 17-valerate (Vetsovate). The preparation which contains betamethazone sodium phosphate has a medium potency corticosteroid (Betsolan eye and eardrops). The preparations which contain hydrocortisone contain still less potent corticosteroids.

Local anaesthetics

Table 17.3 summarizes the topical preparations available which contain local anaesthetics and antibiotics.

Table 17.3 Topical preparations for the eye: antibiotics and local anaesthetics

Generic name	*Product*
Sulphathiazole + amethocaine	Amethozol Ointment
Chloramphenicol, sulphacetamide, neomycin and lignocaine	Ophthaural Ointment

Artificial tears

Hypromellose (Isopto Alkaline; Isopto Plain; Liquifilm)

These agents are used for the treatment of conditions like keratoconjunctivitis sicca where there is an inadequate tear secretion. They are used to lubricate and protect the cornea.

Mucolytics

N-acetylcysteine (20%)

N-acetylcysteine at a concentration of 20% acts to produce a breakdown of the thick mucus which may be present over the cornea in keratoconjunctivitis sicca. An alternative approach is to use bromhexine (Bisolvon) which may be administered by injection and acts as a mucolytic.

Fluorescein

Fluorescein is used as a diagnostic stain to detect the presence of corneal ulceration and blockage of the nasolacrimal duct. It is available as a solution of sodium fluorescein or Fluorets strips as disposable strips.

Antiviral agents

Idoxuridine (Kerecid; Dandrid)

Idoxuridine acts to inhibit thymidylic phosphorylase and the specific DNA polymerase necessary for the synthesis of viral DNA. As a result it will inhibit the multiplication of DNA viruses like herpes. It is applied as an ointment five times daily for periods up to 30 days; it is characterized by poor corneal penetration.

Antifungal agents

Amphotericin B

This drug has broad antifungal activity but does not penetrate the cornea particularly well.

Pimaricin (Natamycin)

A 5% suspension is available for topical ocular use. It is a polyene antibiotic which acts to form an ionophore in the membranes of susceptible fungi. It therefore has a good spectrum of activity but has poor penetration powers.

Muconazole (in Oftentral)

Muconazole is benzimidazole-like and has antifungal and antiyeast actions.

Antiallergic preparations

Sodium cromoglycate (Opticrom)

This drug has a remarkable ability to prevent degranulation of mast cells; thus this preparation, applied as eye drops, will prevent and control conditions like hay fever if applied regularly.

Antazoline (Antistin)

This agent is available in a 0.5% solution for installation in the eye or in tablets of 100 and 200 mg. It has potent H_1 antagonistic actions and is used to control hay fever-like conditions.

Xylometazoline (Octrivine)

This drug is an α-agonist and, applied as a 0.1% solution, acts to produce local vasoconstriction. It may be used in combination with antazoline (Octrivine-Antistin drops).

Therapeutic aspects of some conditions of the eye

Lagophthalmos

This condition arises as a result of an inability of the animal to close an eyelid in some exophthalmic breeds, for example the Pekingese. Treatment may consist of administration of artificial tears (Liquifilm; Isopto Alkaline). Following administration these usually last at least 30 minutes. Surgery is usually required subsequently and may involve shortening of the palpebral fissure at the lateral canthus.

Conjunctivitis

This condition is one of the more common syndromes treated in small animal practice and may arise as a result of:

1. Bacterial infection producing a purulent discharge; this often has an initiating cause like a foreign body or some disturbance in the eyelid.
2. Viral conjunctivitis, which is usually seen in both eyes and is part of a systemic disease like feline herpesvirus or canine adenovirus.
3. Mycoplasma infection in the conjunctiva. This produces a pseudomembrane formation on the conjunctiva.

4. Chlamydia infection which usually causes a conjunctivitis more severe than the other types and produces follicular development after several days.
5. Mycotic conjunctivitis which is often associated with keratitis.
6. An allergic reaction in the conjunctiva.
7. Decreased tear production.

Treatment is aimed at correcting and controlling the underlying causes of the conjunctivitis. For example, it is necessary to remove and eliminate any foreign body from the eye before treatment can be successful. The eye should be cleaned thoroughly for examination and regularly to keep the animal comfortable. Antibiotics are often chosen empirically but generally they are not administered systemically but applied topically. Ointments have one advantage in that, compared with drops, they can be applied with longer intervals between applications. Corticosteroids may be used in combination with the antibacterial agent to reduce the inflammatory response; they should not be used if there is any evidence of corneal ulceration. To establish whether this is present, fluroescein should be used to detect the presence of any ulcer. Obviously irritant and allergic conjunctivitis will respond well to glucocorticoid therapy incorporated into the treatment schedule. This often affects the palpebral conjunctiva and the outer surface of the third eye lid. It can be treated by bursting the follicles with cottonwool on mosquito forceps followed by antibiotic ointment for 5–7 days.

Wet eye (epiphora)

Again, this is a frequently occurring condition seen in the dog. A rust-coloured tear streak with wetting of the hair on the cheek, sometimes associated with dermatitis, is produced when there is an overproduction of tears or inadequate drainage. Fluorescein instilled into the eye with subsequent examination of the patency of the nasolacrimal duct is required. If the duct appears to be blocked, it may be flushed under general anaesthesia, possibly with probing with a dilator. Causes of overproduction of tears must also be investigated. These may include entropion, conjunctivitis, etc. If no underlying cause can be determined, oral tetracycline (50 mg/day) will minimize the staining effect but will not affect the overproduction of tears.

Dry eye (keratoconjunctivitis sicca)

This condition may occur unilaterally or bilaterally in the dog. It is characterized by tacky and profuse mucoid ocular discharges, together with a reddened conjunctiva, alteration of vascularization and, sometimes, pigmentation and opacity of the cornea. There is also a reduction in the movement of the eyelid and a narrowed palpebral fissure and dry nostrils. Eventually blindness will ensue if this condition is untreated. A diagnosis can be confirmed using the Schirmer tear test with 5 ml/minute being diagnostic and above 15 ml/minute considered normal. Although a majority of cases arise through unknown mechanisms it is known that distemper, trauma and sometimes sulphonamide drugs will give rise to this condition. Treatment normally consists of an appropriate combination of the following:

1. Applying artificial tears as often as possible but at least four times a day (Liquifilm; Isopto Plain; Isopto Alkaline). At night, ointments may be used if application of artificial tears is not possible.
2. Natural secretion of tears may be stimulated by the application of topical pylocarpine (Isopto Carpine). Oral pylocarpine (pylocarpine nitrate 2%) may be added to the food at a dose rate of 1–4 drops; care is taken to avoid the side-effects of muscarinic stimulation which include vomiting, salivation and diarrhoea.
3. Any infection which might be present can be controlled with the administration of a broad spectrum antibiotic solution.
4. Acetylcysteine (5%) in artificial tears will act as a mucolytic and help to keep the tears more liquid.
5. Subconjunctival or topical steroids may be used if there is an excessive vascularization or corneal epithelialization.

Medical treatment may be useful in controlling the condition for some time. However, usually the disease progresses so that it is necessary to carry out a parotid duct transposition to act as a source of tears. Despite this, artificial tears may still be required, even if the transplant is successful.

Keratitis

Inflammation of the cornea is common in small animal practice. There is a variety of causes including bacteria, viruses and fungi. Certain breeds of dog show specific types of keratitis;

brachycephalic breeds are more prone to keratitis than other types. The signs consist of vascularization, sometimes corneal opacity, pigmentation, blepharospasm, lacrimation and photophobia. Superficial vascularization is characterized by tree-like branching of the blood vessels in the cornea. Deep vascularization appears as straight, brush-like vessels in the corneal stroma and is sometimes accompanied by oedema. In general, the treatment consists of controlling and removing the aetiological agents; antibiotics and corticosteroids are often applied topically to control bacteria and excessive vascularization.

Chronic superficial keratitis (pannus)

This condition occurs mostly in German shepherd dogs of 3–6 years of age. In most cases the temporal quadrant is affected; it is usually bilateral but not necessarily symmetrical. The condition arises because of the invasion of blood vessels and mononuclear cells into the corneal stroma. After some time pigmentation may follow so that a grey band is often present in the stroma adjacent to the advancing edge of the lesion.

Treatment is symptomatic since the cause is not known. It usually consists of controlling the inflammation by the administration of topical ophthalmic steroids or subconjunctival administration of long-acting steroid preparations (Depomedrone).

Mycotic keratitis

This condition is due to fungi, like aspergillus or fusarium, producing white plaques in the cornea with marked deep vascularization thereof. Often there are satellite lesions in the cornea. The condition is refractory to normal antibacterial chemotherapy and is often chronic. Treatment consists of the topical administration of amphotericin B, pimaracin or miconazole (Oftentral) every four hours for two days and then twice daily. Prolonged treatment for up to six weeks is often required.

Herpes keratitis (feline)

This condition, seen in cats, is characterized by a seromucoid discharge with conjunctivitis and superficial vascularization of the cornea. Sometimes there is mild corneal oedema. Often there are superficial ulcers in the cornea which have a characteristic branching pattern; usually this is a sufficient finding on which to base the diagnosis.

Treatment normally consists of the topical application of antiviral drugs like idoxuridine (Kerecid), using one drop every four hours for two days and subsequently four times a day. Treatment should continue for about 14 days to allow re-epithelialization of the cornea. Any purulent discharge which may be present indicates the action of bacteria which should be controlled with a broad spectrum antibiotic in addition to the antiviral therapy.

Corneal ulceration

A variety of causes including bacterial, viral and fungal infections, together with distichiasis, ectopic cilia, entropion, foreign bodies, trauma, etc. may give rise to ulceration of the cornea. The condition is characterized by the presence of blepharospasm, ocular discharge, conjunctivitis and local corneal opacity. A diagnosis is usually made after an examination of the clinical signs in the history, together with the application of the fluorescein stain (retention) test. An ulcer will retain the stain. A very deep ulcer (Descemet's) will not usually retain the stain; it is a serious sign indicating potential rupture of the cornea. Treatment usually consists of the topical application of the broad spectrum antibiotics to control any bacterial infection. Corticosteroids are contraindicated in most cases since they may inhibit healing. Pain may be relieved by the application of cycloplegic drugs (atropine sulphate 0.5–1%) topically if there is an accompanying anterior uveitis. Chemical cautery with phenol and the removal of epithelial debris from the edge of the ulcer may facilitate and stimulate healing.

Corneal oedema in association with canine adenovirus type 1

This condition known as 'blue eye' is seen in a small number of dogs recovering from infectious canine hepatitis. In many cases the cornea will clear without treatment but prolonged and severe cases may lead to a bullous keratopathy with small vesicles of fluid appearing in the corneal epithelium. Normally, treatment is directed at controlling the anterior uveitis using atropine and glucocorticoids. Sometimes a secondary glaucoma develops so that atropine and the steroids should be discontinued. Artificial tears applied topically may be useful in some cases to help clear the corneal oedema.

Anterior uveitis

The cause of this condition is usually unknown; almost any injury will cause uveal inflammation. The condition is inflammation of the iris and ciliary body (cyclitis) and is synonymous with iridocyclitis. It is characterized by the clinical signs of pain, visual loss, photophobia, inflammation and swelling of the iris, together with the presence of inflammatory material in the aqueous humour. Treatment is usually aimed at controlling the inflammation to minimize damage. Thus corticosteroids are often given, either as drops or injected subconjunctively. If there is also a corneal ulceration, where corticosteroids may be contraindicated, non-steroidal anti-inflammatory drugs may be used (oxphenbutazone; Tanderil ointment). Atropine sulphate applied topically in concentrations of 1 or 2% is also of value in controlling the pain associated with the irideitis and preventing development of synechiae and subsequent glaucoma. Unfortunately atropine is less effective as a mydriatic in the inflamed eye so that its frequency of application must be increased according to the severity of the condition, the aim being to maintain a dilated pupil.

Glaucoma

Medical treatment of glaucoma is really only appropriate for the early and acute stages of glaucoma. Chronic glaucoma due to long-standing increases in intraocular pressure, with irreversible damage, is not susceptible to medical treatment.

Treatment using medicines must begin as soon as the diagnosis of glaucoma is made. The general aim of the therapy is to open the drainage angle of the pupil using miotic agents as well as to decrease the production of aqueous humour. Treatment consists of a combination of the following approaches:

1. Intravenous mannitol as a 20% solution; a dose of 2.5 ml given once only. Water must be withheld for the first few hours after administration.
2. Pilocarpine as a cholinergic agent at a concentration of about 2% is given topically every hour until the pupil constricts; thereafter it is applied three times a day.
3. Potent anticholinesterase drugs like demecarium (Tosmilen) and ecothiopate (Phospholine). These drugs are administered topically in sufficient quantities to produce constriction of the pupil.

4. Carbonic anhydrase inhibitors which act to decrease the formation of aqueous humour by producing a localized acidosis may be given in the form of intravenous acetazolamide at a dose rate of 50 mg/kg once only, or acetazolamide at a dose rate of 7 mg/kg orally three times a day. Alternatively, dichlorphenamide at a dose rate of 2–5 mg/kg orally can be given three times a day. It may be necessary to adjust individual doses to balance the effects of production of aqueous secretion with the side-effects of vomiting and panting.
5. Autonomic blocking agents which include the β-antagonist timolol (Timoptic) and the α-antagonist thymoxamine may be applied topically twice a day.

Once the acute glaucoma has been controlled medically, long-term therapy may be required and frequent reassessment of the animal is necessary. Despite this, however, long-term control of glaucoma is not usually achievable medically in animals. Surgical procedures may be necessary.

Central retinal degeneration in the cat

This condition in the cat arises as a result of taurine deficiency and is seen in cats fed on low quality dog food. The condition is characterized by changes which begin in the central area as small but well-defined increases in granularity and reflectivity and then progress to an area dorsal to the optic disc. The condition will lead to complete retinal degeneration if the diet remains unchanged. A taurine-rich diet which includes fish will stop the progression of the disease but may not correct the existing condition.

Further reading

Gelatt, K. N. (ed.) (1981) *Textbook of Veterinary Ophthalmology*, Lea and Febiger, Philadelphia

Marlin, C. L. (1983) Ophthalmic diseases. In *Current Veterinary Therapy VIII* (ed. R. W. Kirk), Saunders, Philadelphia, p. 530

Potter, D. E. (1981) Adrenergic pharmacology of aqueous humour dynamics. *Pharmacological Reviews*, **33**, 133–153

Chapter 18

Cancer Chemotherapy

Cancer chemotherapy is still a developing field in veterinary science. It is the intention of this chapter to introduce the principles of cancer chemotherapy and to describe the actions and doses of drugs which may be used. Finally, there is a section on the therapy of some specific conditions to illustrate the therapeutic approach.

Chemotherapy is one approach

Cancer was originally treated only by surgical methods: currently, in human practice, surgery is used together with a variety of other supportive therapeutic approaches. These include radiation therapy and chemotherapy. In most veterinary circumstances radiation therapy is not available.

Chemotherapy remains the best method of controlling disseminated cancers; however, it is important to explain to the owner that most drugs used for chemotherapy are toxic to the animal as well as being of therapeutic use. It is the quality of the animal's life that is most important: it is the toxic side-effects of anticancer drugs that limit their capacity to kill cancer cells in the host. Most owners of pets will prefer euthanasia and will only accept limited toxic actions of chemotherapeutic agents. It is important to keep these to a minimum.

The cell cycle

Neoplastic cells may be (1) dividing actively and therefore highly malignant, (2) in a temporary non-dividing stage, or (3) may have differentiated and reached the end stage or non-dividing condition.

The ability of various anticancer drugs to attack these stages varies; it is the actively dividing cells against which cancer chemotherapy is most effective.

During cell division the cell cycle (Figure 18.1) consists of:

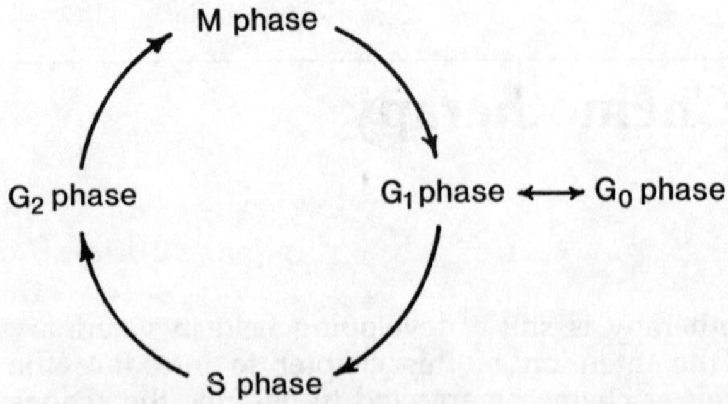

Figure 18.1 The cell cycle during division

1. Mitosis (the M phase; lasts 60 minutes).
2. Gap 1 (the G_1 phase of protein and RNA synthesis; lasts days to weeks).
3. Gap 0 (the G_0 phase; a resting phase that cells can enter from G_1).
4. Synthesis (the S phase; a phase of DNA synthesis lasting hours).
5. Gap 2 (the G_2 phase; a period of tubulin synthesis just before mitosis).

Site of action of chemotherapeutic agents

Therapy consists of attacking one or more of these stages. For example, vinblastine and vincristine attack the G_2 stage during the period of synthesis of tubulin. Alkylating agents (cyclophosphamide, chlorambucil) can react with many enzymes and cell constituents but probably the most sensitive stage is the S phase, during DNA synthesis. The alkylating agents form cross-linkages between the DNA strands and prevent them splitting for replication. Thus DNA strands cannot divide for new DNA synthesis. Alkylating agents affect many cells but cells where replication is occurring rapidly are the most sensitive. Slowly dividing cells may be able to repair the DNA which is damaged by the alkylating agent.

Combination of agents

Successful chemotherapy often involves the combination of several chemotherapeutic agents designed to minimize the toxicity and maximize the killing of cancer cells. Chemotherapy can produce symptomatic cures for varying periods. They do not usually produce a lasting clinical cure.

Chemotherapeutic agents

Calculation of doses

Most anti-cancer drugs are potentially very toxic. It is best to calculate the dose of drug on the basis of body surface area rather than weight. The doses are given are for body surface area in square metres (m^2). The body surface area can be estimated from body weight using Table 18.1.

Table 18.1 Conversion of body weight (kg) to body surface area (m^2) for the dog

kg	*m^2*	*kg*	*m^2*	*kg*	*m^2*	*kg*	*m^2*
1	0.10	13	0.55	25	0.85	37	1.11
2	0.15	14	0.58	26	0.88	38	1.13
3	0.20	15	0.60	27	0.90	39	1.15
4	0.25	16	0.63	28	0.92	40	1.17
5	0.29	17	0.66	29	0.94	41	1.19
6	0.33	18	0.69	30	0.96	42	1.21
7	0.36	19	0.71	31	0.99	43	1.23
8	0.40	20	0.74	32	1.01	44	1.25
9	0.43	21	0.76	33	1.03	45	1.26
10	0.46	22	0.78	34	1.05	46	1.28
11	0.49	23	0.81	35	1.07	47	1.30
12	0.52	24	0.83	36	1.09	48	1.32

Cyclophosphamide (Endoxan)

Cyclophosphamide is a widely used alkylating agent. It is a prodrug and has to undergo activation in the liver; it accumulates gradually in the kidneys, liver and spleen. The dog is not able to tolerate large doses, so it is usual to give small amounts on a continuous low-dose basis. The toxic effects of cyclophosphamide include leucopenia, anaemia, thrombocytopenia (not very common), liver and kidney toxicity, together with gastrointestinal ulceration, alopecia and cardiotoxicity at particularly high dose levels. One other noted effect of cyclophosphamide arises as a result of the excretion of the unchanged drug in the urine; this can give rise to haemorrhagic cystitis with particularly nasty ulceration of the bladder wall.

N-acetylcysteine has been shown to prevent development of cyclophosphamide-induced cystitis in animals under experimental conditions. However, the safest approach is to discontinue cyclophosphamide treatment as soon as any of these signs of toxicity appear.

Dose
50 mg/m^2 orally for four days/week or 200 mg/m^2 intravenously given once weekly.

Uses
Cyclophosphamide can be used for the treatment of lymphoreticular neoplasia, lung and mammary carcinomas, and a variety of sarcomas.

Chlorambucil (Leukeran)

This agent may be used as an alternative to cyclophosphamide if haemorrhagic cystitis has occurred. It does not appear to be as effective as cyclophosphamide on its own but recent evidence suggests that larger doses may be more effective if given in combination with prednisolone. The toxic effects include mild leucopenia, anaemia, thrombocytopenia, occasionally vomiting and nausea.

Dose
2 mg/m^2 orally for 2–4 days/week.

Uses
Lymphoreticular neoplasia and chronic lymphocytic leukaemia.

Triethylene thiophosphoramide (Thiotepa)

This drug has been used as a 0.3% solution applied directly into the bladder (instillation) for the treatment of carcinoma; systemic toxicity is minimized when the drug is applied topically in this manner. Toxicity consists of leucopenia and thrombocytopenia, as well as anaemia.

Dose
9 mg/m^2 as a single dose or divided over 2–4 days or for installation as a 0.3% solution in the bladder for 30 minutes/week.

Uses
Various carcinomas and sarcomas.

Melphalan (Alkeran)

This drug may be used for the treatment of multiple myeloma, lymphoreticular neoplasia and monoclonal gammopathies.

Dose
1.5 mg/m^2 orally for seven days and repeated every three weeks.

Antimetabolites

Antimetabolites resemble natural substrates of the body and block specific enzymes by competing with their receptor sites; some are DNA or RNA analogues and block DNA or RNA synthesis.

Methotrexate (Amethoptrin)

This is a widely used antimetabolite. It acts by competing with the site for folic acid on the enzyme which converts folic acid to folinic acid. Folinic acid is essential for the synthesis of DNA and RNA.

The prime organ for methotrexate toxicity is the bone marrow; the red blood cells, white blood cells and thrombocytes are depressed in number. Additional toxic signs include gastrointestinal ulceration and liver damage. Vomiting may also be a problem. However, it is possible to reverse some of the toxic effects of methotrexate by the administration of a high dose of folinic acid. Thus methotrexate may be given to kill tumour cells in the G_1/S phase and then folinic acid given to minimize the depression of the bone marrow.

Dose
Doses between 0.5 and 2.5 mg/m^2 body weight have been suggested for daily oral administration. However, methotrexate is particularly toxic in the dog (greater than in man). Methotrexate may be given on a continuous low-dose basis, alternating treatment with cyclophosphamide. An example is to use cyclophosphamide or methotrexate for one month and then alternate with the other agent, maintaining therapy for a total of four months. It is suggested that a period of two months may be allowed for rest and a repeat of the dose cycle being given subsequently.

Cytosine arabinoside (Cytosar)

This drug is an antimetabolite which acts by inhibiting the enzyme DNA polymerase. It has been used on veterinary animals, in combination with cyclophosphamide, vincristine and prednisolone, for the treatment of canine lymphosarcoma and mast cell tumours.

Dose
100 mg/m^2 subcutaneously or as an intravenous drip over four days. Toxic symptoms include the usual depression of white and red blood cells together with nausea, vomiting and anorexia.

5-Fluorouracil (Flouro-uracil; Efudix cream)

This drug inhibits the synthesis of thymidylic acid. In dogs and cats it often produces severe CNS side-effects, including convulsions. However, a cream for topical application is available.

Dose
200 mg/m^2 intravenously weekly for the treatment of various sarcomas and carcinomas. The cream is applied topically twice weekly for two to four weeks for the treatment of cutaneous tumours.

Antitumour antibiotics

Actinomycin D (Cosmegen)

This drug is particularly toxic to dogs and cats, producing thrombocytopenia, leukaemia and vomiting. It is suggested that a dose of 1.5 mg/m^2 may be administered intravenously weekly for the treatment of various carcinomas and sarcomas, as well as lymphosarcoma. However, this agent may be too toxic to use. It is often used for experimental studies on antitumour drug actions since it acts by mixing with the DNA helix and inhibiting RNA synthesis.

Doxorubicin (Adinamycin)

This compound is an antibiotic isolated from *Streptomyces peucetius*. It has been used successfully in the human field for the treatment of lymphoreticular neoplasia and is particularly effective against solid tumours of soft tissues, including sarcomas and adenocarcinomas. It acts by placing itself between base pairs of DNA strands and disrupting the helical structure of DNA. Thus RNA synthesis is impaired. It is particularly well bound to the DNA of the heart and this accounts for its myocardial toxicity. This drug possesses the common toxic effects of other cancer chemotherapeutic agents, including suppression of the bone marrow and white blood cells.

Dose

30 mg/m^2 given intravenously once every three weeks. A total dose of 240 mg/m^2 should not be exceeded. This approach minimizes toxic symptoms. The drug is claimed to be most effective when given intralesionally in isolated tumour nodules in man and this approach may be worth trying in animals.

Uses

Lymphosarcoma, carcinoma and osteogenic sarcoma.

Bleomycin (Blenoxane)

A variety of cancers which occur in the skin and lung, as well as other malignant tumours, are effective in their ability to synthesize peptidase enzymes. As a result, complex antibiotics like bleomycin will accumulate in these tissues and in tumour sites. Squamous cell carcinomas are particularly likely to concentrate bleomycin so that this is one of the chief indications in man. It is also useful for the treatment of lymphoreticular malignancies.

Bleomycin has a minimal suppressive effect on the bone marrow, a feature of particular note. At high doses it will cause cutaneous and pulmonary fibrosis. It may cause allergic reactions since it is a polypeptide antibiotic. The action of bleomycin is to inhibit the passage of cells through the G_2/M phase of the cell cycle. Thus, because the drug acts in this way, it may be most effective if given on a continuous low-dose basis.

Dose

Suggested dosages are 10 mg/m^2 intravenously or subcutaneously for 3–9 days followed by 10 mg/m^2 intravenously given weekly. A total dose of 200 mg/m^2 should not be exceeded.

Plant alkaloids

Vinca alkaloids

The drug vincristine (Oncovin) and vinblastine (Velban) are jointly known as the vinca alkaloids. These compounds have been extracted from the periwinkle plant. Their site of action is on the protein tubulin which is involved in separating the chromosomes during mitosis in metaphase.

The main toxic effect of vinblastine is depression of the bone marrow which limits the dose which may be administered. Vincristine is less likely to produce bone marrow depression but more likely to produce a peripheral neuropathy, paraesthesia and constipation.

Dose

Vincristine 0.5 mg/m^2 intravenously weekly. Vinblastine 2.5 mg/m^2 intravenously weekly.

Uses

Vincristine: the treatment of transmissible venereal tumours and lymphosarcoma. Vinblastine: the treatment of a variety of carcinomas and lymphosarcoma.

Hormones

Prednisolone

Prednisolone will depress division of a variety of white blood cells. It is therefore useful for the treatment of lymphoreticular neoplasia, mast cell tumours and, rather interestingly, CNS tumours. Toxic effects include hyperadrenocorticism and secondary adrenocortical insufficiency.

Dose

This varies tremendously; 20 mg/m^2 orally every second day or up to 60 mg/m^2 orally daily.

Diethylstilboestrol

This is useful for the treatment of perianal adenoma or prostatic neoplasia. It acts by suppressing androgen stimulation.

Dose

1.0 mg/kg intramuscularly as a single dose but do not administer more than 25 mg every three days. Possible toxic effects include suppression of the bone marrow and femininization.

Some specific conditions

Canine lymphosarcoma

This condition should still be regarded as terminal but it is possible to obtain remission. One recommended therapy for the multicentric form is:

Week 1

1. Prednisolone 40 mg/m^2 orally/day.
2. Days 1–4 cyclophosphamide 50 mg/m^2 orally on each day.
3. Cytosine arabinoside 100 mg/m^2 by slow intravenous drip or subcutaneously on each of days 1–4.
4. Vincristine 0.5 mg intravenously on day 1 only.

Weeks 2–8

1. Prednisolone 20 mg/m^2 once every other day.
2. Cyclophosphamide and vincristine as in week 1.

If remission has been obtained after eight weeks, maintenance may be obtained with prednisolone at a dose of 20 mg/m^2 once every other day and with chlorambucil at a dose rate of 2 mg/m^2 orally on days 1–4 each week and continued until relapse. Other forms of canine lymphosarcoma, such as the alimentary, cutaneous and renal forms, do not appear to be as responsive as the multicentric forms. It is pointed out that this combination of therapeutic agents may produce suppression of the white and red blood cells. It is important that these should be monitored throughout treatment. It may be possible to produce remissions so that the animal may last for approximately one year. Without treatment survival is limited to about 4–6 weeks.

Mast cell tumours

Canine mast cell tumours may be treated with prednisolone as the single agent and it is suggested that a dose of 60 mg/m^2 is given once daily for two weeks and that this is followed by a dose of 30 mg/m^2 once daily for a further two weeks. This is then followed by a dose of 30 mg/m^2 once every other day for five months. The dose is then tapered off. The feline form of mast cell tumour does not respond well to chemotherapy. In addition to the administration of prednisolone, it maybe useful, if there is a rapid destruction of the mast cell tumours, to counteract the effects of histamine release. Any gastrointestinal signs may be countered using the agent cimetidine (Tagamet, an H_2 blocker) at a dose rate of 5–10 mg/kg three times daily.

Multiple myelomas

The aim of treatment here is to reduce the viscosity of the serum proteins. One recommended therapy is to use melphalan at a dose rate of 1.5 mg/m^2 orally, administered daily for seven days and repeated every three weeks. Usually toxic effects of melphalan are as a result of the leucopenia. This limits the maximum dose which may be given. Survival times of approximately one year have been reported following this treatment schedule.

Venereal tumours (transmissible)

Venereal tumours of the transmissible variety may be cured using chemotherapy. Recommended therapy includes vincristine at a dose rate of 0.5 mg/m^2 intravenously every seven days until there is no sign of disease. This usually requires five treatments. The prognosis for the complete elimination of the venereal tumour of the transmissible type is good.

Mammary tumours

A common tumour in dogs and cats. Epidemiological evidence of canine and feline tumours suggests the presence in some tumours of oestrogen receptors. Ovariectomy before two years of age provides protection against mammary neoplasia in bitches and queens. Ovariectomy at mastectomy has no beneficial effect on survival. Pseudopregnancy in bitches is not related to tumour production. The growth rate of mammary tumours increases during oestrus in bitches.

Further reading

Bostock, D. E. and Owen, L. N. (1972) Chemotherapy of canine and feline neoplasia. *Journal of Small Animal Practice*, **13**, 359

Cohen, H. *et al.* (1975) Combination chemotherapy with vincristine, vinblastine and prednisolone. *American Journal of Veterinary Research*, **36**, 1483

Hamilton, J. M., Else, R. W. and Foreshaw, P. (1977) Oestrogen receptors in canine mammary tumours. *Veterinary Research*, **101**, 258

Pedersen, N. C. (1980) Feline leukaemia virus disease complex. In *Current Veterinary Therapy VII* (ed. R. W. Kirk), Saunders, Philadelphia

Rosenthal, R. C. (1985) Chemotherapy of neoplastic diseases. In *Handbook of Small Animal Therapeutics* (ed. L. E. David), Churchill Livingstone, New York, Edinburgh, London and Melbourne, p. 175

Chapter 19

Vitamins and Minerals

Vitamins and minerals are important in small animal practice for two reasons:

1. Deficiency or an excess gives rise to a number of clinical syndromes.
2. Pet health products in the form of vitamins and minerals are being sold in an increasing amount in small animal practice.

This chapter considers vitamins and some minerals together with deficiency syndromes and the products which may be used to treat those syndromes (Table 19.1).

Vitamin A

Vitamin A_1 (retinol) and vitamin A_2 (3-dehydroretinol) are carotenes. They are found in many fish-liver oils as well as green vegetables and carrots. One of their main functions is in the rods of the retina in the eye. An early symptom of vitamin A deficiency is night blindness. Other roles of vitamin A are less well defined but it seems to be needed for the formation of mucus-secreting cells which synthesize glycoproteins. In vitamin A deficiency there is a hyperkeratinization, xerophthalmia (dryness of the conjunctiva followed by hyperkeratinization), squamous metaplasia of the mucosa of the respiratory tract, bone deformities, retarded growth and impairment of reproductive activity. Deficiency of vitamin A is unlikely in animals fed on conventional diets. However, animals fed exclusively on dried carbohydrate foodstuffs may develop low levels. As a result the cerebrospinal fluid (CSF) pressure rises and low liver and plasma vitamin A levels are found.

Hypervitaminosis A (cervical spondylitis)

This condition is seen in cats which have been exclusively fed on liver and other vitamin A rich sources. As a result extra bone is laid down, particularly in the cervical regions of the neck; this leads to a spondylitis. In addition, extra bone may be laid down

Table 19.1 Vitamin preparations

Abidec capsules	
Vit A	4000 units
Vit B_1	1 mg
Vit B_2	1 mg
Vit B_6	0.5 mg
Vit C	15 mg
Vit D	400 mg
Nicotinamide	10 mg
Dose: 1 daily	
Also Abidec drops	
Biotin tablets	
Biotin	50 µg
Dose: 2 tablets twice daily for 3 days, then 1 tablet twice weekly	
Collo-Cal D	
Colloidal calcium oleate	0.75% w/v
Vit D	70 IU/ml
Uses: osteomalacia, rickets, lactation tetany	
Dose: dogs 1 ml/2 kg	
Jectadine	
Vit A	50 000 units/ml
Vit D_3	25 000 units/ml
Vit E	20 units/ml
Dose: dogs 0.5–4 ml; cats 0.5–2 ml	
Norderm	
Linoleic acid	365.5 mg/ml
Linolenic acid	55 mg/ml
Arachidonic acid	29 mg/ml
Oleic, palmitoleic and clupanodonic acid	280 mg/ml
Lecithins	10.8 mg/ml
Vit A	230 IU/ml
Vit D	54 IU/ml
Vit E	1.8 IU/ml
Sorbitan mono-oleate	37.0 mg/ml
Polysorbate 80	3 mg/ml
Uses: treatment of skin and coat conditions	
Dose: orally 1 ml/5 kg	
Tocovite 50 Tablets	
α-Tocopheryl acid succinate = 50 IU Vit E	
Uses: cardiac disease, muscular dystrophy and geriatric degenerative diseases	
Dose: dogs 50–100 IU daily	
Vi-Sorbin	
Cyanocobalamin	8.24 µg/ml
Pyridoxine	2.0 mg/ml
Ferric pyrophosphate	100 mg/ml
Folic acid	0.5 mg/ml
Sorbitol solution	4.4 ml
Uses: Vit B_{12}, B_6 and iron deficiencies, anaemia	
Doses: dogs 5–15 ml daily (orally); cats 2–5 ml daily	
Bimavite Plus	
Thiamine	35 mg/ml
Riboflavine	0.6 mg/ml
Nicotinamide	22.5 mg/ml
Pyridoxine	7 mg/ml
Ascorbic acid	70 mg/ml
Benzyl alcohol	15 mg/ml
Uses: for the treatment of Vit B and C deficiencies	
Dose: dogs and cats 2–3 ml once or twice weekly	
Parenterovite multidose injection	
Thiamine	35 mg/ml
Riboflavine	0.5 mg/ml
Pyridoxine	7 mg/ml
Nicotinamide	23.0 mg/ml
Ascorbic acid	70 mg/ml
Benzyl alcohol	20 mg/ml
Chlorocresol	0.1 %
Uses: stress, toxicity or deficiency	
Dose: dogs 1 ml/3 kg; cats 1 ml	
Neo-Cytamen 250	
Hydroxycobalamin (B_{12b})	250 µg/ml
Uses: debility, unthriftiness, liver diseases	
Dose: dogs and cats 1–2 ml weekly	

Table 19.1 cont.

Vitamin B_{12} injection Cyanocobalamin 250 μg/ml Dose: 10 μg/5 kg i.m. *Bimeda Vitamin K injection* Menadione 10 mg/ml Dose: 10–30 mg *Tendex injection* 10% iron dextran = 100 mg iron/ml Dose: 0.5–2 ml	*Feed additives* Canovel Dia-Glo Feline Tangies Pet-Tabs Pet-Tabs Feline SA 37 VH 100 Hypernutrient Vitatrace Vitrise LZM

in the joints of the legs. The characteristic signs are pain in the base of the skull with a reluctance and inability to turn the head. Usually there is a general depression and inappetence. Sometimes there are skin and dental changes with bone deformities.

Treatment consists of removing the excess vitamin A source in the diet and the administration of glucocorticoids.

B vitamins

Glucose, fatty acids and amino acids are metabolized in the body by oxidative processes in the cells. Acetyl-coenzyme A is required for the synthesis of new carbohydrate, protein and fat. The various enzymes involved use a number of the B vitamins, i.e. thiamine, riboflavine, nicotinic acid, pyridoxine and pantothenic acid.

Vitamin B_1 (thiamine)

Thiamine or vitamin B_1 was originally known as aneurin. It is found in many cereals, meats and potatoes as well as the germs and pericarp tissues of cereals.

A deficiency syndrome (most common in cats) may arise in animals fed entirely on cooked meats or on diets which contain thiaminase (raw fish or bacterial thiaminase in intestines). Thiamine is used in the form of its pyrophosphate and acts as a coenzyme of carboxylase. This enzyme is involved in the metabolism of pyruvic acid.

A deficiency of vitamin B_1 in dogs or cats may give rise to a subcutaneous oedema or to sudden death.

Vitamin B_2 (riboflavin)

The main sources of riboflavin are milk, meat, cereals and other vegetables, fruit and fish. Rice and maize are poor sources of riboflavin.

Riboflavin acts as an active prosthetic group of the flavoproteins which are used for oxidation in the control of cellular energy processes. A deficiency will therefore interfere with the energy processes and lead to an odd assortment of clinical abnormalities which include angular stomatitis, nasolabial seborrhoea, glossitis and invasion of the cornea by capillary blood vessels. Further, there is a conjunctivitis and corneal opacity. At post-mortem there may be a yellow, fatty liver.

It is unlikely that a riboflavin deficiency alone will be recognized but it may be associated with other deficiencies which will almost certainly be present.

Vitamin B_6 (pyridoxine)

Pyridoxine or vitamin B_6 is the name given to a related group of compounds which includes pyridoxol, pyridoxal and pyridoxamine. Vitamin B_6 is involved in the metabolism of amino acids. Deficiency is unlikely except in circumstances where unusual artificial feeding is given to young animals. Signs include CNS disturbances and convulsions.

Nicotinamide/niacin

Nicotinic acid is a simple derivative of pyridine and normally occurs as the amide in the body. It is involved in cellular oxidation processes in a dehydrogenase system responsible for oxidation in the citric acid cycle.

Nicotinic acid is widely distributed in foodstuffs and its main sources are meat, cereal (especially maize), potatoes and other vegetables, fish and milk. It is found in a bound form and may be biologically unavailable; thus dogs which are fed on a very high maize diet and a very low protein diet (sheepdogs) may develop signs of nicotinamide deficiency (black tongue). Black tongue is characterized by erythema, dermatitis, glossitis, diarrhoea and CNS disturbances with a peripheral neuropathy in severe cases.

Since nicotinic acid itself may cause dilatation of the cutaneous blood vessels it is usual to use preparations of nicotinamide in tablet or injection form.

Vitamin B_{12} (cyanocobalamin)

The name vitamin B_{12} is used to describe various complexes of cyanocobalamins. Vitamin B_{12} has to be synthesized by microorganisms in the tissues and organs of animals since it does not normally occur in plants. It is found in meat and eggs but not vegetables.

The cobalamins are originally bound to protein but are freed by the digestive processes. They then combine with a glycoprotein (the intrinsic factor) secreted by the parietal cells of the stomach. The vitamin B_{12}–intrinsic factor complex passes through the cells of the ileum and eventually reaches the liver as 5′-deoxyadenosylcobalamin. Normal stores in the liver are sufficient to last for 2–3 years. Large doses of vitamin B_{12} taken by mouth may enter the bloodstream independent of the intrinsic factor.

Vitamin B_{12} is essential for the synthesis of nucleic acids and the metabolism of all cells. It is required for fat breakdown and detoxification processes in the liver, haemopoiesis, the integrity of the nervous system, and full utilization of carbohydrates and proteins.

A deficiency of vitamin B_{12} can occur following an increase in demand arising from tissue breakdown disease or failure of absorption. It can also arise as a result of chronic parasitic infection in the gut as well as changes in the gut flora following diet changes or nervous stimuli.

There are four main indications for vitamin B_{12} therapy:

1. Lack of intrinsic factor, as in pernicious anaemia.
2. Malabsorptive disorders or operations involving the lower ileum.
3. Severe dietary deficiency over a long period.
4. Infectious hepatitis.

An interesting and unrelated use for hydroxocobalamin is in the treatment of cyanide poisoning. After injection, hydroxocobalamin is converted to cyanocobalamin as it picks up the cyanide radical. Hydroxocobalamin is also known as vitamin B_{12a}; cyanocobalamin is known as vitamin B_{12b}. Both of these preparations are equally effective for treating vitamin B_{12} disorders but it is hydroxocobalamin, not cyanocobalamin, which should be used for the treatment of cyanide intoxication.

Vitamin C (ascorbic acid)

Vitamin C deficiency was thought to occur only in man and guinea pigs but a syndrome which can be treated by the administration of vitamin C is now recognized in dogs. It is known as Barlow's disease or hypertrophic osteodystrophy.

Vitamin C is required for the synthesis of collagen, since it is involved in the conversion of proline to hydroxyproline. In addition, because it acts as an antioxidant, it may assist in the utilization of iron and decrease the requirements for other vitamins. Large doses of ascorbic acid improve the absorption of iron from the small intestine.

Barlow's disease

In puppies of 2–6 months of age there is a change in the metaphyseal areas of the bone. There is pain and swelling in this region as well as a pyrexia (40–41°C). The puppy is unwilling to move or walk and may cry out in pain when approached or touched. It is dull but its appetite is not reduced except during pyrexic periods. This condition is most commonly seen in large dogs, including the boxer and Dobermann. On X-ray the metaphyseal areas of the long bones present a characteristic picture. In addition, soft tissue swelling may be evident around the metaphysis. There may also be the development of spicules of new bone in subperiosteal haematomas.

Treatment of this condition consists of the administration of large amounts of ascorbic acid (0.5–1 g per day). Often this produces a dramatic remission of the pain and return to a normal temperature. Once the pup reaches six months of age no further attacks of this condition are likely.

Hypertrophic oestodystrophy in giant dogs

This condition is similar to that seen in pups but occurs in dogs such as the Great Dane, St Bernard and Pyrenean mountain dog. However, in these breeds the condition is characterized by the development of extracortical new bone around the metaphysis. It is associated with swelling of the limbs, pain and lameness. Since the animals are often receiving mineral supplements, it appears that the best therapeutic approach is to reduce the mineral and vitamin intake to satisfactory levels, as well as administering vitamin C.

Vitamin D

Vitamin D is the name of the dietary factor known to be involved in the prevention of rickets. Calciferol (vitamin D_2) and cholecalciferol (vitamin D_3) are the two main components of vitamin D. Calciferol is formed by the photochemical ring cleavage of ergosterol in plants, while cholecalciferol is formed by a similar reaction from 7-dehydrocholesterol in animal tissues. Thus, sunlight contributes to the formation of cholecalciferol in animal tissues and contributes significantly to the amount of vitamin D in the body. Vitamin D is stored in the fat and muscle for periods up to six months.

Once cholecalciferol has entered the body some of it is hydroxylated in the liver to calcifediol (25-hydroxycholecalciferol). The amount of calcifediol is regulated and carried in the plasma bound to an α_2-globulin. Calcifediol is then converted when it reaches the kidney to form calcitriol (1,25-dihydroxycholecalciferol). Calcitriol is known to be about ten times as potent as cholecalciferol. It is synthesized only in the kidney and is secreted in increasing amounts when there is a low extracellular calcium activity; it also responds to the stimulation of parathyroid hormone.

Calcitriol accumulates in the nuclei of cells in the intestinal mucosa and renal cortex, and in osteocytes. It then leads to the production, through stimulation of protein synthesis, of a calcium-binding protein. In the gut this produces an increased calcium absorption from the lumen; in the kidney, calcitriol increases tubular reabsorption. In calcium-deficient bone there is a net inflow of calcium into the bone so that it can be mineralized.

Vitamin D preparations made from irradiated yeast or fish-liver oil are usually adequate sources. Vitamin D is soluble and fairly stable in alcohol and oils. It is not soluble in water. If it is more important to affect calcium metabolism immediately, it is more usual to use vitamin D metabolites or analogues. Dihydrotachysterol can be used since it is a closely related compound and undergoes conversion in the liver to produce 25-hydroxydihydrotachysterol. It has less than a hundredth of the activity of calcitriol but unfortunately its production is not regulated and it may cause hypercalcaemia through bone resorption, and toxicity can arise from slight overdosage. The ideal vitamin D substitute is 1α-hydroxycholecalciferol since it is easily synthesized in the laboratory and, following administration, is converted in the liver to calcitriol and so bypasses the renal regulatory system. Since the conversion of 1α-hydroxycholecalciferol to calcitriol in the liver is self-regulated, it is less likely to produce toxicity but can rapidly produce calcitriol, a potent and effective substance.

High doses of vitamin D may produce toxicity and are used commercially as rodenticides. Overdose of vitamin D-like substances will produce hypercalcaemia, bone resorption and metastatic calcification. If this is sufficiently prolonged it will produce death.

Rickets

This is seen in fast-growing pups on unsupplemented feeds. There is a dietary deficiency in calcium and/or vitamin D. The pups show characteristic signs of bowed legs, stunting, painful epiphyses and swollen costochondral junctions. Treatment consists of the provision of 0.25–1% of the diet, on a wet weight basis, of both calcium and phosphorus as well as the addition of vitamin D at the rate of 10 IU/kg body weight daily. Once the rapid period of growth is over after six months of age, rickets is virtually impossible to produce.

Nutritional secondary hyperparathyroidism (juvenile osteoporosis)

This condition is seen in animals fed predominantly on meat which is high in phosphorus without adequate amounts of calcium. Excess or adequate amounts of vitamin D may be present in the diet. The excess phosphorus appears to lead to a hypocalcaemia and stimulates the parathyroid hormone. There is then resorption of the bone to counteract the hypocalcaemia. There are changes in the whole skeleton which are characterized by loss of intramedullary trabeculae, thinning of cortices, increase in the number and size of haversian canals but no change in the rate of bone growth. The bones, which have thin and often rudimentary cortices, are fragile and may fracture. The clinical signs arise as a result of this and include localized lameness, abnormal gait due to laxity of ligaments, and an inability or reluctance to stand or walk. There may be widespread bone pain and pathological fractures of the long bones.

Treatment depends on the correction of the mineral deficiency. In most cases this consists of correcting the abnormally large amount of meat which contains little calcium and too much phosphorus. Regulation of the vitamin D intake may also be necessary if there is an excessive amount given.

Renal hyperparathyroidism (rubber jaw)

This condition arises as a result of failure of the kidney to produce calcitriol. As a result there is an osteomalacia. The condition is characterized by changes in the whole skeleton but the greatest changes are shown in the bones of the head. In the adult dog the mandible becomes demineralized and soft, hence rubber jaw. Treatment is usually unrewarding since the condition is associated with chronic irreversible changes in the kidney. Treatment is therefore palliative, consisting of an increase in the dietary content of calcium.

Vitamin E

There is a family of closely related alcohols known as the tocopherols: α-tocopherol (vitamin E) is the most important since it is twice as active as the others and is the only one which is absorbed to any degree from the diet. The tocopherols are insoluble in water but highly soluble in fats and oil and rapidly inactivated by heat, light and oxygen; they can be stabilized by antioxidants like ascorbic acid.

At a biochemical level, vitamin E is involved in reactions which are characterized by the formation of free radicals. The role of vitamin E is similar to that of selenium and it is involved in tissues like the skeletal muscle and cardiac muscle. The tocopherols are also involved in the safe metabolism of polyunsaturated fatty acids. If there is an increase in the polyunsaturated fatty acids then there is an increased requirement for vitamin E.

Pansteatitis (yellow fat disease)

This condition is seen in cats fed excessive amounts of fat, particularly in canned food where the vitamin E has been destroyed by oxidation; an example is canned red tuna fish. The clinical signs in cats consist of anorexia, pain on palpation and occasionally excitability when handled. The subcutaneous tissue is firm and lumpy to palpate; the abdominal fat may also be palpable. Death will follow in a few weeks if the animal is untreated. Treatment consists of the administration of glucocorticoids to reduce the inflammation, together with vitamin E at a dose rate of 10 mg/kg/day. It is also wise to reduce the amount of polyunsaturated fat in the diet.

Vitamin K

This vitamin complex is fat soluble and is required for the formation of coagulation factors II, VII, IX and X in the liver. There are various forms of vitamin K but those which occur in nature are K_1 (phylloquinone) and K_2 (menaquinone). Menadione (K_3) is a synthetically prepared substance which in itself is virtually inactive but is converted in the liver to the active menaquinone (vitamin K_2).

Bile is required for the absorption of vitamin K and if the liver is diseased (reducing bile production and vitamin K supply) the formation of clotting factors is impaired. The following causes reduce vitamin K absorption:

1. Obstructive jaundice with a lack of bile salts in the small intestine.
2. Malabsorptive disorders.
3. Prolonged disruption of the microflora of the gut; for example, following the use of oral, broad spectrum antibiotics.
4. Chronic diarrhoea.

Vitamin K preparations

Phylloquinone (vitamin K_1) is fat soluble and available in 10 mg tablets or as a colloidal solution in ampoules containing 1 mg in 0.5 ml or 10 mg in 1 ml. Another fat soluble analogue is acetomenaphthone which is available in 5 mg tablets. There is also a water-soluble preparation of menadione (Synkavit) which is in 10 mg tablets or available in ampoules containing 10 mg/ml.

Use of vitamin K

Hypoprothrombinaemia is an indication for the use of the vitamin K group; the K vitamins are also antidotes to the anticoagulants of the warfarin group. In an emergency 10–30 mg phylloquinone (vitamin K_1) should be given intravenously. If it is administered in this manner it can, within 15 minutes, reduce the clotting time in animals poisoned with warfarin. This route of administration should be reserved for real emergencies since there is a high incidence of anaphylactic and haemolytic reactions. Oral and subcutaneous administration is considerably safer in less urgent cases.

Menadione derivatives are water soluble and more easily formulated. However, they are more irritant to the tissues and only adequate for dietary supplementation because the conversion to the active vitamin is insufficiently rapid to be of much benefit to those animals which are suffering from acute warfarin poisoning.

Essential fatty acids

The fatty acids linolenic and linoleic acid are required for the production of arachidonic acid, a component of phospholipid membranes. A deficiency may arise as a result of malabsorption syndromes and liver and pancreatic disease.

A deficiency condition is found in dogs and cats; if dogs are fed less than 3% of fat in a canned diet and less than 8% in a dry diet, they may develop a deficiency syndrome. In cats the requirement is higher, since 35–40% of their calorific intake is normally provided by fats.

The clinical features are lack of lustre coat and the skin may be scaly with areas of alopecia. Later a seborrhoeic oleosa develops with a secondary pyoderma and acanthosis. Treatment consists of supplementing the diet with one teaspoon of a mixture of equal parts vegetable oil and animal fat. It is also important to treat any underlying systemic disease.

Zinc

Two types of zinc deficiency are recognized in dogs: type 1 and type 2.

Type 1

This is recognized in Alaskan malamutes and Siberian huskies; it is also seen in the Dobermann and Great Danes. In the malamute there may be a genetic deficiency in the ability to absorb zinc from the intestine. Other causes of zinc deficiency include an oversupplementation with calcium which binds the zinc and prevents absorption. Further factors which reduce absorption are diets with high phytate which binds the zinc.

The clinical signs of this condition consist of erythema, alopecia, crusting and scaling, together with secondary infection of the mouth, chin, ears and eyes, scrotum and prepuce. Sometimes there may be hyperkeratosis of the foot pads. The skin becomes pigmented if the condition is chronic.

Type 2

This occurs in many breeds, particularly the Great Dane and Dobermann as well as the Alsatian and German pointer. Puppies are particularly affected if given excessive quantities of vitamins and minerals. The condition is recognized as hyperkeratotic plaques over pressure points (foot pads and hock).

Treatment of these conditions consists of the administration of zinc sulphate (Zincomed) at a dose rate of 10 mg/kg/day. Response is usually rapid and is seen within a few weeks. Type 1 cases need life-long therapy, in contrast to type 2 cases which frequently do not require further treatment after the animal has matured.

Iron

Iron is a vital component of myoglobin and haemoglobin. Ionic iron is highly toxic and is not normally present in the tissues or plasma.

Iron is absorbed in the proximal duodenum by a specific receptor which is saturable and can be blocked by chromium, manganese, cobalt and zinc. Only a small proportion of dietary iron (5–20%) is absorbed in the body. This is because iron is excreted very slowly from the body and has an approximate half-life of eight years. Iron deficiency is more likely to occur in very young animals which have not yet gained sufficient iron or in those animals where there is an abnormal loss (haemorrhage). Iron balance is therefore controlled by intestinal absorption. Parenteral administration will bypass this control, allowing overdose or possible waste.

Iron preparations

Ferrous (Fe^{2+}) salts are absorbed more readily than ferric (Fe^{3+}) salts. Simple preparations of ferrous sulphate are an adequate source of iron in the diet.

Iron dextran is the most common parenteral preparation. It is possible to administer this substance intravenously although it is usually given by deep intramuscular injection.

Iron sorbitol injection (iron sorbitol–citric acid complex BP) is also used for intramuscular injection. It must not be given intravenously.

Desferrioxamine (deferoxamine; Desferal)

Desferrioxamine is a highly specific iron chelating agent obtained from *Streptomyces pilosus*. It combines with ferric iron to form a non-toxic chelate which is excreted in the urine. It can be used for treating acute iron poisoning at a dose rate of 20 mg/kg intramuscularly or by slow intravenous injection of 15 mg/kg/ 15 mg/kg/h to a maximum dose of 80 mg/kg in 24 hours.

Further reading

Herbert, V. and Das, K. C. (1976) The role of Vitamin B_{12} and folic acid in hemato- and other cell-poiesis. *Vitamins and Hormones*, **34**, 3–30

Chapter 20

Poisons

This chapter describes treatment of various commonly occurring poisonings in small animal practice. The general approach is described first; this is followed by a description of signs, symptoms and treatment of specific poisons.

Cats are more susceptible than dogs to most poisons for two reasons: (1) they lick their coats and are therefore likely to consume more; and (2) most foreign substances (drugs or poisons) are more slowly metabolized in the cat because cats lack the ability to form glucuronide conjugates (see Chapter 2).

General treatments

Once diagnosis of poisoning has been made the first action is to prevent further absorption by the approach described below.

Washing skin

If an animal has been exposed to a substance like tar, grease or various phenols, and this covers the skin it is important to prevent further cutaneous absorption. Baths with large volumes of water are one way of achieving this by removing the substance from the skin surface. Intensive scrubbing, which can give rise to cuts, and the use of detergents are not desirable since they may actually increase absorption. The use of soap, with mild scrubbing, may be necessary to remove lipid-soluble compounds.

Emesis

In animals that have swallowed the poison (within 2 h) it is often useful to produce emesis to empty the stomach and so minimize further absorption. This may be produced in a variety of ways as illustrated in Table 20.1. Normally, vomiting is produced within about 20 minutes following administration of one of these agents. Severe respiratory depression can be caused by

Table 20.1 Induction of emesis

Substance	*Administration*	*Dose*
Apomorphine	(Dog only) i.m./s.c.	0.1 mg/kg
Ipecac. syrup	Oral	1–2 ml/kg
Salt water	Oral	1–2 teaspoons in a cup of warm water
Mustard water	Oral	2 teaspoons in a cup of warm water
Washing soda crystals	Placed on back of tongue	
H_2O_2	Oral	5–25 ml
Xylazine (cat)	i.m.	0.44 mg/kg

apomorphine but this may be reversed and antagonized by the administration of naloxone; excessive vomiting may be controlled using acepromazine or chlorpromazine as a dopamine antagonist. Ipecac syrup should not be used in association with activated charcoal since the effectiveness of the charcoal is greatly reduced thereby. It may be useful to save the contents of the stomach for further analysis so that confirmation of poisoning may be achieved.

The production of emesis is contraindicated if the poison is a corrosive agent or a volatile hydrocarbon like petrol or a petrol distillate. It is also contraindicated if the animal is unconscious since it may inhale the vomit. The presence of convulsions are a further contraindication for the induction of emesis. If there has been a long period (say 4 hours) between the ingestion of the poison and induction of emesis, little effect will be achieved since most of the poison will already be absorbed.

Gastric lavage

This is indicated if the animal is unconscious or lightly anaesthetized. The technique consists of using an endotracheal tube to prevent inspiration of any gastric contents and a separate, large stomach tube to wash the stomach out. Large volumes of saline (10 ml/kg) are alternately syringed into and out of the stomach. This procedure is continued until the contents of the stomach have been removed as indicated by the presence of a clear solution following evacuation of the stomach contents. Gastric lavage is not likely to be effective if it is carried out more than two hours after the ingestion of the poison. It is contraindicated if there is any known weakening of the stomach wall.

Minimizing absorption

It is possible to minimize absorption of poisons from the gastrointestinal tract by administering nonabsorbable carriers. Activated vegetable charcoal (2–8 g/kg) can be given at a concentration of 1 g/7.5 ml water administered by stomach tube. This is usually followed after 30 minutes by a cathartic solution, unless gastric lavage is being performed. The cathartic solution can consist of sodium sulphate at a dose rate of 1 g/kg to reduce the transit time of the poison in the gastrointestinal tract and so encourage excretion in the faeces. Sodium sulphate is safer than magnesium sulphate and more effective. If fat-soluble poisons like phenol are involved, it is possible to use mineral oil or vegetable oil followed by a saline cathartic to achieve a similar effect.

BCK granules have been specifically recommended for use in toxic conditions and poisonings of the stomach and intestine. A dose of 1–3 teaspoons in dogs and cats has been suggested and should be given as a drench with a little water.

Respiratory support

Some poisons lead to respiratory depression. Examples include accidental overdose of barbiturates and sleeping tablets which belong to the owner. Respiratory support may be achieved by intubation with an endotracheal tube and the administration of artificial respiration as required.

Anticonvulsant drugs

Some poisons like strychnine produce convulsions. It is appropriate in these cases to use anticonvulsants to control the effects of the poison. A variety of compounds can be used and these have already been mentioned and considered in Chapter 7. Most useful compounds are diazepam (Valium) and pentobarbitone, both of which have a selective anticonvulsant action.

Control of pain

One aspect of poisonings is that they are frequently associated with severe pain. Pain can arise as a result of severe damage to the tissues or as a specific effect of the toxin. Potent opiate analgesics would then be indicated; these include morphine and pethidine. However, due care should be taken since these compounds are themselves respiratory depressants and may be contraindicated in particular cases of poisoning.

Increasing elimination

It is possible to increase the elimination of many poisons since they are excreted through the urine via the kidney. Diuretics can be used to increase the excretion rate of poisons in the urine. Mannitol at a dose of 2 g/kg/h or frusemide at a dose of 5 mg/kg every 6–8 hours will be sufficient to produce diuresis. Supportive fluid therapy by itself will also increase urine output and enhance the elimination of the poison. Both of these approaches (diuretics and fluid therapy) are effective for poisons undergoing tubular reabsorption: they act by increasing the clearance rate.

To further increase clearance of various poisons, it may be possible to modify the pH of urine. Thus, for weak acids like aspirin and barbiturates, making the urine alkaline will trap the compounds in the renal tubule in their ionized form and reduce reabsorption: the effect, therefore, of making the urine alkaline is to increase the clearance of acidic drugs. If the urine is acidified it will reduce the clearance of acidic drugs but will increase the clearance of basic drugs like amphetamines, quinidine and morphine. Ammonium chloride is probably the most effective acidifying agent; sodium bicarbonate is probably the most effective alkalinizing agent for this purpose.

Insecticides

Chlorinated hydrocarbons

This group of compounds are very persistent. They are very slowly broken down in the environment or following consumption by the animal. They consist of a large number of compounds like DDT, BHC (lindane), bromocyclen (Alugan) and toxaphene.

These products are found in various sprays and dusting powders for the control of aphids and other garden insects. They are also found in preparations for the treatment of various ectoparasites.

Following consumption, chlorinated hydrocarbons give rise to an increase in excitability, hyperaesthesia, tremors and convulsions. Consumption is more likely in the cat with its particular predisposition towards grooming. Usually treatment in mild cases is not necessary. However, to control convulsions in severe cases, sodium pentobarbitone (10–30 mg/kg) given intravenously initially may be useful. Following intravenous injection further administration of pentobarbitone can be given intraperitoneally. In order to confirm diagnosis of chlorinated hydrocarbon poisoning it is necessary to collect stomach contents; if the animal has died, a liver sample is required. Post-mortem symptoms are variable but can include small haemorrhages on or around the heart and peritoneal cavity, together with congestion and oedema of the lungs.

Organophosphorous compounds

These agents include malathion, parathion, fenitrothion and diazinon. There are many organophosphorous compounds available. The compounds are found in sprays and dusting powders which are used for control of garden insects and various ectoparasites of small animals.

The organophosphorous compounds act by inhibiting cholinesterase and give rise to accumulation of acetylcholine at muscarinic and, later, nicotinic receptor sites. Excessive muscarinic receptor stimulation gives rise to salivation, vomiting, diarrhoea, tremors, dyspnoea and occasionally convulsions. There is also a chronic form of organophosphorous poisoning characterized by a delayed neurotoxicity which may occur with some specific organophosphorous compounds. This is characterized by a demyelination of sciatic nerves.

Treatment of acute organophosphorous poisoning is most effectively carried out using atropine sulphate cautiously at a dose rate of 0.25 mg/kg intravenously. If the organophosphorous compound has been administered or consumed recently, a further compound, pralidoxime (Protopam), may be given at a dose rate of 20 mg/kg i.v. slowly. It is important to realize that pralidoxime is only effective if given soon after exposure to the organophosphorous compound since its main action is to reactivate the acetylcholinesterase enzyme before it becomes 'aged' (the organophosphorous compound becomes permanently fixed to the cholinesterase).

To confirm diagnosis, stomach contents and urine may be collected, as well as blood from the living animal, for cholinesterase estimation. In poisoned animals the cholinesterase levels are very low. Post-mortem signs consist of inflammation of the gastrointestinal tract and sometimes oedema of the lungs and pericardium. Morphine, aminophylline and phenothiazine are contraindicated.

Carbamates

Substances like carbaryl (Sevin) are found in sprays and dusts which are used for horticultural and veterinary purposes for control of insects. Their action is similar to the organophosphorous compounds in that they act by blocking the action of cholinesterase. They give rise to the same symptoms as organophosphorous poisons.

Treatment is with atropine administered cautiously by intravenous injection; pralidoxime is contraindicated.

In order to confirm diagnosis it is usually necessary to demonstrate the consumption of carbamates: analysis of urine and blood is rarely effective since carbamates are not stable. Post-mortem findings include inflammation of the alimentary tract.

Nicotine

Nicotine is used in horticultural sprays as an insecticide. The clinical signs of nicotine poisoning include excitement, rapid respiration, vomiting, diarrhoea and salivation, together with paralysis and coma. These arise as a result of an initial stimulation and then a subsequent depression of nicotinic receptors found on autonomic ganglia and at neuromuscular junctions.

Treatment consists of artificial respiration and the administration of xanthine derivatives (theophylline) as a stimulant. It is not usual for treatment to be successful in acute cases of poisoning.

Stomach contents and liver can be sent for analysis for confirmation of the diagnosis. Post-mortem signs are vague and include inflammation of the alimentary tract.

Herbicides

Sodium chlorate

This compound is an oxidizing agent and a fairly old-fashioned, nonselective weed killer. Following consumption it will produce signs of vomiting, anorexia, inflammation of the throat, and tenderness over the loins. Treatment consists of the administration of reducing agents (1% sodium thiosulphate given by gastric lavage or the intravenous administration of methylene blue at a dose rate of 2 mg/kg using a 1% solution).

Post-mortem findings are dominated by the brown coloration produced by the oxidation of haemoglobin. Thus there is a chocolate-coloured blood and dark-coloured liver, lungs, spleen and muscle.

Paraquat

This agent is found in the herbicide 'Gramoxone' or 'Weedol'. It produces vomiting, jaundice, depression and difficulty in breathing due to pulmonary oedema.

It is said that paraquat poisoning is irreversible and that no antidote is available. Stomach contents or urine may be saved for analysis for confirmation of the diagnosis. Post-mortem signs include haemorrhagic gastritis.

Chlorinated phenoxyacids

These agents include 2,4-D and 2,4,5,-D; they are used as herbicides and act as growth stimulants in plants. The clinical signs of poisoning in small animals are only likely to occur following consumption of massive doses. In these cases, vomiting, respiratory depression and coma are the likely signs. No specific antidote is known and the post-mortem findings consist mainly of a haemorrhagic gastroenteritis.

Rodenticides

Warfarin and warfarin derivatives

This group of compounds includes chlorophacinone, coumachlor and diphacinone which are commonly used as rat poisons.

These agents act by inhibiting the production of vitamin K. As a result, clotting factors are prevented from acting and are gradually depleted over a period of several days. Haemorrhage is found in many areas of the body; this gives rise to pale mucous membranes and haemorrhagic diarrhoea which may be preceded by a lameness as a result of small haemorrhages in joints.

Treatment consists of administering vitamin K_1 intramuscularly at a dose rate of 2 mg/kg or 10–30 mg intravenously. Since the blood of these animals is released into the thoracic cavity, it has been suggested that autotransfusion with this blood, collected from the thoracic cavity, may be a useful adjunct in therapy.

Collection of materials for analysis is rarely practical. Post-mortem signs include multiple haemorrhages in many parts of the body, including the body cavities.

α-Chloralose

This substance is used as a mouse poison (Alphakil) and for killing pigeons. In cats, signs of α-chloralose poisoning consist of a bizarre anaesthetized state which is characterized by a jerky response to tapping of the animal; the animal otherwise appears anaesthetized. Prior to this anaesthesia, symptoms of excitement or aggression may be seen in the dog or cat.

Treatment can usually be carried out by placing the animal in a warm, quiet place to avoid sensory stimulation and allowing the animal to clear and metabolize the α-chloralose itself. The administration of further CNS depressants like sodium pentobarbitone is contraindicated. The animal should be kept warm in cases of hypothermia. Emetics are useful at an early stage.

There are no characteristic macroscopic changes at post-mortem.

Yellow phosphorus

This compound is used as a rat poison and will produce severe abdominal pain, vomiting, jaundice, convulsions and delirium. Treatment may be tried using emetics and gastric lavage but must be attempted early. Since yellow phosphorus causes severe damage to the gastrointestinal tract, glucose saline or other plasma expanders given intravenously may be a useful adjunct for therapy.

The stomach contents can be sent for analysis; liver may be collected for histopathology. Post-mortem findings are characterized by severe inflammation of the gastrointestinal tract together with a fatty degeneration of the liver and kidney.

Zinc phosphide

This substance is used as a rat poison and causes similar signs to yellow phosphorus poisoning. The treatment and post-mortem findings are also similar.

Strychnine

Strychnine is used as a poison for moles and, illegally, for the poisoning of rats and foxes. It is used as a stimulant or tonic in nux vomica bitters.

Strychnine inhibits the action of a natural inhibitory transmitter (glycine) in the spinal cord. The signs and symptoms of poisoning consist of convulsions or exaggerated responses to external stimuli and, in extreme cases, opisthotonos. To control this condition, anticonvulsants can be used (sodium pentobarbitone intravenously or intraperitoneally, or diazepam). It may be possible to minimize the absorption of strychnine by administration of very strong tea (tannic acid) to precipitate the strychnine in the intestine. To confirm the diagnosis, stomach contents and liver may be sent for analysis. Post-mortem signs are not characteristic.

α-Napthylthiourea (ANTU)

This substance acts rapidly to produce a pulmonary oedema which may be preceded by vomiting as a result of gastric irritation. ANTU is an old-fashioned rat poison. There are no specific treatments for poisoning with ANTU but if the animal survives longer than 12 hours it is likely that the outcome will be favourable. Death normally occurs within 4 hours of consuming the poison. Stomach contents can be used for analysis. Post-mortem findings consist of gastrointestinal irritation (hyperaemia) together with pulmonary oedema, hydrothorax and renal hyperaemia. There may be a hydropericardium.

Crimidine

This compound is used as a rodenticide and causes convulsions in the dog and cat. Treatment usually consists of trying to control these convulsions with diazepam or pentobarbitone and the administration of vitamin B (pyridoxine).

Sodium fluoroacetate

This compound is very toxic and will kill dogs or cats which actually consume a poisoned rodent. This phenomenon is sometimes referred to as relay toxicity and has led to a decrease in the use of this compound in recent years. It acts by blocking the tricarboxylic acid cycle by forming fluorocitric acid which inhibits aconitase activity. This means that many cells are unable to obtain enough energy to carry out their normal metabolic tasks.

The signs of sodium fluoroacetate poisoning occur after a period of about 4–5 hours following consumption; the animal becomes restless and often vomits. There is an increase in the gastrointestinal activity; the animal runs aimlessly, barking or crying. There are then consulvions which can last about a minute. In cats, cardiac arrhythmia may follow. Eventually the animal fails to recover from a convulsive episode and passes into a coma. Death usually follows 12 hours after ingestion.

There is no specific antidote for sodium fluoroacetate poisoning. Treatment is usually supportive (controlling the convulsions and giving calcium gluconate for the maintenance of energy). Stomach contents may be saved for analysis. Post-mortem signs consist of an inflamed gastrointestinal tract with few other distinctive features.

Reserpine

This compound is used as a rodenticide and acts by depleting catecholamines (adrenaline and noradrenaline) from sympathetic nerves and the central nervous system. It produces vomiting and CNS depression. Treatment consists of the administration of a methylamphetamine injection as well as nikethamide. The agents act by potentiating the effects of any remaining adrenaline or noradrenaline. To confirm the diagnosis, histology of sympathetic nerve endings or sympathetic ganglia is useful. There are no characteristic gross post-mortem findings.

Thallium

Thallium acetate is used as a rat poison. It produces anorexia, vomiting and colic associated with gastritis, which is usually haemorrhagic. There are usually skin lesions in cases of chronic thallium poisoning (hyperkeratosis and alopecia). Treatment consists of administration of diphenylthiocarbazone given orally at a dose rate of 5 mg/kg daily. Alternatively, Prussian blue at a dose rate of 0.15 mg/kg can be administered three times daily by mouth. It is also useful to treat the skin lesions symptomatically.

Stomach contents and urine are useful for confirmation of the diagnosis. Post-mortem findings consist of a haemorrhagic gastrointestinal tract together with the alopecia and dermatitis.

Molluscicides

Metaldehyde

This compound is found in slug poisons. The poison primarily causes CNS signs of hyperactivity. Thus salivation, hyperaesthesia, nystagmus, tremors and convulsions are seen.

Anticonvulsants (diazepam and pentobarbitone) may be useful. Calcium borogluconate may be administered subcutaneously at a dose rate of 5–25 ml of 10% solution per dog to act to stabilize the membranes of the nervous system and to minimize excitation. Stomach contents of the animal are useful for confirmation of the diagnosis. Post-mortem findings usually consist of a hyperaemia of the liver, kidney and lungs.

Methiocarb

This compound is used as a slug killer; it is a carbamate. Like the previous carbamates described, it acts by blocking cholinesterase. It produces the same signs and can be treated in the same way (atropine).

Miscellaneous organic compounds

Acrolein

This compound is found in foods prepared from overheated fats. The characteristic signs of poisoning are: fever, tonsillitis, cyanosis, difficulty in breathing, collapse and death.

Unfortunately, there are no specific treatments and symptomatic treatment is the only option available.

Aflatoxin

Aflatoxin poisoning occurs in grain which is contaminated with a fungal growth. The characteristic signs produced by this toxin consist of dullness, anorexia and weight loss over a number of weeks, together with gastrointestinal disturbances, ascites, liver damage (jaundice) and death. No specific treatment is available. It is imperative once diagnosis is made that contaminated food is withdrawn. The poison results in a characteristic liver damage which can be diagnosed on histopathology.

Cyanide (HCN)

Cyanide poisoning can arise from consumption of sodium cyanide which is used for industrial processes, or following the consumption of cyanogenetic glycosides which are found in certain plants, including almonds and linseed. The presenting signs usually consist of a sudden death, or possibly excitement, salivation, dilated pupils, convulsion and then death. Treatment is aimed at correcting the histotoxic anoxia which is produced by the cyanide ion interfering with the cytochrome oxidase in mitochondria. There is a specific treatment for cyanide poisoning. It consists of the administration of sodium nitrite at a concentration of 1% and given intravenously at a dose rate of 25 mg/kg. This is then followed by sodium thiosulphate at a concentration of 25% given slowly intravenously at a dose rate of 1.25 g/kg. Oxygen at a concentration of 100% may also facilitate survival of the animal. Stomach contents or blood may be collected for analysis to confirm the diagnosis. There is usually a characteristic almond smell associated with cyanide poisoning. Macroscopic post-mortem findings include haemorrhages in the alimentary tract in subacute cases.

Detergents and disinfectants

These compounds are commonly used for cleansing and disinfection in many domestic and commercial situations. The normal signs of poisoning consist of a moist or purulent dermatitis as a result of skin contact with these necrotic or damaging substances. After consumption, there is irritation of the gastrointestinal tract which produces salivation, vomiting and depression. There are no specific antidotes. Treatment is usually symptomatic.

Cresols and phenols

These substances are found in tar, pitch, creosote and carbolic acid. They are found in various types of disinfectant. Following consumption they will produce a thirst and inappetence, together with pain in the abdomen due to irritation of the gastrointestinal tract. Absorption will lead to incoordination, anaemia, convulsions and jaundice. Death and coma are common sequelae.

Treatment consists of administration of emetics and gastric lavage to minimize the absorption, together with the administration of glucose saline given intravenously to counteract dehydration.

Paraffin oils

These consist of petrol, diesel, white spirit and similar substances. Following consumption or absorption they will produce a depression, weakness, vomiting and collapse. Treatment consists of removing the spirit or oil from the skin and the administration of olive oil by mouth to minimize absorption.

Bee stings

Bee stings occur infrequently and, if there has been a multiple stinging, vomiting, diarrhoea, collapse and death will follow. Treatment consists of administration of corticosteroids and antihistamines for treatment of allergic responses and to minimize shock. Intravenous fluids are also indicated.

Wasp stings

Multiple stingings produce symptoms of vomiting, diarrhoea and collapse. Corticosteroids and antihistamines, together with fluid therapy, are useful for the treatment of this condition.

Toad venom

Most species of toad produce a venom which irritates the gastrointestinal tract. It leads to salivation, vomiting and collapse. Occasionally toxins produce cardiac arrhythmia. Treatment consists of washing the mouth to minimize the irritation of buccal mucous membranes. Atropine sulphate is useful given by intramuscular injection. Corticosteroids are also useful.

Miscellaneous inorganic compounds

Arsenic

Arsenic trioxide and sodium arsenite are used as sheep dips. Lead arsenite is used as a horticultural spray. It is found in some old types of paint, particularly mineral and emerald greens. It was also found in Fowler's solution. Arsenic and its organic derivatives act by inhibiting SH groups in enzymes which are involved in oxidative phosphorylation. Arsenic produces a histotoxic anoxia; the organs affected are the liver, kidney, spleen, lung and skin. The clinical symptoms of arsenic poisoning consist of a sudden onset of haemorrhagic gastro-enteritis; this is associated with restlessness and vomiting together with a bloody diarrhoea. In terminal stages the animal is very weak and debilitated; there is usually an anaemia. If sublethal doses are absorbed, chronic poisoning is possible: this is characterized by toxic nephrosis. The treatment is specific and consists of the administration of dimercaprol (BAL) given intramuscularly at a dose rate of 2.5 mg/kg every four hours for two days; this is then followed by a twice-daily dose until recovery is complete. Supportive therapy, with the administration of fluid and electrolytes, is also very valuable.

Diagnosis of poisoning can be confirmed on the basis of stomach contents or kidney analysis. Post-mortem findings include inflammation of the gastrointestinal tract which is usually severe but only slight in peracute cases.

Lead

This is found in paints, linoleum and car batteries in the form of metallic lead, lead oxide or lead carbonate. The clinical signs of an animal suffering from lead poisoning consist of anorexia and vomiting, sometimes with or without nervous signs, tremor and convulsions. If poisoning is chronic, the animal may simply be losing weight. Treatment consists of the administration of sodium calcium EDTA given intravenously, using a dose rate of 75 mg/kg as a 4% solution administered in divided doses. Blood from a living animal may be collected to confirm the diagnosis; liver or kidney may be used at post-mortem for confirmation. Post-mortem findings consist of a gastroenteritis in acute cases but a degenerative change in the liver and kidney in chronic cases.

Salt poisoning

Sodium chloride is found in a variety of substances in excess (e.g. sea water and whey, a milk product). Salt poisoning gives rise to ataxia, convulsions and blindness. Treatment consists of the intraperitoneal administration of water to permit the cat or dog to secrete excess salt. Post-mortem findings in acute cases consist of congestion and excessive fluid in the alimentary tract.

Aspirin

Aspirin (salicylic acid) poisoning follows the consumption of ordinary aspirin tablets to excess. In the cat this syndrome is characterized by anorexia, vomiting and depression. The cat is particularly susceptible to salicylate poisoning since in this species there is a very long half-life and salicylate is secreted very slowly, compared with the dog and other animals. Treatment consists of gastric lavage with sodium bicarbonate if the cat is conscious. Lactated Ringer can be administered intravenously or intraperitoneally to correct the fluid and pH imbalance. Stomach contents and urine may be collected for analysis to confirm the diagnosis. Post-mortem signs include a haemorrhage of the stomach wall together with a swollen liver.

Benzoic acid

Benzoic acid is used as a food preservative in meat products. In cats which ingest too much benzoic acid there is an ataxia followed by aggression and convulsions. Treatment consists of minimizing the severity of convulsions by keeping the animal in a quiet place. Anticonvulsants like diazepam and pentobarbitone may be given to control the convulsions. The unconsumed food can be sent for analysis. There are no macroscopic changes seen at post-mortem.

Ethylene glycol

This type of poisoning is more commonly seen in dogs since they are more sensitive to ethylene glycol than cats. It is a constituent of antifreeze and is attractive to pets because of its sweet taste. There is an acute acidosis if massive amounts are absorbed. The clinical signs consist of moderate CNS depression, incoordination and ataxia, occasionally with frequent vomiting. This may progress to a paralysis and coma. If the urine is examined after six hours, oxalate crystals will be present.

A subacute uraemic syndrome is also recognized. This occurs following survival of the acute phase and is due to renal failure as ethylene glycol is converted to nephrotoxic metabolites (oxalic acid). Cats metabolize ethylene glycol more slowly and are thus less susceptible to this stage. In the subacute phase animals show a raised serum urea nitrogen, oliguria and anuria. Sometimes there are muscle fasciculations, paddling and episodes of generalized muscle contraction.

Treatment in the acute phase consists of administration of 20% ethanol intravenously at a dose rate of 5.5 mg/kg, followed by 8 ml/kg 5% sodium bicarbonate solution given intraperitoneally to correct for the acidosis. This protocol is best repeated at 4-hour intervals for a day and then at intervals of 6 hours for another one or two days. Another approach is to use ethanol at a concentration of 50% to induce anaesthesia or CNS depression so that the animal becomes insensitive to toe pinch. Pure ethanol must be used for this so that it blocks alcohol dehydrogenase, which would otherwise metabolize ethylene glycol to oxalic acid. Fluid therapy is also given during this stage. Usually prognosis is quite good if the animal responds within 18 hours.

The treatment of the subacute phase consists of trying to control the uraemic state. Usually this is not successful.

Further reading

Clarke, E. G. C. (1973) Lead poisoning in small animals. *Journal of Small Animal Practice*, **14**, 183

Clarke, E. G. C. (1984) *Veterinary Toxicology*, 4th edn, Baillière Tindall, London

Chapter 21

The Law and Medicines

This chapter considers the Medicines Act (1968) and the Misuse of Drugs Act (1971) which are the two main Acts in the United Kingdom which govern the use of therapeutic substances. The Medicines Act provides regulations for the safety, quality and efficacy of therapeutic agents. It controls the manufacture, importation and distribution of medicines. Certain drugs which are capable of misuse are subject to control under the Misuse of Drugs Act. This Act controls drugs like morphine, heroin and LSD. The Poisons Act (1972) which is concerned with non-medicinal products is not considered here.

Medicines Act (1968)

Medicinal products are controlled by this Act and are defined as substances or articles which are manufactured, sold, supplied, imported or exported for use wholly or mainly for administration to human beings or animals for a *medicinal purpose*. A medicinal purpose is then further defined as covering diagnosis, treatment, prevention of disease, contraception, prevention or interfering with the normal operation of a physiological function, and induction of anaesthesia. A product which is exclusively manufactured, sold, supplied, imported or exported for the purpose of being administered to animals but not for the purpose of being administered to human beings is referred to in the Act as a *veterinary drug*.

Committees

Under the Medicines Act the Secretaries of State for Health and Agriculture in the UK are responsible for the administration of the Act. This is carried out under the auspices of the Medicines Commission which has set up a variety of expert committees. These expert committees have members with a broad experience of medicine, veterinary medicine, pharmacy and the pharmaceutical industry. Some of the expert committees include:

1. The Committee on Safety of Medicines which is responsible for medicinal products and clinical trials in man.
2. Committees on prescription-only medicines and general sales lists which have been appointed for the specific purpose of classifying medicinal products into categories for supply.
3. The Veterinary Products Committee which is appointed for veterinary medicinal products and medicinal tests on animals. This committee advises the Minister for Agriculture on safety, quality and efficacy of veterinary medicinal products and promotes the collection and investigation of information related to adverse reactions from veterinary drugs.

Secretaries of State (health and agriculture)

The Secretaries of State for Health and Agriculture are empowered under the Medicines Act to issue licences or certificates in order to promote the safety, efficacy and quality control of medicinal products or veterinary drugs.

Licences

Product licence

A produce licence is required for the sale, supply, import or export of any medicinal product or its manufacture. The regulations which govern the issue of the product licence require the manufacturer to supply details concerning the chemistry, quality control, pharmacological and toxicological studies, arrangements for performance of tests and evaluation of laboratory and clinical studies, and, for veterinary products, possible hazards to man, livestock and wildlife.

Wholesale dealer's licence

This is required for anyone who sells or offers for sale any medicinal product by wholesale dealing.

Manufacturer's licence

This is required for anyone who manufactures or assembles a medicinal product. This licence only allows a manufacturer to make his product if he also has a product licence.

Licences of right

Before 1 September 1971, products which were in use and on the market were issued with licences of right. Eventually, licences of right will be reviewed so that all products will be subject to the same standards of safety, quality and efficacy.

Exemptions for veterinary surgeons

A veterinary surgeon does not require a licence for a medicinal product provided he has specifically prepared it for himself, or another veterinary surgeon, for administration to a particular animal under his care. A pharmacist does not require a licence to prepare a preparation of the medicine or product in accordance with a prescription issued by a veterinarian.

Animal test certificates

These are issued to manufacturers and authorize the sale and supply of medicinal products for the purpose of testing new drugs. Exceptions to the requirement for possessing an animal test certificate include a veterinarian who is testing products on animals under his own care.

In general, an individual veterinarian will not be involved in the licensing system. If, however, he intends to import or export medicinal products or prepare those products not directly under his control (or another veterinarian at his request) then he must obtain the appropriate licences.

Supply and sale of veterinary medicinal products

There are three major legal categories described under the Medicines Act for the sale and supply of medicinal products. These are:

1. General sales list products (GSL).
2. Prescription-only medicines (POM).
3. Pharmacy medicines (P).

A veterinarian can sell and prescribe medicines in all these three legal categories providing the drugs are for 'administration by him or under his direction to an animal or herd which is under his care'. It is illegal and unethical to prescribe drugs for animals 'not under his care'. Prosecution has resulted from ignoring this aspect of the Act. The Royal College has given guidance on the interpretation of the term 'animals under his care'. The college suggests that the following conditions should be met:

1. The veterinary surgeon should have been given responsibility for the health of the animal in question by the owner or his agent.
2. The care of the animal by the veterinary surgeon should be real and not merely nominal.
3. In amplification of (2) above, although circumstances will vary enormously, the veterinary surgeon must at least:
   (a) either have seen the animal for the purposes of diagnosis or prescription and immediately prior thereto, or
   (b) have visited the premises at which the animal is kept sufficiently often, and recently enough, to have acquired from personal knowledge and inspection an accurate picture of the current health state on the premises to enable him to make a diagnosis or prescribe for the animal in question.

This interpretation is also acceptable by the Ministry of Agriculture, Fisheries and Foods.

General sales list

Medicinal products which are subject to a very small hazard to health and do not need special precautions for handling, and where there is a wide sales demand, are subject to general sales regulations. These products may be sold freely without prescription from premises or vans but not from automatic machines. However, the drugs have to be sold in prepacked containers or in unopened containers. A number of drugs are available on the general sales list if they are only used for external use; if they are intended for internal use they may be subject to other regulations. Sometimes there is a maximum limit to the strength of the drug which may be issued under general sales list regulations. Also listed under the regulations are a number of products which are not on the general sales list. These are veterinary drugs marketed for:

1. Use as anthelmintics, except those containing dichlorophen, diethylcarbamazine citrate, piperazine adipate, piperazine calcium edetate, piperazine citrate, piperazine dihydrochloride, piperazine hydrate or piperazine phosphate.
2. Parenteral administration.
3. Use as eye drops.
4. External treatment of ringworm.

It can be seen then that pet shops may sell anthelmintics containing drugs listed in (1) above. These include dichlorophen, diethylcarbamazine and piperazine.

Prescription-only medicines (POM)

Prescription-only medicines are products which are sold or prescribed by a dentist, doctor or veterinary surgeon. A veterinary surgeon must only use these agents on animals under his own care. Prescription only medicines have to be labelled

POM

Drugs which are sold by wholesalers have to show this sign but not when they are dispensed. The list of drugs governed by prescription-only medicine regulations include, in general, antibacterial agents, hormones, antiparasitic agents and anti-inflammatory drugs. The legal category of each veterinary product is given in the compendium of data sheets for veterinary products (ABPI). There is a list of exceptions to those drugs which normally require prescription-only regulations. These include particular preparations below a specified maximum strength, all products intended for a particular use, or products for a particular route of administration.

The parenteral administration of veterinary prescription-only medicines is restricted to veterinary surgeons or persons acting under their directions.

Prescribing prescription-only medicines

A prescription from a veterinary surgeon for medicines must be signed by him in ink with his own name and must contain the following particulars:

1. His address.
2. The date.
3. An indication of his professional qualifications (veterinary surgeon).
4. The name and address of the person to whom the medicine is to be delivered.
5. The declaration 'this prescription is issued in respect of animals under my care'.

It is also good practice to include the total amount of the medicine to be supplied and the dose of the medicine. A prescription must be used within six months of the date of issue and cannot be repeated unless so stated in the prescription. If drugs are subject to Controlled Drugs regulations (under the Misuse of Drugs Act, 1971) more stringent prescription requirements are specified. Figure 21.1 illustrates an example of a POM prescription.

Central Veterinary Hospital
22 Church Street
Leicester

Date: 4.1.87

Person supplied:

(Dog of) J Smith
83 Station Road
Leicester

R_X Kaolin and Morphine mixture B.P.

Mitte 100 ml

Sig 5 ml to be given twice daily

This prescription is issued in respect of an animal under my care.

Signature (of veterinary surgeon)
Qualifications

Figure 21.1 A POM prescription

Pharmacy medicines

In general these drugs may be sold only by a registered pharmacist. They are labelled with the symbol

P

when they are sold, or supplied for retail, for administration to animals. There is no requirement for prescriptions for medicines sold under the pharmacy medicines regulations.

Labelling of medicinal compounds

Standard labelling is required by manufacturers under appropriate regulations. This comprises the name of the product, pharmaceutical form, quantitative details of composition, quantity in the containers, directions for use, contraindications, warnings and precautions, special requirements for storage, expiry date, name and address of the product licence holder, product licence and manufacturer's licence numbers, batch number and the statement 'for animal treatment only' (unless the container or package is too small), purpose of the product, restrictions for which the product licence specifies, withdrawal period, and the statement 'keep out of reach of children' or words with a similar meaning. The general provisions in the regulations require that labelling is carried out in an indelible manner and that the writing is legible.

Warnings for compounds containing aloxiprin, aspirin or salicylamide

There are specific requirements for warning labelling which must appear on the containers or packages of certain veterinary products supplied to a veterinary surgeon for particular animals under his care. These requirements are:

1. Veterinary medicines containing aloxiprin must be labelled with the words 'unsuitable for cats' and 'contains an aspirin derivative'.
2. Veterinary medicines containing aspirin must be labelled with the words 'unsuitable for cats' and 'contains aspirin' (unless the name of the product includes the word 'aspirin').
3. Veterinary medicines containing salicylamide must be labelled with the words 'unsuitable for cats'.

These warnings must be placed in a prominent position on the container and enclosed in a complete rectangle, so that there is no matter other than the warning contained in the rectangle.

Dispensing medicinal products

Veterinarians can dispense general sales list medicines, merchant's or farmer's list medicines, pharmacy medicines and prescription-only medicines, for animals under their care. All dispensed drugs, including antibiotics, Controlled Drugs, vitamin tablets and medicated shampoos, must be labelled according to the regulations for dispensed medicinal products. These requirements apply to bulk stock and stock dispensed in smaller packets. The labelling must be clear, indelible and legible. It must contain the following:

1. The name of the person who has possession or control of the animal and the address of the premises where the animal is kept.
2. The name and address of the veterinary surgeon.
3. The date of dispensing.
4. The words 'for animal treatment only' unless the container or package is too small.
5. The words 'keep out of reach of children'.
6. The words 'for external use only' if the product is an embrocation, liniment, lotion, liquid antiseptic or other liquid preparation for external use. The statement 'for external use only' must be surrounded by a complete rectangle. No other matter other than the warning must appear in the rectangle.

When a veterinary surgeon issues a prescription he can request that the labelling should bear the following particulars:

1. The name of the product.
2. Directions for use.
3. Precautions relating to the use of the product.

Liquid products for external use should be dispensed in fluted bottles unless their capacity is greater than 1.14 litres or if they are ear or eye drops supplied in plastic containers. External application is defined as 'application to skin, hair, fur, feathers, scales, hoof, horn, ear, eye, mouth, mucosa, the throat or prepuce'. Records for recording the use of medicinal products are only required for Schedule 2 Controlled Drugs (see below, Misuse of Drugs Act, 1971).

Adverse reactions

The medicines unit of the Ministry of Agriculture, Fisheries and Foods, Central Veterinary Laboratory, New Haw, Weybridge, Surrey KT15 3NB should be notified if adverse reactions in animals are seen. This permits the Veterinary Products Committee to collect and investigate information about adverse reactions of veterinary medicines.

The supply of stilbenes and thyrostatic substances for administration to animals

The demonstration of high residues of diethylstilboestrol in veal-based baby foods in Italy, following its illicit use in veal calves, was the cause of EEC legislation preventing the marketing of stilbenes intended for use in animals of all species.

Stilbenes are defined as benzoestrol, dienoesterol, hexoestrol or stilboestrol and its salts and esters. This prohibition does not apply if steps are taken prior to administration to ensure that the animals are unavailable for human or animal consumption. This exception presumably includes the use of drugs to inhibit thyroid hormone production.

Phenacetin prohibition

Phenacetin is banned under a Medicines Act regulation for use in veterinary medicinal products.

Sale of veterinary drugs under the merchants' list

Many orders and restrictions under the medicines act apply to drugs sold under the merchants' list or the farmers' list. They are primarily intended to govern, control and regulate the medication of animal feedstuffs, as well as administration of specific products for large animal use. They are not considered further here.

Misuse of Drugs Act (1971)

This Act now governs the use of dangerous drugs which are referred to as Controlled Drugs. The Act controls the purpose, possession and supply of drugs to authorized persons. Thus, veterinary surgeons and practitioners can possess, prescribe, administer and supply most of the Controlled Drugs under this Act. They may only do so providing the drugs are for professional use. This means that a veterinary surgeon may only use these drugs for the treatment of animals but not for human beings, himself or his family. Since most Controlled Drugs are also prescription-only medicines, they are also subject to the Medicines Act (1968).

Classification of Controlled Drugs

Over 100 compounds with their derivatives are controlled under the Misuse of Drugs Act. There are two ways of classifying the Controlled Drugs under the Act. The first method divides the drugs into three classes (A, B and C). This provides for maximum penalties which are applied for offences. The other basis of classification is the use of four schedules which controls their legitimate use.

Schedule 1 includes drugs such as cocaine, morphine and opium of less than a specified amount which do not constitute a major health risk. Most preparations of codeine are included in this schedule. Schedule 1 drugs are mainly exempt under the Misuse of Drugs Act and require no special record-keeping or safe custody arrangements. They are only controlled at the level of manufacture and supply. However, they are mainly classified as prescription-only medicines under the Medicines Act.

Schedule 2 includes morphine, diamorphine (heroin), cocaine, methodone, etorphine (Immobilon), pethidine, fentanyl and stimulants like amphetamines. It does not include pentazocine or buprenorphine. Schedule 2 drugs are strictly controlled under the Misuse of Drugs Act and are only available to the public on prescription. They are subject to strict record keeping and safe custody arrangements.

Schedule 3 drugs include a few minor stimulants subject to controls similar to Schedule 2 drugs. They are not frequently used in veterinary practice; the main difference is that they are exempt from record-keeping requirements.

Schedule 4 drugs are not used in veterinary practice and include drugs like cannabis and hallucogenic drugs like LSD and mescaline. These compounds have no therapeutic use.

Authority for the possession, prescription, administration and supply of Controlled Drugs

Qualified veterinary practitioners can process, prescribe, administer and supply all drugs in Schedules 1, 2 and 3 under the Act. The requirement is that they are for professional use only. If a practitioner is convicted of an offence under the Misuse of Drugs Act, the Home Secretary has the power to withdraw authority for the use of these compounds. Veterinary surgeons have no authority in law to make Controlled Drugs available for human use.

Purchase of Controlled Drugs for professional use

A veterinary surgeon may obtain Schedule 2 drugs from a pharmacist, wholesaler or manufacturer, by requisition. The requisition must contain the following particulars:

1. Signature of the veterinarian.
2. His name, address and profession.
3. The purpose for which the drug is required.
4. Total quantity required.

If he sends a messenger to collect the drug, he must also provide a written requisition and a signed letter of authorization, so that the messenger can receive the drug on his behalf.

Safe custody arrangements for Controlled Drugs

Controlled Drugs must be kept in a 'locked receptacle' which can only be opened by the veterinary surgeon or authorized person. It is recommended that keys to the Controlled Drug receptacle be limited to one key per veterinary surgeon in the practice. This key should be kept on his person so that he may open the receptacle himself or so that he may give the key specifically to a trusted member of staff to open it and withdraw the necessary amount of the Schedule 2 drug. The 'locked receptacle' is not defined by law except that case history does not accept a locked motor car as a 'receptacle'. Thus, the view is that veterinary surgeons should not keep their stocks in locked cars. It also implies that appropriate precautions should be taken to safeguard Schedule 2 drugs on visits. Locked receptacle requirements do not apply for Schedule 1 drugs.

Controlled Drugs records

Veterinary surgeons must record the purchase and administration of Schedule 2 drugs in a register within 24 hours. Records must be kept in a register (in the form of a bound book) which is used solely for entries relating to Controlled Drugs. The regulations require that:

1. A separate register must be kept for each set of premises where the Controlled Drugs are used. Thus, a separate register must be kept at each branch surgery if Controlled Drugs are stored there. Only one register must be kept for each premises.
2. A separate part of the register must be used for each class of drug, e.g. morphine and pethidine require a separate part of the register.
3. The class of drug to which the entries relate must be specified at the head of each page of the register.
4. Entries must be made in chronological order.
5. Entries must be indelible.
6. Entries must not be cancelled or altered. Corrections, if necessary, must be made by means of a marginal note or footnote which must specify the date on which the correction was made.

7. The register must be kept for a period of two years from the date of the last entry.

Printed registers with subdivisions for the main classes of drugs in use in the UK are available commercially. They are easy to use. Figure 21.2 illustrates an example record for the purchase of a Controlled Drug. Figure 21.3 illustrates two examples of the register for dispensing Controlled Drugs.

Date on which supply received	Name and address of person or firm from whom obtained	Amount obtained	Form in which obtained
1.4.87	F Smith 4, Great Street, Leicester	20 mg anhydrous etorphine	Small animal Immobilon

Figure 21.2 Purchase of a Controlled Drug

Date on which transaction was effected	Name and address of person or firm supplied	Particulars as to licence or authority of person or firm supplied to be in possession	Amount supplied	Form in which supplied
1.4.87	F Smith-Jones 80 Park Lane, Leicester	Dispensed	6 x 50 mg	Pethidine tabs
2.4.87	L Simpson 3 Leicester Road, Birstall	Direct administration	25 mg anhydrous Pethidine	Pethidine injection 1 ml

Figure 21.3 Dispensing Controlled Drugs

Prescribing Controlled Drugs

A prescription for a Schedule 2 Controlled Drug must be in ink and contain the following particulars provided by the veterinary surgeon:

1. His usual signature.
2. The date.
3. His address.
4. An indication of his professional qualifications.

5. The words 'for animal treatment only'.
6. The name and address of the client.
7. The dose.
8. The total quantity in *words* and *figures* and, in the case of a preparation, the form and, where appropriate, the strength of preparation, e.g. 10 (ten) pethidine tablets, each 50 mg (fifty).
9. A declaration that the drug is prescribed for an animal under his care (for example 'this prescription is issued in respect of animals under my care').

Requirements (6), (7) and (8) must be completed by the veterinarian in his own handwriting. A prescription issued for Controlled Drugs under Schedule 2 must not be dispensed later than 13 weeks after the date of issue. Figure 21.4 illustrates a prescription for a controlled drug.

Central Veterinary Hospital
22 Church Street
Leicester

Date: 4.1.87

Client J Smith
83 Station Road, Leicester
R_x Pethidine tablets 50 (fifty) mg.
Mitte 10 (ten)
Sig 1 (one) tablet to be given twice daily
(For animal treatment only).
This prescription is issued in respect of an animal under my care.

R.J. Martin
Signature (of veterinary surgeon)
Qualifications BVSc, MRCVS

Figure 21.4 A prescription for a Controlled Drug

The destruction of Controlled Drugs

If Schedule 2 Controlled Drugs are no longer required, they may only be destroyed in the presence of an authorized person. Such persons include drugs squad officers and Home Office inspectors. A record of the destruction must be kept in the register and include the signature of the authorized person who witnessed the destruction, together with the date of the destruction and the quantity destroyed. Schedule 1 and Schedule 3 drugs do not need to be destroyed in this manner since no record of them needs be kept.

Further reading

Knifton, A. and Edwards, B. R. (1987) Controlled drugs and medicinal products. In *Legislation Affecting the Veterinary Profession in the United Kingdom*, 5th edn, R.C.V.S., London, pp. 43–74

Medicines and Poisons Guide (1982) The Pharmaceutical Press, 1 Lambeth High Street, London SE1 7JN

Index